Advances in Drug Research

Volume 11

Advances in Drug Research

Series Editors

N. J. HARPER

Weddel Pharmaceuticals Ltd
St Albans, Hertfordshire, England

and

ALMA B. SIMMONDS

Chelsea College
University of London, England

Volume 11

edited by Alma B. Simmonds

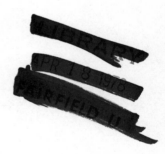

1977

ACADEMIC PRESS
LONDON   NEW YORK   SAN FRANCISCO

A Subsidiary of Harcourt Brace Jovanovich, Publishers

ACADEMIC PRESS INC. (LONDON) LTD.
24–28 Oval Road
London NW1

US edition published by
ACADEMIC PRESS INC.
111 Fifth Avenue,
New York, New York 10003

Library of Congress Catalog Card Number: 64-24672
ISBN: 0-12-013311-3

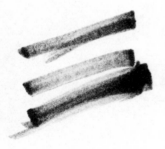

MADE AND PRINTED IN GREAT BRITAIN BY
THE GARDEN CITY PRESS LIMITED
LETCHWORTH, HERTFORDSHIRE
SG6 1JS

Contributors to Volume 11

T. R. BOSIN, PhD
Department of Pharmacology, School of Medicine, Indiana University, Bloomington, Indiana, USA

P. BRESLOFF, BSc, PhD
The Boots Co Ltd, Research Department, Pennyfoot Street, Nottingham, England

E. E. CAMPAIGNE, PhD
Department of Chemistry, Indiana University, Bloomington, Indiana, USA

J. F. HOWES, BPharm, PhD
SISA Incorporated, Concord Avenue, Cambridge, Massachusetts, USA

H. G. PARS, PhD
SISA Incorporated, Concord Avenue, Cambridge, Massachusetts, USA

R. K. RAZDAN, PhD
SISA Incorporated, Concord Avenue, Cambridge, Massachusetts, USA

K. M. SHAW, MA, MRCP
Medical Unit, University College Hospital, London, England

A. J. THODY, PhD
Department of Dermatology, University of Newcastle upon Tyne, Newcastle upon Tyne, England

Contents

Miscellaneous Antirheumatic Drugs and their Possible Modes of Action

P. BRESLOFF, BSc, PhD

The Boots Co Ltd, Research Department, Pennyfoot Street, Nottingham, England

1 Introduction

Antiinflammatory drugs of the aspirin and corticosteroid types have proved to be very useful agents in the treatment of rheumatoid arthritis. However, in spite of the development of increasingly potent drugs of these types, none have proved to be effective inhibitors of the underlying chronic inflammatory processes which are accompanied by synovial proliferation and degeneration of the organized connective tissues of the rheumatoid joints. There is a great need for the development of a new generation of drugs whose actions may alter fundamentally the disease process and its destructive course, but these are unlikely to be found using existing classical pharmacological screening techniques.

There is an interesting group of miscellaneous nonsteroidal, nonaspirin-like compounds which, though failing to show reproducible activity in most classical screening tests, except perhaps under exceptional conditions, have proved to be efficacious in the treatment of rheumatoid arthritis. The most important of these agents are probably gold compounds, chloroquine

1

and, more recently, penicillamine. Unfortunately, the use of these compounds is usually restricted to the treatment of more advanced disease because of the associated side effects, which can often be severe and require very careful monitoring of the patient.

The purpose of this chapter is to review actions of these compounds which may be relevant to their antirheumatic activity and possibly provide a basis for seeking new antirheumatic drugs.

2 Gold compounds

Gold compounds are particularly interesting since there is evidence that they can significantly retard joint destruction when given on a long-term basis. In a major study by the Empire Rheumatism Council (1961), treatment with the gold compound sodium aurothiomalate (1) was shown to have a beneficial effect on all the disease parameters measured, with the exception of radiological progression where improvement was suggested but was not significant. Further studies by Sigler *et al.* (1972 and 1974), however, did show significant inhibition of the radiologically assessed progression of bone and cartilage destruction in patients treated with sodium aurothiomalate. The most important difference between the studies of the Empire Rheumatism Council and Sigler *et al.* appears to be in the dosing schedules. In the former study, patients received a total dose of 1000 mg of sodium aurothiomalate spread over a five-month period and were assessed radiologically eighteen months after entry to the study without further gold being given. In the latter study, Sigler *et al.* gave "tissue loading" doses of gold in an initial twenty-two-week period and then maintenance doses at increasing intervals up to two years.

(1) Sodium aurothiomalate

Although the absorption of gold from injection sites appears to be rapid (Mascarenhas *et al.*, 1972) the onset of a clinical response is slow and appears to bear no obvious relationship to the blood levels achieved (Gerber *et al.*, 1972; Mascarenhas *et al.*, 1972; Rubinstein and Dietz, 1973).

The precise mode of action of gold compounds remains unknown but they do have a number of activities which may be relevant to their efficacy in rheumatoid arthritis. These activities are considered below.

2.1 ANTIMICROBIAL ACTIVITY

The role of infective agents in the initiation of rheumatoid arthritis has been a source of argument for many years with evidence having been put forward to suggest that the agent responsible is either bacterial, viral or mycoplasmal (Gardner, 1972). Although different workers have apparently isolated a variety of infective agents from rheumatoid joints, none have been demonstrated reproducibly in a high percentage of joints and by different workers. Perhaps this failure to isolate infective organisms is due to their lack of persistence in viable form but, remaining as antigenic components which cannot be identified (Barland, 1973), they are responsible for a subsequent series of immunological events leading to rheumatoid arthritis. Brostoff *et al.* (1973), for example, reported that leucocyte migration inhibition in the presence of *Mycoplasma fermentans* membranes correlated with the severity of the disease in rheumatoid arthritis, suggesting possible previous exposure to this agent.

The relationship between gold compounds, rheumatoid arthritis and infective agents has an historical basis. Gold compounds appear to have first been used in the treatment of rheumatoid arthritis in the mistaken belief that the disease was related to tuberculosis. As early as 1890 Koch had shown that tubercle bacilli were sensitive to gold cyanide. Landé (1927) reported that aurothioglucose (2) relieved joint pains when used to treat bacterial endocarditis and this early work suggested that the effectiveness of gold compounds was due to an antimicrobial activity.

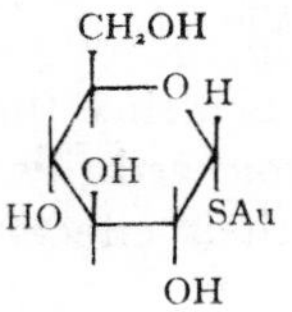

(2) Aurothioglucose ((D-glucosylthio)gold)

The ability of gold compounds to suppress arthritis induced in rodents by infective agents has also been known for many years. Activity was shown against haemolytic streptococci (Rothbard, 1941), mycoplasmas (Findlay *et al.*, 1939; Sabin and Warren, 1940) and other infective agents (Jasmin, 1957). More recently Thomas (1973) discussed several models of arthritis induced in laboratory animals by mycoplasma and suggested that these models might be useful for studying the therapeutic activity of gold compounds. Thomas *et al.* (1966) had found previously that aurothiomalate was effective therapeutically against *M. gallisepticum* infections in turkeys and chickens.

The studies of Sabin and Warren (1940), however, suggested that gold was not acting directly through an antimicrobial activity. These authors found that neither aurothiomalate, nor the blood of mice treated with it, could prevent the growth of the mycoplasma they had used to induce arthritis. Further support for an indirect effect of gold compounds in mycoplasma-induced arthritis was provided by the study of Wiesinger (1965) using rats. In these experiments allochrysine (3) did not inhibit the growth of *M. arthritidis* although it has an apparent antiarthritic effect, as judged by inhibition of the swelling of the rat's paw.

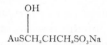

OH
|
AuSCH₂CHCH₂SO₃Na

(3) Allochrysine: sodium 3-aurothio-2-hydroxypropanesulphonate

The lack of direct effect of gold compounds on some of the micro-organisms that cause experimental arthritis suggests that they might work through some other mechanism. Further, until active infective organisms can be proven to be responsible for a high percentage of the cases of rheumatoid arthritis, the antimicrobial activity of gold compounds must remain unlikely to explain their therapeutic efficacy.

2.2 ACTIONS ON THE IMMUNE SYSTEM

It is obvious from a weight of evidence that immunological processes are intimately involved in rheumatoid arthritis and it has been suggested that gold compounds could exert their effects by interfering with immuno-logical behaviour.

In the clinical situation, although Mourisden *et al.* (1974) reported that they could not find statistically significant changes in IgG or IgM metabolism in patients treated with sodium aurothiosulphate for three months, Gottlieb *et al.* (1975) did find significant decreases in the serum levels of these immunoglobulins after treatment with sodium aurothiomalate for six and twelve months. Reductions in IgG, IgA, IgM and rheumatoid factor titres appeared to correlate with the clinical response to treatment in the study of Gottlieb *et al.* However, decreases in immunoglobulin levels may reflect either direct effects of gold on the metabolism of immuno-globulins or a beneficial effect on the disease process. Gold was reported to be heavily concentrated in the reticulo-endothelial system, especially the lymph nodes, of a patient on gold thioglucose (Gottlieb *et al.*, 1972) and this could suggest that lymphocytes are target cells. A direct effect of gold on lymphocytes was suggested by the finding that the lymphocytes of patients receiving gold therapy were unresponsive to the effects of streptolysin S, a blastogenic agent (Fikrig and Smithwick, 1968). However, these authors suggested that this effect might be mediated by an inhibition of lysosomal enzymes and this may be related to the mode of action of gold (section 2.4).

Animal studies also suggest that the reticulo-endothelial system is a site of accumulation of gold (Swartz *et al.*, 1960) though most evidence does not support a direct effect of gold on the lymphocytes. In an attempt to determine the effect of sodium aurothiomalate on immune responses, Persellin *et al.* (1967) measured circulating antibody levels in rabbits following hyperimmunization with bovine serum albumin, typhoid-paratyphoid vaccine and *E. coli*. Gold had no effect on the antibody levels suggesting that it did not have a direct effect on immunoglobulin production by lymphocytes. Further, Persellin *et al.* also demonstrated a lack of effect of sodium aurothiomalate on delayed hypersensitivity to diphtheria toxoid and dinitrochlorobenzene in the guinea pig.

The ability of gold compounds to inhibit the development of rat adjuvant arthritis, a complex disease involving delayed (cell-mediated) hypersensitivity, is debatable. Jessop and Currey (1968) found that sodium aurothiomalate failed to affect the progress of adjuvant arthritis. They also found that primary antibody responses to sheep erythrocytes and delayed skin reaction to tuberculin were not affected in these same animals, even when gold was given prophylactically and in high doses. In contrast, Walz *et al.* (1971), Sofia and Douglas (1973) and Arrigoni-Martelli and Bramm (1975) all reported that sodium aurothiomalate did significantly inhibit adjuvant arthritis. It is possible that the differing results in these studies might be related to differences in absorption from the injection site, since Jessop and Currey gave the gold subcutaneously whilst the other workers gave it intramuscularly. Unfortunately, the blood levels of gold were not measured in the former study so that adequacy of absorption from the subcutaneous injection site cannot be confirmed. Walz *et al.* (1972 and 1974) used rat adjuvant arthritis to evaluate an orally active gold compound, SKF 36914 (4), and found it to be as effective as intramuscularly injected sodium aurothiomalate.

Although sodium aurothiomalate appeared to suppress both the non-immune (primary lesion) and immune (secondary lesion) stages of adjuvant arthritis in some experiments, it did not appear to inhibit antibody production to sheep erythrocytes or cutaneous hypersensitivity to purified protein derivative in these same animals (Walz, 1974). Both Walz (1974) and Gerber

(1972) showed that sodium aurothiomalate delayed but did not inhibit rat allergic encephalomyelitis, suggesting that it did not inhibit cell-mediated hypersensitivity. Aspirin-like drugs have also been shown to delay rat allergic encephalomyelitis whilst immunosuppressive drugs, such as cyclophosphamide and methotrexate, can inhibit it completely.

$$(C_2H_5)_3 P \longrightarrow AuCl$$

(4) Triethylphosphino-gold chloride (SKF 36914)

On the basis of the evidence available, it must be concluded that gold compounds probably do not have a direct immunosuppressive action on either immediate or delayed (cellular) responses and that other actions are responsible for their activity in immunologically based diseases.

2.3 INTERACTIONS WITH PROTEINS

The apparent ability of gold to inhibit the heat-induced aggregation of human gamma-globulin *in vitro* (Gerber, 1971) could be of relevance to its action *in vivo*.

Complexes of IgG and IgG + rheumatoid factors (IgG or IgM) have been found in rheumatoid synovial fluids and synovial tissues. Their presence was associated with a marked decrease in synovial fluid complement levels (Zvaifler, 1974) following activation of the complement system and complement activation products could contribute to persistent articular inflammation. Further, indigestible immune complexes can be taken up by phagocytically active cells within the inflamed joint (polymorphs, macrophages and synovial lining cells) and this could result in the release of lysosomal enzymes which may cause further inflammatory changes and connective tissue destruction (Allison and Davies, 1975). Recent experiments with cultured cell lines derived from rabbit synovium showed that stimulation of phagocytosis by these cells could also lead to the secretion of nonlysosomal enzymes which can digest connective tissue (Reynolds and Werb, 1975).

It can be seen that if gold compounds did in fact slow down or inhibit the formation of immune complexes or aggregates in the joints (or other sites) they could modify both inflammatory changes and connective tissue degradation. However, an *in vivo* effect of gold on immune complex formation at synovial sites remains to be demonstrated.

The antirheumatic activity of gold may be associated with its interaction with collagen. Adam *et al.* (1965, 1968) studied the uptake of gold by collagen fibres of rat tail tendon following regular administration of sodium aurothiosulphate and found that the collagen fibres showed distinct staining bands of gold. These authors suggested that, initially, negatively charged gold thiosulphate complexes were bound to collagen molecules by electrostatic forces but these subsequently decomposed forming new coordinate cross-links through the gold resulting in cross striations. It was also suggested that the course of rheumatoid arthritis might be influenced by an increase in the stability of the collagen structure and by the occupation of immunologically active sites on collagen molecules or their breakdown products. However, the relationship of these animal studies to the binding of gold to collagen in the rheumatoid joint remains to be clarified.

2.4 INHIBITION OF ENZYMES

Gold compounds have been shown to inhibit a number of enzymes of both lysosomal and nonlysosomal origin *in vitro*. As already mentioned in section 2.3, the release of lysosomal and non-lysosomal enzymes in the inflamed joint can promote further inflammatory changes and degrade the connective tissue matrix components which are mainly proteoglycans and collagen.

In rheumatoid arthritis, inflamed swollen granulation tissue (pannus) covered with proliferating lining cells grows over the cartilage and into the subchondral bone (Fig. 1).

The major destruction of articular cartilage takes place where the pannus and cartilage are in intimate contact (Ball, 1968) with little breakdown occurring randomly over the cartilage surface except for some loss of proteoglycans (Hamerman, 1969). This suggests that the enzymes necessary for degrading cartilage come either from the pannus, probably the lining cells, or that the pannus releases substances which stimulate the chondrocytes of the articular cartilage to degrade their own matrix. Although the polymorphs which migrate into the synovial fluid and the macrophages which line the synovial cavity can release into the synovial fluid a number of proteolytic enzymes which are active at neutral pH, these enzymes are probably prevented from random attack on the articular cartilage surface by the naturally occurring plasma protein enzyme inhibitors α_2-macroglobulin and α_1-antitrypsin (Ohlsson and Delshammar, 1975).

Amongst the enzymes which gold compounds have been shown to inhibit are the lysosomal acid hydrolases, acid phosphatase, β-glucuronidase (Persellin and Ziff, 1966; Ennis *et al.*, 1968), cathepsin D and cathepsin B (Barrett, 1975), the neutral proteases collagenase and elastase from polymorphs (Janoff, 1970) and collagenase from human rheumatoid synovium (Woolley, 1975).

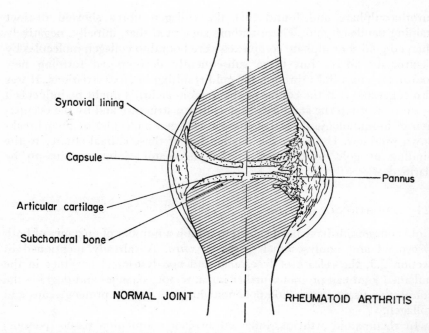

Fig. 1. Changes in the rheumatoid joint. Inflamed swollen granulation tissue (pannus) covered with proliferating lining cells grows over the articular cartilage and into the subchondral bone.

Although the elastase of polymorphs has an exceptionally broad specificity and is the only mammalian enzyme known to degrade all the major structural macromolecules of connective tissues (Barrett, 1975), the relevance of its inhibition by gold to the ability of gold to slow down joint destruction is questionable. As already mentioned, the polymorphs accumulate in synovial fluid which contains natural plasma protein enzyme inhibitors, and very few polymorphs appear in the invasive pannus. The ability of gold to inhibit rheumatoid synovial collagenase may be far more relevant since this enzyme is being produced by cell types which do lie in intimate contact with the articular cartilage and bone where the pannus invades these tissues and natural proteolytic enzyme inhibitors in the synovial fluid are excluded. Further, the free macrophages within the inflamed synovium contain enzymes whose release could be responsible for maintaining the chronicity of inflammation (Allison and Davies, 1975). Inhibition of some of these enzymes, either intracellularly or extracellularly, could account for moderation of inflammatory changes within the synovium by gold.

Although the concentrations of gold compounds required to inhibit some enzymes *in vitro* appear quite high, gold accumulates in endocytically active cells and the concentrations achieved within these cells may eventually be very high. Perhaps this explains why gold compounds take such a long time to exert a demonstrable antiinflammatory and antirheumatic effect.

2.5 INHIBITION OF PROSTAGLANDIN SYNTHESIS

In the past five years it has been shown that prostaglandins are important mediators of inflammation, pain and pyrexia and that aspirin-like non-steroidal antiinflammatory drugs inhibit their synthesis (for a review see Flower, 1974). These discoveries have made a major contribution towards explaining the mode of action of this group of drugs and some workers have considered whether unrelated drugs with apparent antiinflammatory activity such as gold might have similar actions.

Deby *et al.* (1973) found that Allochrysine (3) and gold chloride could inhibit bull seminal vesicle prostaglandin synthetase *in vitro* at 10^{-4} and 10^{-5}M. Similarly, Penneys *et al.* (1974) found that aurothiomalate could inhibit prostaglandin synthesis by a sheep seminal vesicle preparation with an ID_{50} of 5×10^{-5}M. In contrast, Stone *et al.* (1975), also using a sheep seminal vesicle PG synthetase, found that the inhibitory effect of aurothiomalate and aurothioglucose appeared to be specifically on $PGF_{2\alpha}$ synthesis with simultaneous stimulation of PGE_2 synthesis, though the latter results may differ from those of Penneys *et al.* because of addition of copper and glutathione to the *in vitro* system.

Although these studies do suggest that the inhibition of prostaglandin synthesis by gold compounds is a possible explanation of some of their antiinflammatory activities, inhibition of prostaglandin synthesis *in vivo* in the rheumatoid joint has yet to be demonstrated. Further, since much more potent inhibitors of prostaglandin synthesis such as indomethacin do not appear to have the same antirheumatic actions as gold, it suggests that gold works principally through other mechanisms.

*   *   *

It is apparent that much remains to be clarified about the relevance of the apparent actions of gold compounds, especially *in vitro*, to their antirheumatic activity. However, further studies are worth while to establish a basis for seeking "gold-like" compounds devoid of many of the side effects of existing drugs.

3 Chloroquine

Although the principal use of chloroquine (5) has been in the chemotherapy
of malaria, for which the drug was originally developed, it has also been
used in the treatment of rheumatoid arthritis for almost twenty-five years.
Unfortunately, its use in rheumatoid arthritis remains somewhat limited
by its toxic side effects, mainly retinopathy. Chloroquine is similar to gold
compounds in that the onset of its antirheumatic effects is slow and seldom
noted for at least two months; it appears to slow down joint erosion in
long-term treatment (Young, 1959) and its effects continue after drug
withdrawal. It does not behave as an antiinflammatory agent in the same
way as aspirin-like drugs but appears to affect some of the more basic
features of the disease.

(5) Chloroquine

A notable characteristic of chloroquine is its accumulation in tissues and
very high concentrations have been found in the liver, spleen, kidney and
lungs after administration to many species (Grundmann et al., 1972).
Information on the persistence of chloroquine in man varies. Zvaifler and
Rubin (1962) found measurable amounts of chloroquine and metabolites in
plasma and urine three and a half years after the last administration. Rubin
et al. (1963) found detectable amounts of chloroquine in urine, erythrocytes
and plasma of patients with chloroquine retinopathy five years after the
last known ingestion of chloroquine. In contrast, McChesney and Rothfield
(1964) reported that significant plasma and urinary levels were not found
later than eight weeks after discontinuation of therapy, regardless of the
duration of original treatment.

Although chloroquine and related antimalarials have been reported to
have effects in a number of biological systems, there is no biological assay
agreed upon as being predictive of the utility of this class of agents for the
treatment of rheumatoid arthritis (Scherrer, 1974). There is general
agreement that chloroquine is not effective in adjuvant arthritis (Newbould,
1963; Graeme et al., 1966; Perrine and Takesue, 1968) or other experimental immunologically based diseases, nor does it appear to affect
primary or secondary antibody responses (Kalmanson and Guze, 1965)

and cellular transfer of delayed hypersensitivity or immune complex mediated reversed passive Arthus reactions (Goldlust and Schreiber, 1975).

Some of the activities of chloroquine which do seem of possible relevance to its antirheumatic activity are discussed below.

3.1 EFFECTS ON LEUCOCYTE CHEMOTAXIS

Inflammation within the joint involves both an influx of inflammatory cells from vessels into the local tissues and local cell proliferation. Theoretically, drugs which inhibit the chemotaxis of cells into the inflammatory site, especially macrophages, might have a modifying effect on chronic inflammation in the rheumatoid joint. There have been reports that chloroquine can inhibit rabbit polymorphonuclear leucocyte chemotaxis *in vitro* (Ward, 1966; 1968). However, Perper *et al.* (1974), using a technique involving the adoptive transfer of ^{51}Cr-labelled isologous rat leukocytes and measurement of their accumulation in a carrageenan-induced inflammatory reaction, failed to find any effect of chloroquine at 100 mg kg^{-1} on either polymorphonuclear or mononuclear leucocyte cell chemotaxis. Whether chloroquine has any effect on leucocyte chemotaxis in man is unclear.

3.2 LYSOSOMOTROPIC ACTIVITY AND EFFECTS ON LYSOSOME FUNCTION

Although the precise mode of action of chloroquine is obscure, the relationship between chloroquine and the lysosomal system seems to be central to explaining many of its actions. The possible role of lysosomes and their enzymes in inflammation and connective tissue destruction in the joints has already been referred to in the section on gold compounds and there is evidence that chloroquine might exert its therapeutic effects through inhibition of lysosome function.

Many cells exposed to chloroquine take it up avidly and achieve much higher intracellular concentrations than in the surrounding medium. This rapid uptake is accompanied by a high degree of cytoplasmic vacuolation and there is substantial evidence that the site of accumulation of the drug is in the lysosomes (Allison and Young, 1969; Fedorko *et al.*, 1968). Autophagy, a mechanism whereby cells sequester and digest, within vacuoles, portions of their own cytoplasm, is associated with a high degree of vacuolation and has been shown to be induced by chloroquine in leukocytes of man (Fedorko, 1967), pancreatic cells of rats (Fedorko, 1968), cultured fibroblasts (Gaddioni *et al.*, 1964) and macrophages (Fedorko *et al.*, 1968). The latter authors suggested that these effects could conceivably be the basis, at least in part, for some of the toxic complications of long-term chloroquine treatment in man. However, similar effects might also explain the drug's antimalarial and possibly other therapeutic activities.

Erythrocytes containing chloroquine-sensitive malaria parasites concentrate the drug to high levels and the drug produces typical vacuolation and autophagy in the parasite indicating a lysosomal localization similar to that found in mammalian cells. Homewood et al. (1972) proposed that chloroquine may act by inhibiting intralysosomal haemoglobin digestion in the parasite either by raising the intralysosomal pH or directly by inhibiting proteolytic enzymes. The reduced ability of the parasite to digest haemoglobin, essential for its nutrition, inhibits its growth.

The concentrations of chloroquine achieved within mammalian lysosomes are probably also adequate to inhibit directly a number of hydrolytic enzymes. Evidence of enzyme inhibition was provided by the inability of human fibroblasts exposed to chloroquine in vitro to digest proteins and mucopolysaccharides (Lie and Schofield, 1973), an effect similar to that seen on raising the medium pH (Lie et al., 1972). De Duve et al. (1974) also showed that chloroquine inhibited the breakdown of exogenous proteins by macrophages in vitro. Of direct relevance to the effects of chloroquine on enzymes involved in connective tissue degradation, in vitro experiments have shown that chloroquine inhibited a chondromucoprotease of cartilage (Barrett, 1975; Cowey and Whitehouse, 1966), a cathepsin B in cartilage (Ali et al., 1967) and collagenases from rat skin and bovine cartilage (Cowey and Whitehouse, 1966). Since collagenases have not been shown to be lysosomal in origin, it is not known if the concentrations of chloroquine achieved in vivo at the site of collagenase action would be high enough for it to have an inhibitory activity.

Although many antiinflammatory drugs and chloroquine stabilize the leakage of enzymes from isolated lysosomes (Filkins, 1969; Hyttel and Jorgensen, 1970; Abraham and Hendy, 1970; Ignarro, 1971), much of this in vitro work, especially with liver lysosomes, is of doubtful relevance to the behaviour of lysosomes in intact cells of the types found in the rheumatoid joint. As already described in the section on gold compounds, the in vivo stimulus for enzyme release from lysosomes may well involve the uptake of indigestible immunological or other materials and require the combined responses of the intact cell to achieve lysosomal enzyme secretion. Indeed, in contrast to the results with isolated lysosomes, Ringrose et al. (1975), using cultured mouse peritoneal macrophages, showed that chloroquine at concentrations in excess of 10^{-4}M tended to stimulate release of lysosomal enzymes induced with zymosan. In another model involving stimulated cells, in this case human leukocytes in contact with aggregated IgG immobilized on cartilage discs, Perper and Oronsky (1974) found that chloroquine did not inhibit directly the nonphagocytic release of neutral protease. It did, however, inhibit the enzyme directly in a manner similar to but less effective than sodium aurothiomalate. These results provide little evidence to support a stabilizing effect of chloroquine on lysosomes in intact cells.

3.3 EFFECTS ON CARTILAGE AND COLLAGEN

In vivo, chloroquine has been found to have either protective or destructive effects on damaged articular cartilage depending upon the concentrations to which it is exposed. Volastro *et al.* (1973) administered chloroquine either intraperitoneally or intraarticularly to rabbits with experimentally scarified articular cartilage. When the chloroquine was given intraperitoneally at 4 mg kg^{-1} there was promotion of the healing of the cartilage clefts in addition to greater metachromasia of the ground substance (proteoglycans). However, the same weekly amount given intraarticularly in two divided doses caused extensive cartilage damage and an inflammatory synovitis, though the noninjected contralateral joint showed healing of the clefts similar to that seen following intraperitoneal administration. Although intraarticular administration confirmed the toxic effects of high concentrations of chloroquine on cartilage seen *in vitro* (Whitehouse and Boström, 1962), the protective effect of chloroquine *in vivo* has also been demonstrated in another model. Teitz and Chrisman (1975) induced a synovitis and articular cartilage changes (loss of mucopolysaccharide staining) in rabbit knees by injection of prostaglandin E$_1$. Daily intramuscular injections of chloroquine (10 mg kg^{-1}) were found to prevent the synovitis and cartilage changes, though oral sodium salicylate was ineffective.

The above studies suggest that high concentrations of chloroquine are cytotoxic to cartilage though low concentrations promote cartilage healing and/or have a protective effect on proteoglycans degradation. Chloroquine also appears capable of interfering with disturbances of collagen in connective tissue at other sites in experimental animals. Trnavská and Trnavský (1968a) found that chloroquine protected skin collagen from lathyritic changes induced by β-aminoproprionitrile, i.e. prevented the inhibition of collagen maturation (cross linking) caused by this agent. In contrast, Trnavský and Trnavská (1968a) found that chloroquine failed to inhibit changes induced in bone collagen of lathyritic chick embryos. Further, the protective effects of chloroquine on skin collagen were not specific for this drug but were also found with sodium salicylate and phenylbutazone, two drugs which are antiinflammatory but do not appear to modify connective tissue changes in the rheumatoid joints. The relevance of the protective effects of chloroquine in the lathyritic rat to a possible effect of chloroquine on the metabolism of collagen in the connective tissues of the rheumatoid joint is therefore unclear.

*   *   *

It has already been pointed out that there is no predictive screening test for the antirheumatic activity of chloroquine or its analogues. However, perhaps further studies of the relationship between chloroquine and the lysosomal system and its enzymes in intact cells may provide a basis for such tests. Another area worthy of further exploration would appear to be the protective effects of chloroquine on cartilage degradation.

4 D-Penicillamine

Although D-penicillamine (**6**) is a chelating agent that has been in use for the treatment of heavy metal poisoning for some twenty years, its use in rheumatoid arthritis is more recent and its mode of action possibly even less well understood or investigated than that of gold or chloroquine.

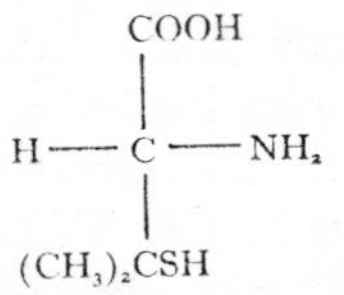

$$
\begin{array}{c}
\text{COOH} \\
|　　　　　　　 \\
\text{H} - \text{C} - \text{NH}_2 \\
|　　　　　　　 \\
(\text{CH}_3)_2\text{CSH}
\end{array}
$$

(**6**) D-Penicillamine (D-ββ-dimethylcysteine)

D-Penicillamine was first used tentatively in rheumatoid arthritis in 1960 (Griffin *et al.*, 1960; Dresner and Trombly, 1960) and in 1964 Jaffe reported a favourable effect of this drug in a case of rheumatoid arthritis with arteritis. However, it is as a result of more recent clinical studies that its use in rheumatoid arthritis has been encouraged. In 1973 a British twelve month double-blind multicentre controlled trial reported that D-penicillamine was undoubtedly of benefit in acute severe rheumatoid arthritis (Andrews *et al.*, 1973). All the parameters measured in this trial were improved by penicillamine treatment except for radiographic changes, but since the erosive changes were so severe in these patients, minor pre and post treatment changes were unlikely to have been seen. Day *et al.* (1974), in a further report on penicillamine including some patients who had received up to five years' treatment, found that penicillamine was undoubtedly an effective antirheumatic drug but, unlike Jaffe (1970), thought that its toxic effects on bone marrow were more important than its nephrotoxicity. In a recent multicentre trial comparing D-penicillamine with gold in rheumatoid arthritis (Huskisson *et al.*, 1974), these two drugs were considered to be of equivalent efficacy and, although adverse effects were more common with penicillamine, gold was associated with more frequent withdrawal of treatment.

Most trials have been carried out with D-penicillamine prepared by acid hydrolysis of benzylpenicillin. Recently Dixon *et al.* (1975) used synthetic D-penicillamine which again confirmed the therapeutic value of D-penicillamine in rheumatoid arthritis with little effect on radiographic changes during three months of treatment. Side effects were similar to those seen in earlier trials and, though proteinuria was infrequent, this may have been related to the short duration of the trial.

It remains to be shown whether D-penicillamine, if given early enough and for long enough, can affect bone and cartilage damage as has been found in the long-term therapy of rheumatoid arthritis with gold and chloroquine.

Although most of the studies on the mode of action of D-penicillamine are recent, probably stimulated by the demonstration of the drug's efficacy, two activities which appear of possible relevance have been investigated.

4.1 EFFECTS ON THE IMMUNE SYSTEM

D-Penicillamine was first used in rheumatoid arthritis in the belief that it might dissociate rheumatoid factor macroglobulins *in vivo*, as had been demonstrated previously *in vitro* (Deutsch and Morton, 1957). Attempts to achieve a fall in rheumatoid factor levels by systemic administration of D-penicillamine were initially unsuccessful: dissociation could only be achieved by instilling relatively large amounts directly into synovial effusions (Jaffe, 1962). When D-penicillamine was given for prolonged periods, however, a fall in rheumatoid factor titre was found (Jaffe, 1963) and despite the rapid excretion of D-penicillamine, the reduced titre persisted for many weeks after drug administration. This suggested that perhaps a mechanism other than macroglobulin dissociation might be responsible for D-penicillamine's antirheumatic effect, an idea further supported by the considerable latent period necessary to obtain initial clinical improvement.

Bluestone and Goldberg (1973) reporting on the British multicentre trial (Andrews *et al.*, 1973) noted that in addition to a fall in rheumatoid factor levels, D-penicillamine also caused a significant fall in serum IgG and IgM levels though not IgA levels. Because this effect on the immunoglobulin population seemed to be selective, Bluestone and Goldberg suggested that the ability of D-penicillamine to disrupt the interchain disulphide bonds of macroglobulins was unlikely to account for the decrease in circulating immunoglobulins and that some other mechanism, possibly a selective immunosuppressive activity at the cellular level, might be responsible.

In contrast to the results of Bluestone and Goldberg, Huskisson and Berry (1974), reporting on a comparative trial of penicillamine and gold, found that D-penicillamine caused a fall in IgG, IgM and IgA levels, They also found that responses to intradermal injection of tuberculin and key-hole limpet haemocyanin were not suppressed by D-penicillamine, suggesting that the drug did not affect delayed or primary immune responses. Further, there was no effect on antibody production in response to Salmonella T antigen. Therefore, the authors found that D-penicillamine did not exert its actions in rheumatoid arthritis by suppressing immune responses and suggested that its effects on immunoglobulins and rheuma-toid factor might well be due to some nonspecific effect such as inhibition of protein synthesis.

In animal experiments, Liyanage and Currey (1972) failed to find an effect of oral D-penicillamine on rat adjuvant arthritis or immune responses, even at doses up to ten times those used clinically. Since adjuvant arthritis is sensitive to immunosuppressant drugs, these results suggest that D-penicillamine does not have immunosuppressant properties, at least of the type seen with standard immunosuppressive drugs such as cyclo-phosphamide and methotrexate. Although Baumgartner et al. (1974) have reported that D-penicillamine does appear to be partially effective in pyridoxine deficient rats with adjuvant arthritis, L-penicillamine was remarkably more effective and perhaps these experiments add little to our understanding of how D-penicillamine works.

Studies on the effects of D-penicillamine on humoral and cellular immune responses in mice have been reported by Schumacher et al. (1975a). Doses up to 200 mg kg^{-1} had no effect on primary immune responses to immunization with sheep red blood cells and the authors suggested that the action of D-penicillamine is mainly directed against T lymphocytes. Pursuing this idea, Schumacher et al. (1975b) looked at the effects of D-penicillamine on cultured lymphocytes obtained from patients with active tuberculosis and stimulated in vitro by various agents. The drug inhibited lymphocyte stimulation by these agents in a dose-dependent manner confirming similar results by Roath and Wills (1974) with human lymphocytes. Further investigations into the effects of D-penicillamine on lymphocyte stimulation may prove to be a fruitful area of research.

4.2   EFFECTS ON COLLAGEN SYNTHESIS

Perhaps the most striking effects of penicillamine are on collagen, an essential structural component of connective tissues. Harris and Sjoerdsma (1966) found that penicillamine treatment of patients with Wilson's disease, cystinuria and rheumatoid arthritis produced an accumulation of poorly cross-linked collagen in skin. Similar effects have been reported on the collagen of sclerodermatous skin, joint capsule of osteoarthritic patients (Herbert et al., 1974) and rat bone (Deshmukh et al., 1973).

The stability of collagen depends on the formation of specific lysine-derived intermolecular cross-links between tropocollagen molecules which make up the fibres (Bailey and Peach, 1968). The initial cross-links are labile aldimine bonds which can be cleaved by D-penicillamine (Bailey, 1968) though, during maturation, these bonds are replaced by more stable bonds which cannot be cleaved by this drug. Therefore, tissues which are rapidly synthesizing collagen with these labile cross-links are susceptible to the action of D-penicillamine.

As well as the effects of D-penicillamine on collagen cross-linking, Herbert et al. (1974) have found that this drug can inhibit partially the synthesis of collagen in sclerodermatous skin when cultured in vitro. These authors have suggested that it could have similar effects on the rapidly proliferating collagen in other tissues such as the joint capsule of osteo-arthrosis subjects and the invading pannus tissue of rheumatoid arthritis, providing they are rapidly synthesizing collagen at the time. Articular cartilage has a relatively low rate of collagen synthesis and D-penicillamine would presumably have relatively little effect on its collagen, though this remains to be shown especially in long-term treatment.

5 General conclusions

Gold compounds and chloroquine have much in common as anti-rheumatic drugs. They both take a long time to produce measurable clinical effects on the disease and yet have persistent effects following withdrawal. They are useful drugs whose effect on the disease appears to be more basic than that produced by nonsteroidal (aspirin-like) and steroidal drugs. They might be considered as marginally effective "true antirheumatic drugs" as opposed to the "antiinflammatory" nonsteroidal drugs in that they appear to moderate the disease process causing joint degradation, if given in large enough doses and for long enough. Unfortunately, both chloroquine and gold compounds are also similar in their highly toxic nature requiring very careful and limited use.

There seems little doubt that drugs such as gold and chloroquine (and penicillamine) would be applied more widely and at an earlier stage in the disease process were it not for their toxic effects. As we have seen, it is unfortunately not possible to select any single in vivo or in vitro activity and say that if one could find a drug with this activity and with low toxicity, it would be very useful for the treatment of rheumatoid arthritis. Hopefully, however, further thought and investigation with these drugs may lead us to discover which activities are desirable for a "true anti-rheumatic drug" and into designing new experimental systems to seek drugs with these activities.

D-Penicillamine is a relatively new drug for the treatment of rheumatoid arthritis, though it holds much promise. As already pointed out, it remains to be shown whether, if given in the right doses and for long enough, it can slow down joint destruction. Nevertheless, further investigation of its mode of action would be worth while since it does appear to have some similarities to gold and chloroquine in affecting some of the basic features of rheumatoid arthritis.

References

Abraham, R. and Hendy R. (1970). *Experimental and Molecular Pathology*, **12**, 148.

Adam, M. (1968). *Zeitschrift für Rheumaforschung*, **27**, 102.

Adam, M., Bartl, P., Deyl, Z. and Rosmus, J. (1965). *Annals of the Rheumatic Diseases*, **24**, 378.

Adam, M., Fietzek, P. and Kühn, K. (1968). *European Journal of Biochemistry*, **3**, 411.

Ali, S. Y., Evans, L., Stainthorpe, E. and Lack, C. H. (1967). *Biochemical Journal*, **105**, 549.

Allison, A. C. and Davies, P. (1975). *In* "The Immunological Basis of Connective Tissue Disorders" (Ed. L. G. Silvestri), p. 155. North Holland, Amsterdam and London.

Allison, A. C. and Young, M. R. (1969). *In* "Lysosomes in Biology and Pathology" (Eds J. T. Dingle and H. B. Fell), vol. 2, p. 600. North Holland, Amsterdam and London.

Andrews, F. M., Golding, D. N., Freeman, A. M., Golding, J. R., Day, A. T., Hill, A. G. S., Camp, A. V., Lewis-Fanning, E. and Lyle, W. H. (1973). *Lancet*, **i**, 275.

Arrigoni-Martelli, E. and Bramm, E. (1975). *Agents and Actions*, **5**, 264.

Bailey, A. J. (1968). *Biochimica et Biophysica Acta*, **160**, 447.

Bailey, A. J. and Peach, C. M. (1968). *Biochemical and Biophysical Research Communications*, **33**, 812.

Ball, J. (1968). *In* "Rheumatic Diseases" (Eds J. J. R. Duthie and W. R. M. Alexander), p. 123. University Press, Edinburgh.

Barland, P. (1973). *American Journal of Medicine*, **54**, 143.

Barrett, A. J. (1975). *In* "Dynamics of Connective Tissue Macromolecules" (Eds P. M. C. Burleigh and A. R. Poole), p. 189. North Holland, Amsterdam and London.

Baumgartner, R., Obenaus, H. and Stoerk, H. C. (1974). *Proceedings of the Society for Experimental Biology and Medicine*, **146**, 241.

Bluestone, R. and Goldberg, L. S. (1973). *Annals of the Rheumatic Diseases*, **32**, 50.

Brostoff, J., Freedman, A. and Roitt, I. M. (1973). *International Archives of Allergy and Applied Immunology*, **45**, 690.
Cowey, F. K. and Whitehouse, M. W. (1966). *Biochemical Pharmacology*, **15**, 1071.
Day, A. T., Golding, J. R., Lee, P. N. and Butterworth, A. D. (1974). *British Medical Journal*, **1**, 180.
Deby, C., Bacq, Z. M. and Simon, D. (1973). *Biochemical Pharmacology*, **22**, 3141.
DeDuve, C., DeBarsy, T., Poole, B., Trouet, A., Tulkens, P. and Van Hoof, F. (1974). *Biochemical Pharmacology*, **23**, 2495.
Deshmukh, K., Just, M. and Nimni, M. E. (1973). *Clinical Orthopaedics and Related Research*, **91**, 186.
Deutsch, M. F. and Morton, J. I. (1957). *Science*, **125**, 600.
Dixon, A. St. J., Davies, J., Dormandy, T. L., Hamilton, E. B. D., Holt, P. J. L., Mason, R. M., Thompson, M., Weber, J. C. P. and Zutshi, D. W. (1975). *Annals of the Rheumatic Diseases*, **34**, 416.
Dresner, E. and Trombly, P. (1960). *Clinical Research*, **8**, 16.
Empire Rheumatism Council (1961). *Annals of the Rheumatic Diseases*, **20**, 315.
Ennis, R. S., Granada, J. L. and Posner, A. S. (1968). *Arthritis and Rheumatism*, **11**, 756.
Fedorko, M. E. (1967). *Journal of Clinical Investigation*, **46**, 1932.
Fedorko, M. E. (1968). *Laboratory Investigation*, **18**, 27.
Fedorko, M. E., Hirsch, J. G. and Cohn, Z. A. (1968). *Journal of Cell Biology*, **38**, 377.
Fikrig, S. M. and Smithwick, E. M. (1968). *Arthritis and Rheumatism*, **11**, 478.
Filkins, J. P. (1969). *Biochemical Pharmacology*, **18**, 2655.
Findlay, G. M., MacKenzie, R. D., MacCallum, M. D. and Klieneberger, E. (1939). *Lancet*, **ii**, 7.
Flower, R. J. (1974). *Pharmacological Reviews*, **26**, 33.
Gaddioni, G., Carraro, P. R. and Capitani, G. (1964). *Archivio Italiano di Dermatologia, Venerologia e Sessilogia*, **33**, 397.
Gardner, D. L. (1972). *In* "The Pathology of Rheumatoid Arthritis" (Ed. D. L. Garder), p. 188. Edward Arnold, London.
Gerber, D. A. (1971). *Arthritis and Rheumatism*, **14**, 383.
Gerber, R. C., Paulus, H. E., Bluestone, R. and Pearson, C. M. (1972a). *Annals of the Rheumatic Diseases*, **31**, 308.
Gerber, R. C., Whitehouse, M. W. and Orr, K. J. (1972b). *Proceedings of the Society for Experimental Biology and Medicine*, **140**, 1379.
Goldlust, M. B. and Schreiber, W. F. (1975). *Agents and Actions*, **5**, 39.
Gottlieb, N. L., Smith, P. M. and Smith, E. M. (1972). *Arthritis and Rheumatism*, **15**, 16.
Gottlieb, N. L., Kiem, I. M., Penneys, N. S. and Schultz, D. R. (1975). *Journal of Laboratory and Clinical Medicine*, **86**, 962.
Graeme, M. L., Fabry, E. and Sigg, E. B. (1966). *Journal of Pharmacology and Experimental Therapeutics*, **153**, 373.
Griffin, S. W., Ulloa, A., Henry, M., Johnston, M. L. and Holley, H. L. (1960). *Clinical Research*, **8**, 87.
Grundmann, M., Vrublovský, P., Demková, V., Mikulíková, I. and Pěgřimová, E. (1972). *Arzneimittel-Forschung*, **22**, 82.
Hamerman, D. (1969). *Clinical Orthopaedics*, **64**, 91.
Harris, E. D. Jr. and Sjoerdsma, A. (1966). *Lancet*, **ii**, 996.
Herbert, C. M., Jayson, M. I. V., Lindberg, K. A. and Bailey, A. J. (1974). *Postgraduate Medical Journal*, **50**, August Supplement, 27.

Homewood, C. A., Warhurst, D. C., Peters, W. and Baggaley, V. C. (1972). *Nature*, **235**, 50.

Huskisson, E. C. and Berry, H. (1974). *Postgraduate Medical Journal*, **50**, August Supplement, 59.

Huskisson, E. C., Gibson, T. J., Balme, H. W., Berry, H., Burry, H. C., Grahame, R., Dudley-Hart, F., Henderson, D. R. F. and Wojtulewski, J. A. (1974). *Annals of the Rheumatic Diseases*, **33**, 532.

Hyttel, J. and Jorgensen, A. (1970). *European Journal of Pharmacology*, **11**, 383.

Ignarro, L. J. (1971). *Biochemical Pharmacology*, **20**, 2861.

Ignarro, L. J. (1973). *Biochemical Pharmacology*, **22**, 1269.

Jaffe, I. A. (1962). *Journal of Laboratory and Clinical Medicine*, **60**, 409.

Jaffe, I. A. (1963). *Annals of the Rheumatic Diseases*, **22**, 71.

Jaffe, I. A. (1964). *Annals of Internal Medicine*, **61**, 556.

Jaffe, I. A. (1970). *Arthritis and Rheumatism*, **13**, 436.

Janoff, A. (1970). *Biochemical Pharmacology*, **19**, 626.

Jasmin, G. (1957). *Journal of Pharmacology and Experimental Therapeutics*, **120**, 349.

Jessop, J. D. and Currey, H. L. F. (1968). *Annals of the Rheumatic Diseases*, **27**, 577.

Kalmanson, G. M. and Guze, L. B. (1965). *Journal of Laboratory and Clinical Medicine*, **65**, 484.

Koch, R. (1890). *Deutsche Medizinische Wochenschrift*, **16**, 756.

Landé, K. (1927). *Muenchen Medizinische Wochenschrift*, **74**, 1132.

Lie, S. O., McKusik, V. A. and Neufield, E. F. (1972). *Proceedings of the National Academy of Sciences, U.S.A.* **69**, 2361.

Lie, S. O. and Schofield, B. (1973). *Biochemical Pharmacology*, **22**, 3109.

Liyanage, S. P. and Currey, H. L. F. (1972). *Annals of the Rheumatic Diseases*, **31**, 521.

Mascarenhas, B. R., Granda, J. L. and Freyberg, R. H. (1972). *Arthritis and Rheumatism*, **15**, 391.

McChesney, E. W. and Rothfield, N. F. (1964). *Arthritis and Rheumatism*, **7**, 328.

Mourisden, H. T., Barentsen, O., Rossing, N. and Jensen, K. B. (1974). *Arthritis and Rheumatism*, **17**, 391.

Newbould, B. B. (1963). *British Journal of Pharmacology and Chemotherapy*, **21**, 127.

Ohlsson, K. and Delshammar, M. (1975). *In* "Dynamics of Connective Tissue Macromolecules" (Eds P. M. C. Burleigh and A. R. Poole), p. 259. North Holland, Amsterdam and London.

Penneys, N. S., Ziboh, V., Gottlieb, N. L. and Katz, S. (1974). *Journal of Investigative Dermatology*, **63**, 356.

Perper, R. J. and Oronsky, A. L. (1974). *Arthritis and Rheumatism*, **17**, 47.

Perper, R. J., Sanda, M., Chinea, G. and Oronsky, A. L. (1974). *Journal of Laboratory and Clinical Medicine*, **84**, 394.

Perrine, J. W. and Takesue, E. I. (1968). *Archives Internationales de Pharmacodynamie et de Therapie*, **174**, 192.

Persellin, R. H. and Ziff, M. (1966). *Arthritis and Rheumatism*, **9**, 57.

Persellin, R. H., Hess, E. V. and Ziff, M. (1967). *Arthritis and Rheumatism*, **10**, 99.

Reynolds, J. J. and Werb, Z. (1975). *In* "Extracellular Matrix Influences on Gene Expression" (Eds H. C. Slavkin and R. C. Greulich), p. 225. Academic Press, New York and London.

Ringrose, P. S., Parr, M. A. and McLaren, M. (1975). *Biochemical Pharmacology*, **24**, 607.

Roath, S. and Wills, R. (1974). *Postgraduate Medical Journal*, **50**, August Supplement, 56.
Rothbard, S. Angevine, D. M. and Cecil, R. L. (1941). *Journal of Pharmacology and Experimental Therapeutics*, **72**, 164.
Rubin, M., Berstein, H. N. and Zvaifler, N. J. (1963). *Archives of Opthalmology*, **70**, 474.
Rubinstein, H. M. and Dietz, A. A. (1973). *Annals of the Rheumatic Diseases*, **32**, 128.
Sabin, A. B. and Warren, J. (1940). *Journal of Bacteriology*, **40**, 823.
Scherrer, R. A. (1974). *In* "Antiinflammatory Agents—Chemistry and Pharmacology" (Eds R. A. Scherrer and M. W. Whitehouse), vol. 1, p. 3. Academic Press, New York and London.
Schumacher, K., Maerker-Alzer, G. and Schaaf, W. (1975a). *Arzneimittel-Forschung*, **25**, 600.
Schumacher, K., Maerker-Alzer, G. and Preuss, R. (1975b). *Arzneimittel-Forschung*, **25**, 603.
Sigler, J. W., Bluhm, G. B., Duncan, H., Sharp, J. T., Ensign, D. C. and McCrum, W. R. (1972). *Arthritis and Rheumatism*, **15**, 125.
Sigler, J. W., Bluhm, G. B., Duncan, H., Sharp, J. T., Ensign, D. C. and McCrum, W. R. (1974). *Annals of Internal Medicine*, **80**, 21.
Sofia, R. D. and Douglas, J. F. (1973). *Agents and Actions*, **3**, 335.
Stone, K. J., Mather, S. J. and Gibson, P. P. (1975). *Prostaglandins*, **10**, 241.
Swartz, H. A., Christian, J. E. and Andrews, F. N. (1960). *American Journal of Physiology*, **199**, 67.
Teitz, C. C. and Chrisman, O. D. (1975). *Clinical Orthopaedics and Related Research*, **108**, 264.
Thomas, L. (1973). *Federation Proceedings*, **32**, 143.
Thomas, L., Davidson, M. and McCluskey, R. (1966). *Journal of Experimental Medicine*, **123**, 897.
Trnavská, Z. and Trnavský, K. (1968a). *Biochemical Pharmacology*, **20**, 564.
Trnavský, K. and Trnavská, Z. (1968b). *Journal of Pharmacy and Pharmacology*, **20**, 564.
Volastro, P. S., Malawista, S. E. and Chrisman, O. D. (1973). *Clinical Orthopaedics and Related Research*, **91**, 24.
Walz, D. T. (1974). *In* "Antiinflammatory Agents—Chemistry and Pharmacology" (Eds R. A. Scherrer and M. W. Whitehouse), vol. 1, p. 217. Academic Press, New York and London.
Walz, D. T., DiMartino, M. J. and Misher, A. (1971). *Annals of the Rheumatic Diseases*, **30**, 303.
Walz, D. T., DiMartino, M. J., Sutton, B. and Misher, A. (1972). *Journal of Pharmacology and Experimental Therapeutics*, **181**, 292.
Ward, P. A. (1966). *Journal of Experimental Medicine*, **124**, 209.
Ward, P. A. (1968). *Biochemical Pharmacology*, **17** (Supplement), 99.
Whitehouse, M. W. and Boström, H. (1962). *Biochemical Pharmacology*, **11**, 1175
Wiesinger, D. (1965). *In* "Non-steroidal Antiinflammatory Drugs"—Proceedings of an International Symposium, Milan 1964, p. 221. Excerpta Medica Foundation.
Woolley, D. (1975). Personal communication.
Young, J. P. (1959). *Annals of Internal Medicine*, **51**, 1159.
Zvaifler, N. J. (1974). *Arthritis and Rheumatism*, **17**, 297.
Zvaifler, N. J. and Rubin, M. (1962). *Arthritis and Rheumatism*, **5**, 330.

The Significance of Melanocyte-stimulating Hormone (MSH) and the Control of its Secretion in the Mammal

A. J. THODY, Phd.

*Department of Dermatology, University of Newcastle upon Tyne,
Newcastle upon Tyne, England*

1 Introduction

The melanocyte-stimulating hormones (MSHs) are a group of polypeptides secreted by the pars intermedia of the pituitary gland. They were first identified by their ability to darken the skin of the lower vertebrates and it was this property which provided the name, melanocyte-stimulating hormone (Lerner et al., 1954). This pigmentary effect of MSH is now well understood and in the lower vertebrates MSH clearly has an important role in the adaptive colour changes that these animals undergo in response to environmental influences (see Bagnara and Hadley, 1973). MSH also promotes melanogenesis in the mammal but it is unlikely that this effect has any physiological significance and MSH has often been dismissed as an evolutionary vestige. During the course of evolution, however, MSH has acquired various extra-pigmentary effects and certain of these may be of significance in the mammal. This possibility has revived new interest in the control of MSH secretion and it now appears that MSH secretion in the mammal is closely controlled by the central nervous system as it is in the lower vertebrates.

The purpose of the present review is to outline our current knowledge concerning the control of MSH secretion and its possible significance in the mammal. Before discussing these points it is proposed to give a brief description of the different MSH peptides that have been found in mammalian species.

2 The MSH peptides and their occurrence

At least two distinct forms of MSH exist and these are known as α- and β-MSH. Both are small polypeptides containing a heptapeptide sequence which is also present in adrenocorticotrophin (ACTH) and the lipotrophins (LPH) (Fig. 1) and is essential for melanocyte-stimulating activity.

2.1 α-MSH

Mammalian α-MSH, the most potent melanocyte-stimulating peptide known, is a basic acetyl tridecapepeptide whose amino acid sequence is identical to the 1-13 portion of ACTH (Fig. 1). Its high potency is probably due to the presence of the acetyl-Ser-Tyr-Ser N-terminal which protects the biologically active heptapeptide core from enzymatic degradation (Lowry and Chadwick, 1970a). The high potency of α-MSH, together with its small size, constant amino acid sequence in all mammals so far studied and its similarity to dogfish MSH (Lowry and Chadwick, 1970b) suggests that it is the more primitive MSH (Lowry and Chadwick, 1970a).

It has recently been proposed that ACTH serves as the precursor of α-MSH in the pars intermedia (Scott *et al.*, 1974). For some years it has been known that ACTH is present in the posterior lobe (Miahle-Voloss, 1958a; Rochefort *et al.*, 1959; Hess *et al.*, 1968; Baker and Drummond, 1972) and has a different role from that in the anterior lobe (Kraicer *et al.*, 1973). Scott *et al.* (1974) considered that the pars intermedia contains a trypsin-like enzyme that cleaves the ACTH molecule between residues 13 and 18 to give α-MSH and the 18-39 portion of ACTH, commonly referred to as corticotrophin-like intermediate lobe peptide or CLIP. Support for this idea was the finding of equivalent amounts of α-MSH and CLIP in pituitary extracts (Scott *et al.*, 1973, 1974) and the strong immunostaining of pars intermedia cells with an anti α(17-39)ACTH serum (Phifer and Spicer, 1970; Kraicer *et al.*, 1973). This cleavage of ACTH is presumably confined to the pars intermedia since only traces of α-MSH have been found in the pars anterior of several mammalian species (Dubois, 1971; Baker and Drummond, 1972; Dubois, 1972; Stefan and Dubois, 1972; Thody *et al.*, 1975a; 1975b).

2.2 β-MSH

Several different forms of β-MSH occur. All are larger than α-MSH and display less melanocyte-stimulating activity. Two forms have been found in the sheep, ox and pig (Geschwind *et al.*, 1956, 1957). One of these contains a glutamyl residue at position 2 and is sometimes known as β-glutamyl MSH, whilst the other has a seryl residue and is referred to as β-seryl MSH (Fig. 1). Another β-MSH has been found in the horse and this is similar to β-glutamyl MSH, but has arginine in position 16 in place of proline (Dixon and Li, 1961) (Fig. 1). Two further variants have been isolated from the pituitary of the monkey (Lee *et al.*, 1961). These are similar to β-glutamyl and β-seryl MSH but contain arginine in position 6 in place of lysine. Human β-MSH has the same substitution but, unlike other forms of β-MSH which are octadecapeptides, contains an additional four amino acids at its N-terminal (Fig. 1).

The structural differences between the β-MSHs and ACTH make it extremely unlikely that β-MSHs are formed in the same way as α-MSH. The β-MSHs are more closely related to the LPHs and it is reasonable to suppose that these pituitary hormones act as precursors for β-MSH. LPHs have been isolated from the pituitary glands of various mammals (Li, 1964; Li *et al.*, 1965; Chrétien and Li, 1967a, 1967b; Lohmar and Li, 1967; Graf *et al.*, 1969) including man (Cseh *et al.*, 1968). So far two main types have been found, β- and γ-LPH consisting of ninety-one and fifty-eight amino acids respectively. The 41–58 sequence of these two molecules

	1 2 3		11 12 13 39
ACTH	Ser-Tyr-Ser		Lys-Pro-Val ....Phe
α-MSH	CH₃CO-Ser-Tyr-Ser	Met-Glu-His-Phe-Arg-Try-Gly	Lys-Pro-Val-CONH₂
β-MSH (ox, pig, sheep)	Asp-Ser-Gly-Pro-Tyr-Lys		Ser-Pro-Pro-Lys-Asp
β-MSH (ox, pig, sheep)	Asp-Glu-Gly-Pro-Tyr-Lys		Ser-Pro-Pro-Lys-Asp
β-MSH (horse)	Asp-Glu-Gly-Pro-Tyr-Lys		Ser-Pro-Arg-Lys-Asp
β-MSH (monkey)	Asp-Glu-Gly-Pro-Tyr-Arg		Ser-Pro-Pro-Lys-Asp
β-MSH (human)	Ala-Glu-Lys-Lys-Asp-Glu-Gly-Pro-Tyr-Lys		Ser-Pro-Pro-Lys-Asp
γ-LPH (sheep)	Glu . . . Ala-Glu-Lys-Lys-Asp-Ser-Gly-Pro-Tyr-Lys		Ser-Pro-Pro-Lys-Asp
β-LPH (sheep)	Glu . . . Ala-Glu-Lys-Lys-Lys-Asp-Ser-Gly-Pro-Tyr-Lys		Ser-Pro-Pro-Lys-Asp . . . Glu
	1 . . . 37 38 39 40 41 42 43 44 45 46		54 55 56 57 58 . . . 90

Fig. 1. Amino acid sequences of MSH peptides and their relationship to ACTH and ovine γ- and β-LPH.

is identical to β-glutamyl MSH and this led to the suggestion that β-MSH is formed by the enzymatic cleavage of β-LPH with γ-LPH occurring as an intermediate component (Chrétien and Li, 1967a, 1967b; Chrétien, 1973).

2.3 OCCURRENCE

MSH peptides have been isolated from the pituitary glands of various mammals including the ox (Geschwind et al., 1957; Li, 1959), pig (Lerner and Lee, 1955; Porath et al., 1955; Geschwind et al., 1956; Li, 1959), sheep (Li, 1959), horse (Dixon and Li, 1960, 1961), monkey (Lee et al., 1961) and man (Harris, 1959; Dixon, 1960) and in most of these mammals more than one form of MSH has been found. In the ox, pig and sheep three forms have been identified as α-, β-seryl and β-glutamyl MSH (see Geschwind, 1966) and these same three forms may also occur in the horse, deer (Burgers, 1963) and rat (Thody, 1969a; Hoekstra and Van der Wal, 1971).

Other workers, however, have failed to identify MSHs in the pituitary of the rat and other rodents (Shapiro et al., 1972) and it now appears that the major MSH in the rat is α-MSH (Shapiro et al., 1972; Scott et al., 1972; Baker, 1973; Thody et al., 1975a, 1975b). In man, the predominant MSH is thought to be a β-MSH (Abe et al., 1967a) (but see section 5) and only trace amounts of α-MSH have been found in human pituitary tissue (Abe et al., 1967b).

Melanocyte-stimulating activity has also been found in the brain of several mammals (Miahle-Voloss, 1958b; Guillemin et al., 1962; Schally et al., 1962) with the highest concentration occurring in the hypothalamus. Guillemin et al. (1962) and Schally et al. (1962) considered this activity to be due to α- and β-MSH, but whether these peptides are conveyed from the pituitary or are synthesized in situ in the hypothalamus is not clear. Immunoreactive α-MSH has been found in the hypothalamus of the rat and to persist after removal of the pituitary (Oliver et al., 1976). The presence of α-MSH in the brain of hypophysectomized rat is not conclusive evidence for its synthesis by neural tissue since it could be produced by the pars tuberalis and the rostral zone of the pars intermedia which often remain intact after hypophysectomy (Oliver et al., 1976).

Other MSH peptides may be present in the brain and Rudman et al. (1973) consider that most of the melanocyte-stimulating activity in neural tissue is attributable to a peptide which they refer to as IIF. This peptide is unlike other known MSHs in that it contains no methionine or tyrosine.

3   Control of MSH secretion in experimental mammals

3.1   HYPOTHALAMIC CONTROL

3.1.1   *Removal of hypothalamic influence*

There have been many reports that the pars intermedia undergoes hypertrophy and hyperplasia after section of the pituitary stalk (Brooks, 1938; Uotila, 1939; Barrnett and Greep, 1951; Daniel and Prichard, 1958; Holmes, 1961, 1962; Vincent, 1969), lesions of the hypothalamus (Stutinsky *et al.*, 1950; Bogdanove and Halmi, 1953; Greer and Erwin, 1956; Kordon and Bachrach, 1959; Howe and Thody, 1969a; Ooki *et al.*, 1973) or transplantation of the pituitary (May and Stutinsky, 1947; Siperstein and Greer, 1956). Changes in pituitary MSH content have also been reported after removal of the hypothalamic influence (Kastin and Ross, 1964; Bal and

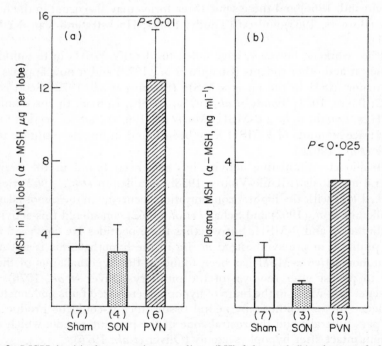

FIG. 2. MSH in (a) the neurointermediate (NI) lobe and (b) plasma of sham-operated rats and after lesions of the supraoptic (SON) and paraventricular nuclei (PVN). MSH activity was measured by bioassay and is expressed in terms of synthetic α-MSH. The number of rats in each group is given in parenthesis. The P value refers to the significant difference when compared with the sham-operated group. (Modified from Thody, 1974.)

Smelik, 1967; Taleisnik *et al.*, 1967; Howe and Thody, 1969a; Thody, 1974).

Changes in hormonal content of a gland without corresponding changes in plasma levels are, however, difficult to interpret because they reflect the balance between hormonal synthesis and release. Increases in plasma MSH levels have been found in rats after large lesions involving the medial basal hypothalamus (Carrillo *et al.*, 1973), although no changes were found in the MSH content of the pituitary. More recently, Thody (1974) reported an increase in plasma and pituitary MSH levels after lesions of the paraventricular nuclei (PVN) (Fig. 2). Destruction of the PVN therefore produces an increase in MSH release and because of this the raised MSH levels in the pituitary gland presumably reflect an enhanced synthesis.

The evidence therefore suggests that the pars intermedia becomes hypersecretory after the removal of the hypothalamic influence. Although it would appear that the hypothalamus normally has an inhibitory effect it may also exert an excitatory control on the pars intermedia and MSH secretion (Howe and Thody, 1969a; Thody, 1969b). This view is supported by an earlier observation that the pars intermedia is reduced in size and apparently hypoactive after small, discrete lesions in the region of the PVN (Olivecrona, 1957). Figure 3 summarizes the areas where lesions have been found to affect MSH secretion.

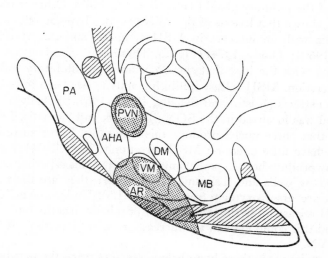

FIG. 3. Diagram of the hypothalamus showing areas (stippled) where lesions have been reported to affect MSH secretion. PA, preoptic area; AHA, anterior hypothalamic area; PVN, paraventricular nucleus; DM, dorsomedial nucleus; VM, ventromedial nucleus; AR, arcuate nucleus; MB, mamillary body.

3.1.2   *The paraventricular and supra-optic nuclei*

Although the precise hypothalamic area concerned with MSH control has not been defined it has been suspected for some years that a functional relationship may exist between the hypothalamo-neurohypophysial system and the pars intermedia. Numerous workers have shown that activation of the neurohypophysis by administration of hypertonic saline or dehydration is accompanied by changes in the histological appearance of the pars intermedia (Selye and Hall, 1943; Legait and Legait, 1961, 1962; Duchen, 1962; Roux, 1962; Legait, 1963; Ziegler, 1963; Kobayashi, 1964; Soboleva, 1964; Howe and Thody, 1970) and its MSH content (Howe and Thody, 1970). Suckling has also been reported to affect the MSH content of the pituitary (Taleisnik and Tomatis, 1968). These observations support the idea that the PVN and supraoptic nuclei (SON), besides being involved in the synthesis and secretion of neurohypophysial hormones, also participate in the control of MSH (Taleisnik *et al.*, 1967; Thody, 1969b).

Extracts of the PVN have been shown to decrease the MSH content of the pituitary and it was suggested that these nuclei are responsible for the production of an MSH releasing factor (MRF) (Taleisnik and Orías, 1965; Taleisnik *et al.*, 1966). Destruction of the PVN results in a loss of MRF activity in the median eminence and neural lobe and a decrease in the MSH content of the pituitary gland (Talesnik *et al.*, 1967). Other workers have, however, shown that lesions of the PVN produce hyperactivity of the pars intermedia with an increase in MSH synthesis and release (Howe and Thody, 1969a; Thody, 1974) (Fig. 2). These latter observations are more in keeping with the idea that the PVN have an inhibitory influence on MSH secretion. MSH release inhibiting activity has been found in hypothalamic extracts (Kastin and Schally, 1966a, 1967a; Schally and Kastin, 1966) and was localized in the SON (Taleisnik and Tomatis, 1967a). It is unlikely that these nuclei produce this inhibitory factor since lesions in the SON have little effect on MSH secretion (Thody, 1974) (Fig. 2). The PVN may produce both hypothalamic factors and this is perhaps likely if, as suggested by Celis and Taleisnik (1971, 1973), they are derived from a common precursor oxytocin (see section 3.1.5). Under normal conditions the MSH release inhibiting factor (MIF) probably has the more dominant effect and this could explain the increase in MSH secretion after ablation of the PVN.

It is not clear how these hypothalamic factors reach the pars intermedia. Unlike the pars anterior the pars intermedia in most mammals is relatively avascular (see Howe, 1973) and is not served by capillaries of the hypothalamo-hypophysial portal system. A possibility is that these factors are released from neurosecretory fibres that directly innervate the cells of the pars intermedia (see Fig. 6). Neurosecretory fibres have been found in the pars intermedia of several mammalian species (Bargmann and Knoop, 1960; Kurosumi *et al.*, 1961; Ziegler, 1963; Kobayashi, 1964, 1965; Howe and Maxwell, 1966, 1968; Vincent, 1969; Vincent and Kumar, 1968, 1969; Cameron and Foster, 1971) and in some cases were seen to make direct contact with cells of the pars intermedia. Since these neurosecretory fibres may originate in the PVN and SON (see Howe, 1973) they could provide a functional link between these hypothalamic nuclei and the pars intermedia.

3.1.3 *MSH release inhibiting factor (MIF)*

Extracts prepared from the hypothalami of a number of species, including man, have been shown to increase the MSH content of the rat pituitary gland and to lighten frogs previously darkened by removal of the hypothalamus (Kastin and Schally, 1966b, 1967a). These findings were taken to indicate the presence of a hypothalamic factor that inhibits MSH release, now commonly known as MSH release inhibiting factor of MIF (Schally and Kastin, 1966). Taleisnik and Tomatis (1967a, 1967b) also found hypothalamic extracts to have MIF activity, but these workers claim that MIF acts by blocking the action of an MSH-releasing factor (MRF) that is present in the hypothalamus (see section 3.4).

MIF was first purified from bovine hypothalami (Schally and Kastin, 1966) and two peptides with MIF activity have now been isolated and identified as Pro-Leu-Gly-NH_2 (Nair *et al.*, 1971) and Pro-His-Phe-Arg-Gly-NH_2 (Nair *et al.*, 1972).

The former, which happens to be the side chain of oxytocin, was found to be more potent in its ability to lighten frogs previously darkened by destruction of the hypothalamus (Nair *et al.*, 1972). Pro-Leu-Gly-NH_2 has also been shown to block the depletion of rat pituitary MSH and the rise in plasma MSH induced by MRF or median eminence lesions (Celis *et al.*, 1971, 1972, 1973). This rise in plasma MSH was also inhibited by Pro-Lys-Gly-NH_2 and Pro-Arg-Gly-NH_2 (Celis *et al.*, 1972) and it would be of interest to know whether these tripeptides are effective in other MIF assays.

Not all workers agree that Pro-Leu-Gly-NH_2 is an MIF and there have been reports that it has no effect on MSH release from incubated pituitaries (Bower *et al.*, 1971; Hruby *et al.*, 1972; Hadley *et al.*, 1973; Grant *et al.*, 1973). Other workers have failed to demonstrate any effect in the intact rat (Kastin *et al.*, 1973; Thody and Shuster, 1973a). Kastin *et al.* (1973)

Sequences	References
Oxytocin Cys-Tyr-Ile-Glu-(NH$_2$)-Asp-(NH$_2$)-Cys-Pro-Leu-Gly-(NH$_2$)	Nair et al. (1971); Celis et al. (1971, 1972)
MIF I Pro-Leu-Gly-(NH$_2$)	Celis et al. (1972)
Pro-Lys-Gly-(NH$_2$)	Celis et al. (1972)
Pro-Arg-Gly-(NH$_2$)	Celis et al. (1972)
Tocinoic acid Cys-Tyr-Ile-Glu-(NH$_2$)-Asp-(NH$_2$)-Cys	Bower et al. (1971); Hruby et al. (1972); Hadley et al. (1973)
MIF II Pro-His-Phe-Arg-Gly-(NH$_2$)	Nair et al. (1972)

FIG. 4. Various peptides which have been reported to inhibit the release of MSH. The amino acid sequence of oxytocin is given as a comparison.

offer the possibility that Pro-Leu-Gly-NH$_2$ is unstable and have attempted to overcome this problem by infusing the tripeptide directly into the pituitary portal system of the rat. This approach produced no significant changes in MSH release. The lack of effect may have been due to the fact that the pars intermedia of the rat is relatively avascular and is probably not served by the hypophysial portal system (see Howe, 1973).

It has been reported that tocinoic acid, the ring structure of oxytocin, and its amide tocinamide, are active in inhibiting MSH release from incubated pituitary glands of several species (Bower et al., 1971; Hruby et al., 1972; Hadley et al., 1973). Others, however, have found tocinoic acid to have no effect on the release of MSH from intact rats (Celis et al., 1972, 1973; Grant et al., 1973).

There is obviously much controversy concerning the identity of MIF. Several peptides have been shown to have MIF activity and these are listed in Fig. 4. Part of the problem could be the question of species specificity and the use of different procedures for the assay of MIF activity. The lack of a standard MIF assay makes it extremely difficult to compare the findings of different workers and until a suitable method is available the nature of MIF must remain open.

3.1.4 *MSH-releasing factor (MRF)*

There is evidence that the hypothalamus is also responsible for a substance that stimulates the release of MSH (Taleisnik and Orías, 1965; Kastin and Schally, 1966b). The proposed MRF has not been identified, although Celis et al. (1971b) have shown that the opened ring portion of oxytocin, H-Cys-Tyr-Ile-Gln-Asn-OH, stimulates MSH release from the rat pituitary gland.

3.1.5 *Formation of MIF and MRF*

An interesting possibility is that both MIF and MRF are formed from a common precursor, oxytocin. It has been proposed that two competing hypothalamic peptidases are concerned with the formation of MIF and MRF (Celis and Taleisnik, 1973). These workers postulate that one enzyme found in the median eminence and designated E_1 favours the formation of MIF, while the other E_2, possibly occurring in the PVN, forms MRF and in so doing prevents the formation of MIF. Whether MRF or MIF is formed depends upon the relative activity of the two peptidases. The amount of the precursor, oxytocin, may also be important, high concentrations favouring the formation of MIF (Celis and Taleisnik, 1973).

Further studies are now required to show that MSH secretion can be affected by changes in the activity of these hypothalamic peptidases. Although the concentration of MIF in the hypothalamus has been shown to vary under different conditions known to affect MSH secretion (Taleisnik and Tomatis, 1968, 1969, 1970; Tomatis and Taleisnik, 1968a) it is not clear whether these changes reflect synthesis or release of MIF.

3.1.6 Biogenic amines and MSH secretion

a. *Effect of drugs.* Drugs such as reserpine, haloperidol and the phenothiazines which deplete catecholamines or block their action have been reported to stimulate MSH secretion (Tomatis and Taleisnik, 1968; Kastin and Schally, 1966b; Kastin et al., 1969; Thody, 1969b; Scott and Stillings, 1972; Peaslee and Milburn, 1973; Thody and Shuster, 1973a; Thody et al., 1975a, 1975b; Penny and Thody, 1976). The effect of trifluoperazine on pituitary and serum MSH levels in the rat is shown in Fig. 5. α-Methyl-p-tyrosine, a drug that inhibits catecholamine synthesis, may also stimulate the release and possibly the synthesis of α-MSH (Fig. 5). On the other hand, the dopaminomimetic drug, bromo-α-ergocryptine (CB154), would appear to inhibit the release of α-MSH in the rat (Fig. 5).

b. *Monoamines and MIF release.* Injection of noradrenaline or dopamine into the third ventricle has been shown to prevent the release of MSH that occurs after the intravenous injection of hypertonic saline (Taleisnik et al., 1972). Since noradrenaline was ineffective when implanted into the pituitary gland it was considered that catecholamines influence MSH secretion at the hypothalamic level through the control of MIF release (Taleisnik et al., 1972). This was supported by the finding that noradrenaline implants in the third ventricle deplete hypothalamic MIF stores (Taleisnik et al., 1972).

Neurosecretory neurones that produce MIF may be innervated by the catecholaminergic fibres whose nerve endings have been found in the PVN (Fuxe and Hökfelt, 1969) (see Fig. 6). The origin of these fibres is not known. Under normal conditions these catecholaminergic fibres may have a tonic activating effect on the release of MIF, thus suppressing the secretion of MSH.

Stimulation of MSH secretion may be affected by a second system that operates by suppressing the activity of the catecholaminergic neurones (Taleisnik et al., 1974). This second system may involve serotoninergic neurones (see Fig. 6) since the effect of MSH releasing stimuli was blocked by p-chlorophenylalanine and methysergide while injection of

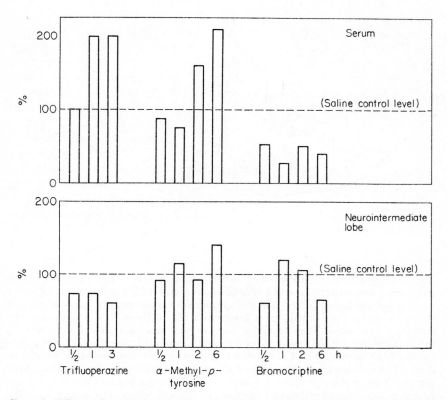

FIG. 5. Effect of a single injection of trifluoperazine, α-methyl-p-tyrosine and bromo-α-ergocryptine (bromocriptine) on α-MSH levels in serum and the neurointermediate lobe of the rat. α-MSH was measured by a radioimmunoassay method (Thody *et al.*, 1975a, 1976a). The results are expressed as a percentage of the value obtained in control rats that received a single injection of 0.9 per cent saline in place of the drug. TFP increased the release of α-MSH and this was reflected by a decrease in the α-MSH content of the neurointermediate lobe. α-MT also increased α-MSH release and the increased α-MSH content of the neurointermediate lobe could suggest a stimulation of hormone synthesis. Bromocriptine had a variable effect on neurointermediate lobe levels of α-MSH, but the decreased serum levels would suggest an inhibition of α-MSH release. (From Penny and Thody, unpublished observations.)

5-hydroxytryptamine into the third ventricle produced a depletion of pituitary MSH (Taleisnik *et al.*, 1974). These same workers consider that γ-aminobutyric acid (GABA) is involved as a transmitter in this system and may mediate the inhibitory effect on the catecholaminergic neurones.

Taleisnik and Celis (1972) have proposed that this neurogenic control of MIF release would allow rapid changes in the secretion of MSH and

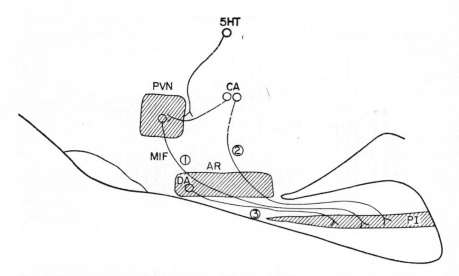

Fig. 6. Diagrammatic representation of the hypothalamus to show possible neural pathways involved in the control of MSH secretion. (1) MIF may be formed in the paraventricular nuclei (PVN) and transported via neurosecretory fibres which end either in direct contact with pars intermedia (PI) cells or in blood vessels that supply these cells. These neurosecretory neurones may be innervated by catecholaminergic (CA) neurones which exert a tonic stimulatory effect, thus maintaining MIF release. The CA neurones in turn may be innervated by serotoninergic (5-HT) fibres which suppress the CA neurones and thus inhibit MIF release. The origins of these CA and 5-HT neurones are not known. (2) CA neurones may also directly innervate the PI cells and control the release of MSH. The origin of these CA neurones is not known. Such a control is thought to exist in amphibia. (3) Dopaminergic fibres with origins in the arcuate nucleus (AR) also innervate the PI and may impose a direct inhibitory control on MSH release.

furthermore, by affecting MIF synthesis, could promote more prolonged changes in MSH secretion. This scheme makes no provision for MRF and it is not clear whether this releasing factor is affected by monoaminergic neurones. Whilst MIF has the more dominant effect and controls normal changes in MSH secretion, larger fluctuations might be mediated by MRF (Taleisnik et al., 1972; Thody and Shuster, 1973a).

c. *Direct catecholaminergic control of MSH release.* Catecholaminergic neurones have been found in the pars intermedia (Smelik, 1966; Fuxe and Hökfelt, 1949; Vincent and Kumar, 1969; Baumgarten et al., 1972; Nobin et al., 1972; Björklund et al., 1973) and it is possible that a direct neural control of MSH release exists, as has been suggested in amphibia (Enemar and Falck, 1965; Iturriza, 1969) (see Fig. 6). Incubation of the rat or frog pituitary resulted in a rapid release of MSH into the incubation medium and this was completely inhibited by the presence of adrenaline, noradrenaline or dopamine (Bower et al., 1974). Since the inhibitory effect of adrenaline was blocked by dibenamine it was suggested that catecholamines inhibit MSH release through α-adrenergic receptors present in the pars intermedia cells (Bower et al., 1974). These workers, however, did not dismiss the possibility that dopaminergic receptors might also be involved.

Evidence for a dopaminergic control of MSH release has come from the recent studies of Tilders and his co-workers. Tilders and Mulder (1974) noticed that a high K^+ concentration in the medium prevented MSH release from incubated pituitaries and that this effect could be abolished by the presence of a dopaminergic receptor blocker (haloperidol). The K^+-induced inhibition of MSH release was also absent in pituitaries from rats that had been pretreated with reserpine or in pituitaries that had been denervated by lesions in the median eminence (Tilders and Mulder, 1974; Tilders et al., 1975). Dopaminergic fibres that terminate in the pars intermedia have been shown to originate in the arcuate nucleus of the hypothalamus (Björklund et al., 1973), and it is suggested that these fibres may impose a direct inhibitory control on the release of MSH (Tilders et al., 1975) (see Fig. 6).

3.2 AUTOREGULATION OF MSH RELEASE

An intravenous injection of MSH has been shown to cause an increase in the MSH content of the pituitary gland and Kastin and Schally (1967b) concluded that circulating levels of MSH may inhibit the release of MSH. This feedback control may operate through an effect on the hypothalamus (Kastin and Schally, 1967b), although evidence from in vitro studies suggests that MSH may act directly on the pars intermedia (Kastin et al., 1971b). This effect has, however, been disputed by other workers (Hadley et al., 1973; Huntington and Hadley, 1974).

3.3 THE GONADS AND MSH SECRETION

There have been several reports that gonadal steroids affect the pars intermedia. Prolonged treatment for several months with oestrogen has been shown to cause hypertrophy and hyperplasia of the pars intermedia in the hamster (Vasquez-Lopez, 1944; Koneff et al., 1946; Racadot, 1958). Such changes were recently found to be accompanied by an increase in pituitary MSH content (Hamilton, et al., 1976). Long-term treatment with oestrogen also enlarges the pituitary gland of the guinea pig with signs of increased secretory activity in the pars intermedia (Barbarossa and

Pende, 1950). Similar changes have been found in the rat (Meddis and Thody, unpublished observations) and Geschwind and Huseby (1966) have described the development of a MSH secreting pituitary tumour in the mouse after chronic administration of oestrogen.

Lower doses of oestrogen given for shorter periods of time also appear to affect MSH secretion. Karkun and Sen (1965) reported increased pituitary levels of MSH in ovariectomized rats after oestrogen treatment for thirty days. We have found similar changes and, furthermore, noticed that ovariectomy reduced MSH levels in the pituitary (Plummer and Thody, unpublished observations). The exact reverse has been reported by Taleisnik and Tomatis (1969). These workers found increased pituitary MSH levels after ovariectomy with restoration to normal levels after oestrogen treatment. Progesterone also reduced MSH activity in the pituitary gland of the ovariectomized rat (Taleisnik and Tomatis, 1970).

Despite the inconsistency of some of these findings it would appear that gonadal hormones influence MSH secretion in some way and may account for the changes in pituitary MSH found in late pregnancy (Karkun and Sen, 1965), pseudopregnancy (Taleisnik and Tomatis, 1970) the oestrous cycle in the rat (Tomatis and Taleisnik, 1968b; Celis, 1975) and constant oestrous in the ferret (Norman et al., 1972). Although the exact nature of this influence is not known it has been suggested that oestrogen and progesterone block the synthesis of MIF (Taleisnik and Tomatis, 1970) and presumably stimulate MSH secretion. However, Celis and Taleisnik (1974) have since demonstrated that oestrogen activates MIF formation in extracts of the hypothalamus. As well as affecting MIF synthesis ovarian steroids may also be necessary for the inhibition of MIF release that occurs after neurogenic stimuli such as suckling and vaginal stimulation (Taleisnik and Tomatis, 1970).

3.4 THE ADRENAL GLANDS AND MSH SECRETION

Adrenalectomy and administration of glucocorticoids have little effect on plasma (Gosbee et al., 1970; Thody and Hinks, 1973) and pituitary MSH levels (Forgacs, 1956; Sulman and Eviatar, 1956; Ivy and Albert, 1957; Gosbee et al., 1970). Adrenalectomy has, however, been reported to produce histological changes in the rat pars intermedia suggestive of increased activity (Gosbee et al., 1970). These findings were consistent with those obtained from electron microscopic studies (Kobayashi, 1965). Since these changes were accompanied by an increase in the ACTH content of the pituitary and no histological changes were evident in the pars anterior it was concluded that the cells of the pars intermedia were concerned with ACTH synthesis (Gosbee et al., 1970). The ACTH in the pars intermedia probably has a different role from that in the pars anterior (Kraicer et al., 1973) and it has been considered to be a precursor of α-MSH (Scott et al., 1974) (see section 2.1).

3.5 LIGHT AND MSH SECRETION

It is well known that light affects MSH secretion in the lower vertebrates. Light may also affect MSH secretion in the mammal. Long daily photo-periods have been reported to darken the hair in short-tailed weasels (Bissonnette and Baily, 1944; Rust and Meyer, 1968). Short daily photo-periods, on the other hand, induced the growth of depigmented hairs in short-tailed weasels (Bissonnette and Baily, 1944; Rust and Meyer, 1968). These pigmentary effects were thought to be mediated by changes in the secretion of MSH.

Alterations in environmental lighting have been reported to produce changes in the MSH content of the pituitary gland. Kastin et al. (1967a) found increased pituitary MSH levels in rats exposed to constant illumina-tion and long daily photo-periods produced similar changes in ferrets (Norman et al., 1972). The stimulus of light may also have caused the sudden increase in the MSH content of the neurointermediate lobe found in young rats 24 hours after the opening of the eyes (Howe and Thody, 1969b; Thody, 1969b).

Darkness, on the other hand, produced a decrease in the MSH content of the pituitary gland (Kastin et al., 1967a). Since this effect did not occur in pinealectomized rats it was considered to be mediated through the pineal gland, possibly by the release of melatonin (Kastin et al., 1967b). Melatonin has been shown to decrease the MSH content of the pituitary gland and may stimulate MSH secretion either by inhibiting MIF or by a direct action on the pituitary gland (Kastin and Schally, 1967b). Thus darkness may enhance MSH secretion through the stimulation of the pineal and hence melatonin release (Kastin et al., 1967b). Conversely, suppression of melatonin activity by constant illumination or by pineal-ectomy would lead to a decrease in MSH release (Kastin et al., 1967a; 1967b). Kastin et al. (1969), however, failed to find changes in plasma MSH levels in rats exposed to dark or light conditions and after pinealectomy. More recently, Tilders and Smelik (1975) found no changes in the MSH content of the rat pituitary gland after administration of melatonin and only slight changes after pinealectomy. Furthermore, neither melatonin or pinealectomy had any effect on the diurnal variation of pituitary MSH levels (Tilders, 1973) and it was concluded that this rhythm, like resting MSH levels, was not related to the light–dark cycle or controlled by melatonin from the pineal gland (Tilders and Smelik, 1975).

3.6 STRESS AND MSH SECRETION

The secretion of MSH, like that of other pituitary hormones, is affected by stress. Short-term stress such as exposure to ether vapours decreases pituitary MSH levels (Kastin *et al.*, 1967c, 1969; Thody *et al.*, 1976a) and increases plasma MSH (Kastin *et al.*, 1969; Thody *et al.*, 1976a).

Exposure to prolonged sound has been reported to produce hyperplasia and an increase in the stainability of pars intermedia cells in the rat (Werner, 1959). Werner considered these changes to indicate increased secretory activity of the pars intermedia although no MSH assays were carried out. Other workers have found increased pituitary MSH levels in rats and mice subjected to such long-term stress as constant illumination (Kastin *et al.*, 1967c), tannic acid feeding (Peaslee and Einhellig, 1973) and DDT administration (Peaslee *et al.*, 1972).

More recently Francis and Peaslee (1974) have investigated the effects of social stress on pituitary MSH levels in mice. Mice that were repeatedly attacked by more aggressive cage mates were found to have larger adrenal glands and increased levels of pituitary MSH. Although it was considered that social stress might cause an increased production of MIF and hence a decrease in MSH release another explanation of the increased pituitary MSH levels might be an enhanced MSH synthesis.

4 MSH in man

4.1 ASSAY OF HUMAN MSH

The control of MSH secretion in man has received relatively little attention. One reason for this has undoubtedly been the failure to recognize a physiological role for MSH in man, but a real problem has also been the absence of a reliable assay for human MSH. Although the melanophore response in lower vertebrates has been used for the bioassay of blood levels of MSH in experimental animals (Geschwind and Huseby, 1966; Kastin *et al.*, 1969; Björklund *et al.*, 1972; Thody and Hinks, 1973; Thody, 1974) it has not proved particularly suitable for the routine measurement of circulating MSH in man. One disadvantage is the lack of sensitivity and in order to detect the low circulating levels of MSH in man elaborate extraction methods are necessary. A variety of extraction methods have been used and because of this and differences in standards it has been difficult to compare findings from various groups. Another major criticism of these bioassay methods is that they are unable to distinguish between various forms of MSH and other hormones that stimulate the melanophores, such as ACTH.

Some of these problems have been overcome by the introduction of sensitive and specific radioimmunoassays for human MSH. Since the predominant MSH in man has been considered to be a β-MSH consisting of twenty-two amino acids (Harris, 1959) radioimmunoassays have been designed to measure this peptide.

4.2 β-MSH LEVELS IN NORMAL SUBJECTS

With the development of such methods and the purification of MSH peptides it has been possible to express MSH concentrations in terms of their weight. The mean plasma β-MSH in normal subjects was found to be 50 pg ml^{-1} (range 20–110 pg ml^{-1}) by Abe et al. (1967). Similar values have been reported by Donald and Toth (1973) and Thody and Plummer (1973).

In normal subjects plasma immunoreactive β-MSH levels were found to be higher in the morning than in the evening (Abe et al., 1969; Thody et al., 1974a) and it has been suggested that β-MSH secretion parallels the diurnal rhythm of ACTH (Abe et al., 1969).

4.3 MSH AND PIGMENTATION

Because of the pigmentary properties of the MSH peptides it is perhaps not surprising that most studies have been concerned with MSH secretion in clinical conditions where pigmentation is a feature. Some of the findings are listed below.

4.3.1 *Menstrual cycle*

Changes in skin pigmentation have been reported to occur during the menstrual cycle (Snell and Turner, 1966) and it is possible that these are related to the variation in urinary levels of bioassayable MSH which have been found during the menstrual cycle (Dahlberg, 1961). These urinary levels may not, however, reflect changes in the secretion of pituitary MSH and this would be supported by the recent finding that plasma immuno-reactive β-MSH levels are no different at the beginning and end of the menstrual cycle (Thody et al., 1975c).

4.3.2. *Pregnancy*

The hyperpigmentation of the skin that often occurs in pregnancy is generally thought to be due to MSH and several workers have reported increased bioassayable MSH both in blood and urine during pregnancy

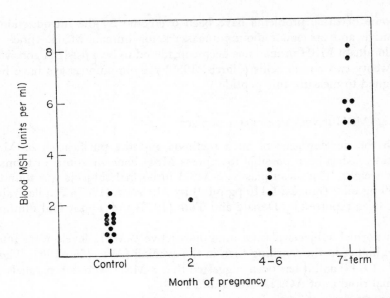

FIG. 7. Bioassayable MSH activity in the blood during pregnancy. (Modified from Shizume and Lerner, 1954.)

(Shizume and Lerner, 1954; Dahlberg, 1961; McGuinness, 1963) (Fig. 7). Plasma β-MSH levels as measured by radioimmunoassay, on the other hand, were not abnormally high in late pregnancy (Thody et al., 1974b) (Fig. 8) and we considered it unlikely that β-MSH is responsible for the increased circulating melanocyte-stimulating activity in pregnancy. Other workers have, however, reported increased plasma β-MSH levels in late pregnancy (Ances and Pomerantz, 1974).

While MSH peptides might be increased in pregnancy it is known that steroid hormones have pigmentary effects (Lerner and Takahashi, 1956; Snell and Bischitz, 1960; Wilson and Spaziani, 1973) and the possibility should be considered that these hormones may contribute to the hyper-pigmentation of pregnancy.

4.3.3 Oral contraceptives

Plasma immunoreactive β-MSH levels were found to be on the low side of normal in subjects taking oral contraceptive therapy (Smith et al., 1977a). The chloasma that sometimes occurs in subjects receiving oral contraceptives is therefore unlikely to be due to increased circulating levels of β-MSH. The steroidal content of the contraceptive pills could be

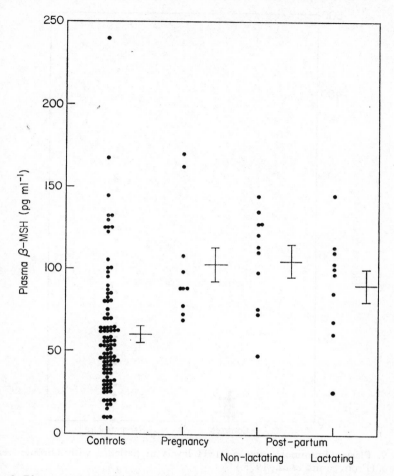

FIG. 8. Plasma immunoreactive β-MSH levels in late pregnancy, after parturition and in control subjects. (From Thody *et al.*, 1974b.)

important since oestrogens and progesterone have pigmentary properties and may account for the pigmentary changes that occur during pregnancy (see section 4.3.2).

4.3.4 *Hypoadrenalism*

It has been considered that the pigmentation occurring in hypoadrenalism was the result of an increase in ACTH secretion (Marks, 1959; Nelson *et al.*, 1960), although the degree of pigmentation did not always correlate with the plasma ACTH levels (Davies, 1964). Other workers using

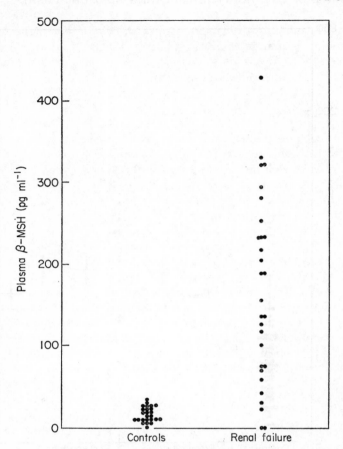

FIG. 9. Plasma immunoreactive β-MSH levels in patients with chronic renal failure. (From Smith *et al.*, 1975.)

bioassay methods suggested that the pigmentation was the result of an increase in MSH secretion (Johnsson and Högberg, 1952; Shizume and Lerner, 1954; Lerner *et al.*, 1954; Sulman, 1956; Lerner, 1961). More recently Abe *et al.* (1967b) have compared bioassayable and radioimmuno-assayable MSH levels in hypoadrenalism and concluded that β-MSH is the main pigmentary hormone in man.

4.3.5 *Ectopic ACTH syndrome*

Abnormally high levels of MSH activity have been found in the plasma of patients with hyperpigmentation associated with the ectopic ACTH syndrome (Island *et al.*, 1965; Shimizu *et al.*, 1965). The major MSH in such tumours is immunologically similar to β-MSH although immunoreactive α-MSH (Abe *et al.*, 1967a, 1967b; Abe *et al.*, 1969) and other unidentified MSH peptides have been found.

4.3.6 Renal failure

Increased levels of plasma immunoreactive β-MSH have been found in patients with chronic renal failure (Gilkes *et al.*, 1975a; Smith *et al.*, 1975) (Fig. 9). These findings may explain the skin pigmentation that is commonly seen in chronic renal failure although no correlation was found between the plasma β-MSH levels and the degree of pigmentation as measured by a reflectance method (Smith *et al.*, 1975). This lack of correlation may have been due to the severity of the renal failure and Smith *et al.* (1975) have suggested that plasma β-MSH levels may relate to the degree of pigmentation in patients with less impairment of renal function.

There could be several explanations for the high levels of plasma immunoreactive β-MSH in renal failure. While β-MSH secretion may be increased the raised levels could also be due to decreased excretion. Recent observations, however, suggest that the increased plasma immunoreactive β-MSH levels in renal failure are the result of an impairment in the metabolism of the hormones by the kidney (Smith *et al.*, 1976).

4.3.7 Other pigmentary conditions

Although increased urinary levels of MSH activity have been found on isolated occasions in patients with Hodgkin's disease, retinitis pigmentosum, alopoecia areata, and primary thyrotoxicosis (Shizume and Lerner, 1954; McGuinness, 1963) plasma β-MSH concentrations in these conditions are quite normal (Abe *et al.*, 1969; Plummer and Thody, unpublished observations).

4.3.8 Hypopituitarism

Low levels of bioassayable MSH have been found in the blood and urine of patients with hypopituitarism (Shizume and Lerner, 1954; McGuinness, 1963), and the depigmentation seen in hypopituitarism has naturally been attributed to a diminished MSH secretion (Lerner *et al.*, 1954). Immunoreactive β-MSH levels are also low in hypopituitarism (Abe *et al.*, 1969; Plummer, 1974) and were undetectable in plasma from patients who had undergone hypophysectomy (Thody and Plummer, 1973). Nevertheless, normal plasma levels of β-MSH have been found in hypopituitarism (Abe et al., 1969; Plummer, 1974). The level of plasma β-MSH obviously depends upon the degree of hypopituitarism and if functional pituitary tissue is present normal β-MSH secretion may continue.

4.4   PARKINSONISM AND β-MSH SECRETION

Increased plasma β-MSH levels have been found in patients with Parkinson's disease, especially when the disease was bilateral (Shuster et al., 1973). A characteristic feature of parkinsonism is a depletion of dopaminergic activity in the mid-brain (Calne, 1970) and the increased secretion of β-MSH may be related to this change (Shuster et al., 1973).

A defect in β-MSH regulation may be important in the pathogenesis of parkinsonism, for exogeneous MSH aggravates Parkinson's disease (Cotzias et al., 1967). The situation therefore arises in which MSH exacerbates parkinsonism yet the disease itself leads to an increase in MSH secretion. Inhibition of MSH secretion might therefore prove useful in the treatment of Parkinson's disease. With this in mind Kastin and co-workers (Kastin et al., 1972a; Kastin and Barbeau, 1972) examined the therapeutic possibilities of MIF (Pro-Leu-Gly-NH$_2$) in parkinsonism. Although preliminary results were disappointing (Kastin et al., 1972a), later studies have been more promising (Kastin and Barbeau, 1972). The action of Pro-Leu-Gly-NH$_2$ may be a direct one on the CNS and not through the inhibition of β-MSH secretion (Kastin et al., 1972a). Indeed we have recently found that Pro-Leu-Gly-NH$_2$ has no effect on the secretion of β-MSH in man (Thody et al., 1974c) (see Fig. 10).

4.5   REGULATION OF MSH SECRETION

4.5.1   *ACTH-like control*

Perhaps the most well-known fact about MSH secretion in man is that it parallels that of ACTH. Thus increased levels of bioassayable MSH have been found in conditions of hypoadrenalism and stress, and suppressed levels after glucocorticoid treatment (Johnsson and Högberg, 1952; Sulman, 1956; Shizume and Lerner, 1954; Lerner et al., 1954; McGuinness, 1963). Plasma β-MSH levels as measured by radioimmunoassay showed similar changes (Abe et al., 1967b, 1969; Donald and Toth, 1973; Thody and Plummer, 1973). A diurnal variation in plasma β-MSH levels has also been found (Abe et al., 1969; Thody et al., 1974a) and, like ACTH, peak values were found during early morning. Liddle (1973) has therefore concluded that "human β-MSH appears to be regulated by the same factors that regulate ACTH secretion".

There are some reports that human MSH and ACTH are not always secreted together (Lerner, 1961; Sawin *et al.*, 1970; Kastin *et al.*, 1973b;

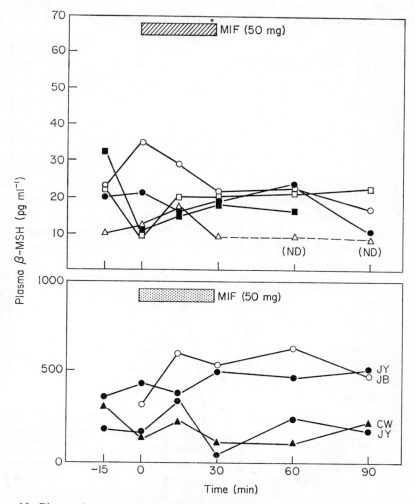

FIG. 10. Plasma immunoreactive β-MSH levels in (a) five normal subjects and (b) three subjects with high resting levels of β-MSH before, during and after infusion of MIF (Pro-Leu-Gly-NH₂). Two of the subjects with high β-MSH levels had Nelson's syndrome (JY, JB) and the third had Addison's disease (CW). JY was examined on two occasions. ND, not detectable.

Donald and Toth, 1973). Further studies are obviously required to investigate the relationship between ACTH and MSH secretion in man.

4.5.2 *Inhibitory control*

Although MIF activity has been found in the human hypothalamus (Kastin and Schally, 1967a) Pro-Leu-Gly-NH$_2$, the most potent MIF in

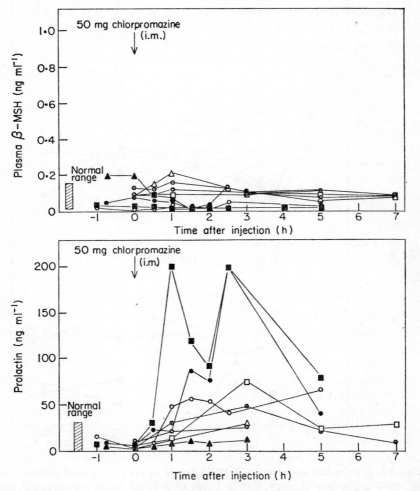

FIG. 11. Plasma immunoreactive β-MSH and prolactin levels in eight subjects before, during and after a single intramuscular injection of 50 mg chlorpromazine. (From Plummer *et al.*, 1975.)

experimental animals, had no effect on bioassayable MSH levels in patients with Nelson's syndrome or Addisons disease (Kastin et al., 1972a). Radio-immunoassayable β-MSH levels in normal subjects (Thody et al., 1974c) and in patients with high β-MSH levels were also unchanged after Pro-Leu-Gly-NH$_2$ infusion (Fig. 10). This may suggest the lack of a hypothalamic inhibitory control of MSH secretion in man but the possibility cannot be ruled out that Pro-Leu-Gly-NH$_2$ shows species specificity.

Further evidence to support the view that MSH secretion in man is not under hypothalamic inhibition has come from studies with chlorpromazine. Acute treatment with chlorpromazine had no effect in plasma β-MSH levels, yet plasma levels of prolactin, a pituitary hormone known to be under hypothalamic inhibition, were greatly increased (Plummer et al., 1975) (Fig. 11). Similar treatment with phenothiazines increases the secretion of MSH in other mammals (see section 3.1.6 and Fig. 5).

More prolonged treatment with chlorpromazine did, however, produce a small increase in plasma β-MSH levels (Thody and Shuster, 1973a). The reason for this is not clear but perhaps it is significant that chronic chlorpromazine administration sometimes produces symptoms of parkin-sonism (Kase, 1967) and elevated plasma β-MSH levels have been found in this neurological disorder (Shuster et al., 1973) (see section 4.4). The increase in β-MSH section after chronic chlorpromazine may therefore be related to disturbances in catecholamine metabolism in the mid-brain, and this suggests the presence of an extra-hypothalamic inhibitory control for human β-MSH.

5   Comparison of MSH secretion in man and other mammals

From the evidence mentioned above it is clear that the control of MSH secretion in man is different from that in other mammals. Some of these differences are summarized below and in Table 1.

a. While there is good evidence that MSH secretion in experimental animals is under an inhibitory control by the hypothalamus (see section 3) there is no evidence for such a control in man. In the first place infusion of Pro-Leu-Gly-NH$_2$, the most potent MIF in experimental animals, has no effect on plasma β-MSH levels in normal subjects or in patients with increased β-MSH levels (see section 4.5.2). Secondly, acute administration of chlorpromazine has no effect on plasma β-MSH and only a slight increase occurred when given orally over several weeks (see 4.5.2).

b. The secretion of MSH in man seems to parallel that of ACTH. Thus both hormones show a diurnal rhythm, are increased by stress and during conditions of hypoadrenalism and are decreased by glucocorticoid treatment

TABLE 1

Differences between β-MSH secretion in man and MSH secretion in other mammals

Treatment or condition	β-MSH secretion in man	References	MSH secretion in other mammals	References
1. MIF	No effect	Thody et al. (1974)	Inhibitory effect reported	Celis et al. (1972, 1973)
2. Phenothiazines	No effect	Plummer et al. (1975)	Increased	Kastin and Schally (1966); Kastin et al. (1969); Scott and Stillings (1972); Peaslee and Milburn (1973); Thody et al. (1975, 1976)
3. Hypoadrenalism	Increased	Abe et al. (1967, 1969); Thody and Plummer (1973)	No effect	Gosbee et al. (1970) Thody and Hinks (1973)
4. Glucocorticoids	Decreased	Abe et al. (1967, 1969); Thody and Plummer (1973)	No effect	Gosbee et al. (1970) Thody and Hinks (1973)
5. Oestrogen and progesterone	No effect	Smith et al. (1977)	Increased?	Taleisnik and Tomatis (1969, 1970)
6. Pregnancy	Slightly increased	Thody et al. (1974); Ances and Pomerantz (1974)	Increased?	Karkun and Sen (1965)

(see section 4.3.4). In the rat, on the other hand, MSH secretion is apparently unaffected by adrenal function (see section 3.4) although it is increased by stress (Kastin et al., 1967c; Kastin et al., 1969; Thody et al., 1975b) and may follow a diurnal rhythm (Tilders, 1973; Tilders and Smelik, 1975).

c. Oestrogen and progesterone appear to increase the secretion of MSH in experimental animals (see section 3.3) yet plasma β-MSH levels in women receiving oral contraceptives are, if anything, slightly lower than normal (see section 4.3.3).

d. MSH secretion appears to be increased during pregnancy in the rat

(Karkun and Sen, 1965). Recent evidence suggests that human plasma β-MSH levels are not abnormally high in late pregnancy (see section 4.3.2).

The control mechanism for MSH secretion in man may therefore be different from those in other mammals. This is perhaps not surprising when it is considered that man, unlike most other mammals, has no distinct pars intermedia and MSH is thought to be produced in the anterior lobe by the same cells that produce ACTH (Phifer et al., 1974). They may explain why, in man, MSH and ACTH are often secreted together.

In the second place the predominant MSH in man is a β-MSH and this is not only different to α-MSH, which is a common peptide in most other mammals, but is also different from other forms of β-MSH (see Fig. 1). In fact recent evidence suggests that a β-MSH does not normally occur in man and the β-MSH present in human pituitaries and plasma is either an LPH or an extraction artefact resulting from its breakdown (Bloomfield et al., 1974; Scott and Lowry, 1974). This would agree with reports from Lerner's group (Lerner and Lee, 1973) that when strong acid conditions are employed β-MSH cannot be isolated from human pituitaries.

Previous results obtained from β-MSH radioimmunoassays may therefore be more relevant to the LPHs. This is quite possible since human β- and γ-LPH completely cross-react with human β-MSH in some radioimmunoassays (Gilkes et al., 1975b). This could explain why the control of human β-MSH secretion is so different from that of MSH peptides in other mammals.

6 Some effects of the MSH peptides

6.1 PIGMENTARY EFFECT

The most well-known effect of the MSH peptides is their pigmentary action. Such an effect is especially obvious in the lower vertebrates where MSH serves an important function in the control of colour change.

The MSH peptides also have a pigmentary effect in mammals. Prolonged treatment with either α- or β-MSH produces darkening of the skin in man and guinea pigs (Lerner and McGuire, 1961; Snell, 1962, 1964). Although microscopic evidence suggests a dispersion of melanin granules into the dendritic processes of the melanocyte (Snell, 1962, 1964; Lerner et al., 1966) the major response would appear to be an increase in melanogenesis (Lerner et al., 1966). This is presumably brought about through the activation of tyrosinase. MSH has been shown to induce tyrosinase activity in skin and malignant melanocytes (Pomerantz and Chuang, 1970; Lee et al., 1972; Wong and Pawelek, 1973; Lee and Lee, 1973; Wong et *al.*, 1974) and this effect is mediated by cyclic AMP (Bitensky and Demopoulos, 1970; Wong and Pawelek, 1973; Wong *et al.*, 1974). MSH increases cyclic AMP levels in mouse melanoma cells (Wong and Pawelek, 1973, Wong, 1974) and these cells are especially sensitive to MSH in the G2 phase of their cell-cycle (Wong *et al.*, 1974). MSH also acts in the G2 phase to induce melanoblasts into melanocytes in organ cultures of caudal fins from goldfish (Chen *et al.*, 1973) and it is possible that vertebrate melanocytes are, in general, responsive to MSH in the G2 phase of the cell cycle (Wong *et al.*, 1974).

With the evolution of hair in the mammal adaptive colour changes in the skin are not important and the MSH peptides may have lost their significance as pigmentary hormones. Some workers, however, believe that MSH has retained a pigmentary role in the regulation of hair colour in certain rodents. Geschwind and Huseby (1966) noticed an increase in hair pigmentation in mice bearing an MSH-secreting tumour and injections of α-MSH have been shown to darken the hair of mice (Geschwind and Huseby, 1968) and guinea pigs (Clive and Snell, 1967). Other observations suggest that in the short-tailed weasel MSH is involved in the seasonal variation of coat colour (Rust, 1965; Rust and Meyer, 1968, 1969).

β-MSH probably has no physiological function as a pigmentary hormone in man. Indeed, recent evidence suggests that β-MSH does not normally occur in man (see section 5) and the hyperpigmentation of the skin sometimes seen in man could be attributed to other factors. For instance, in conditions of adrenal insufficiency an increased secretion of ACTH and the LPHs could cause pigmentation. The human pituitary contains small amounts of α-MSH and in certain circumstances this peptide could be released and thus cause pigmentary changes. This possibility requires further study.

6.2 NATRIURETIC EFFECT

The MSH peptides have many extra pigmentary effects. One such effect is their stimulation of natriuresis (Orías and McCann, 1972). Although this effect is not thought to be mediated through the adrenals (Orías and McCann, 1972) α-MSH has recently been shown to influence aldosterone production (Page *et al.*, 1974).

The significance of this natriuretic effect is not known, but one possibility is that the MSH peptides along with other hormones are concerned with osmoregulation. There have been many reports that the pars intermedia responds to osmotic stress and although these changes could be secondary to changes in the neurohypophysis a definite relationship appears to exist between the development of the pars intermedia and the ability of the animal to resist dehydration (Legait and Legait, 1962).

6.3 LIPOLYTIC EFFECT

The MSH peptides, in common with other pituitary hormones, have the ability to stimulate the release of free fatty acids from adipose tissue. The effect, however, seems to vary in different animals. For instance with rat tissue α- and β-MSH possess little or no lipolytic activity (Raben et al., 1961; Rudman et al., 1963) but in the rabbit they are powerful lipolytic agents (Raben et al., 1961; Rudman et al., 1963).

The effects of α- and β-MSH on free fatty acids in the blood of man has not been determined.

6.4 CARDIOVASCULAR EFFECT

It has been reported that MSH increases the heart rate in the heart–lung preparation of the dog and in intact dogs pretreated with reserpine (Krayer et al., 1961). The heart rate in human beings was also found to be increased after purified preparations of α- and β-MSH (Kastin et al., 1968). More recently Aldinger et al. (1973) observed that α-MSH increased the ventricular contractile force and heart rate of anaesthetized dogs. β-MSH had a similar effect but was slightly less potent. Neither peptide affected blood pressure (Aldinger et al., 1973). ACTH4-10 the heptapeptide sequence common to all MSH peptides, also failed to affect blood pressure, but has been shown to increase the threshold of a centrally induced pressure response (Bohus, 1974).

The cardiovascular effects of the MSH peptides were not blocked by propanolol and were not therefore mediated through the action of catecholamines (Aldinger et al., 1973). These workers therefore considered the possibility that MSH has a direct action on the myocardium. ACTH4-10, on the other hand, is thought to affect the cardiovascular control system through a central action (Bohus, 1974) and it is possible that related MSH peptides act in a similar manner.

6.5 EFFECT ON FOETAL GROWTH

α-MSH has been reported to increase foetal body weight and placental weight in the rat (Honnebier and Swaab, 1974). How α-MSH acts is not known, but it is unlikely to be through a lipolytic effect since other lipolytic agents such as ACTH and TSH fail to stimulate foetal growth (Swaab and Honnebier, 1974). It is not yet known whether MSH has a role in foetal development but such a possibility is supported by the presence of MSH in the foetal pituitaries at an early stage of development (Enemar, 1963; Kastin *et al.*, 1968; Levina, 1968; Silman *et al.*, 1976).

6.6 EFFECTS ON ENDOCRINE GLANDS

6.6.1 *Adrenals*

Although it has been reported that α-MSH depletes adrenal gland ascorbic acid in the rat (Steelman and Guillemin, 1959) this has not been confirmed (Karkun *et al.*, 1963) and it is now generally considered that the MSH peptides have little or no corticotrophic activity in the rat (Dixon and Stack-Dunne, 1955; Dixon, 1960). No changes in the histological appearance or weight of rat adrenal glands have been found after α- or β-MSH administration (Karkun *et al.*, 1963; Thody and Shuster, 1973b, 1975) and the presence of these peptides produced only a very slight steroidogenic response in isolated rat adrenal cells (Seelig and Sayers, 1971; Lowry and McMartin, 1972). Rudman *et al.* (1970) have also reported that β-MSH has no effect on serum costicosterone levels in the rat. On the other hand, in the rabbit β-MSH was found to be as equipotent as ACTH in raising costicosterone levels (Rudman *et al.*, 1970). This is in contrast to the work on isolated rabbit adrenal cells where β-MSH and α-MSH were found to have no effect on steroidogenesis (Lowry and McMartin, 1972).

6.6.2 *Thyroid*

Administration of α- or β-MSH to various mammals has been shown to produce changes in the thyroid indicative of hyperactivity (Courrier and Cehovic, 1960; Cehovic, 1962; Karkun *et al.*, 1963; Yamazaki *et al.*, 1963; Bowers *et al.*, 1964; Werner *et al.*, 1964). Although MSH may act by stimulating TSH release it is active after hypophysectomy (Yamazaki *et al.*, 1963) and it is therefore possible that MSH possesses intrinsic thyrotrophic activity.

6.6.3 *Gonads*

Both α- and β-MSH have been shown to inhibit spermatogenesis in the rat, mouse, and guinea pig (Karkun *et al.*, 1963; Cehovic, 1965a, 1965b). However no changes in testicular size occurred (Karkun *et al.*, 1963; Cehovic, 1965a, 1965b; Thody and Shuster, 1975) although it has been reported that β-MSH reduces ovarian weight (Karkun *et al.*, 1963).

Menstrual bleeding has been reported to occur in five out of six women with secondary amenorrhoea after the administration of highly purified MSH (Kastin *et al.*, 1968). Although the possibility was considered that MSH was acting directly on the ovary this is now thought to be unlikely (Kastin *et al.*, 1972b).

6.6.4 *Pituitary*

In addition to the possibility that MSH may control its own release from the pars intermedia (Kastin *et al.*, 1971) (see section 3.2) there is evidence that MSH peptides may affect the secretion of other pituitary hormones. For example Privat de Garilhe *et al.* (1960) and Li *et al.* (1961) reported that MSH has corticotrophin-releasing activity. However, Guillemin (1964) was unable to confirm this.

More recently Strauch *et al.* (1973) found that α-MSH increased growth hormone secretion in eighteen out of twenty-three human male subjects. Human β-MSH, on the other hand, has been reported to have no effect on growth hormone release (Zahnd and Von Mulhendahl, 1971). The way in which α-MSH stimulates growth hormone release is not known but it is unlikely to be through a direct action on the pituitary since Schally *et al.* (1973) found that α-MSH inhibited the release of growth hormone from rat pituitaries *in vitro*.

6.7 SEBOTROPHIC EFFECT

With the development of hair in the mammal MSH peptides may have acquired a role concerned with the maintenance of hair lipid. A sebotrophic effect of MSH was first indicated in 1971 when it was found that α-MSH stimulated sebum secretion in the rat (Thody and Shuster, 1971a). Soon afterwards it was found that removal of the neurointermediate lobe of the pituitary gland, the site of MSH production, led to a decrease in sebum secretion to a level almost as low as after total hypophysectomy (Thody and Shuster, 1972a, 1973b) and complete restoration to normal levels occurred after replacement therapy with α-MSH (Thody and Shuster, 1973b) (Fig. 12). Skin lipid synthesis, and in particular wax–ester synthesis, was similarly decreased after removal of the neurointermediate lobe and restored to normal after α-MSH (Cooper *et al.*, 1974). This effect on lipogenesis may be specific to sebaceous glands since α-MSH is not lipogenic in rat adipose tissue (Goodman, 1965) but, on the contrary, is slightly lipolytic (Raben *et al.*, 1961).

β-MSH has not yet been examined for its sebotrophic activity. In view of the fact that β-LPH, a hormone structurally related to β-MSH (see

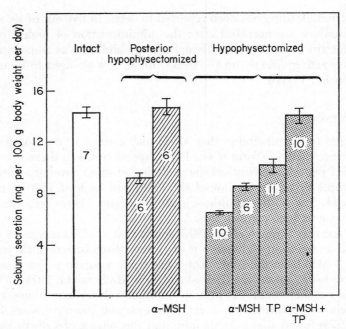

FIG. 12. Sebum secretion in intact, posterior hypophysectomized and completely hypophysectomized rats. Posterior hypophysectomy (removal of the neuro-intermediate lobe) decreased sebum secretion to a level almost as low as complete hypophysectomy. Treatment with α-MSH (30 μg per 100 g body weight per day) for fourteen days restored sebum secretion to normal in posterior hypophysec-tomized, but not in completely hypophysectomized rats. Restoration to normal levels occurred in completely hypophysectomized rats when α-MSH treatment was accompanied by testosterone propionate (TP) (0.2 mg per 100 g body weight per day).

section 2.2) shows sebotrophic activity (Thody and Shuster, 1971c) it might be expected that β-MSH has a similar effect.

In addition to its independent action on the sebaceous glands, α-MSH also acts synergistically with testosterone to stimulate sebum secretion (Shuster and Thody, 1974; Thody and Shuster, 1975) (Fig. 12) and sebaceous gland lipogenesis (Thody et al., 1975d, 1976). Although other hormones are known to affect sebaceous gland activity including ACTH and β-LPH (Thody and Shuster, 1970, 1971b, 1971, 1972b) it would seem that normal sebaceous gland activity can be maintained by α-MSH and testosterone (Thody and Shuster, 1975) (Fig. 12) and these may be two important sebotrophic hormones in the rat.

Modified sebaceous glands such as the preputial glands also respond to α-MSH and testosterone in a synergistic manner (Krähenbühl and Desaulles, 1969; Cooper et al., 1975; Thody and Shuster, 1975; Thody et al., 1975d, 1976).

It has been recently shown that α-MSH influences sebaceous gland activity in the adult rat when administered during foetal or early postnatal life (Thody et al., 1977). Thus sebum secretion was found to be significantly increased in eight-week-old adult rats whose mothers had received α-MSH on days fifteen, seventeen and nineteen of pregnancy. Sebum secretion was similarly increased at eight, eleven and fifteen weeks of age in rats that had received α-MSH for the first few weeks of postnatal life. It is not yet known whether these effects are through a direct action on the sebaceous glands or whether they are secondary to some other action of MSH.

6.8 EFFECTS ON THE CNS

6.8.1 *General effects*

Krivoy and Guillemin (1961) were among the first workers to demonstrate a neurogenic effect of MSH. These workers noticed that β-MSH produced a potentiation of spinal reflexes in the cat and postulated that MSH may be involved in central neural control (Krivoy and Guillemin, 1961; Long et al., 1961). At about the same time Ferrari and his co-workers (1961, 1963) noticed that an intracisternal injection of α-MSH induced drowsiness and stretching in dogs. The same effect occurred with ACTH and ACTH4-10, the heptapeptide sequence essential for MSH activity. Drowsiness also occurred in rabbits after a subcutaneous injection of α-MSH (Dyster-Aas and Krakau, 1965) and in rats after β-MSH (Sakamoto, 1966). In mice, on the other hand, α- or β-MSH produced a state of hyperactivity (Sakamoto, 1966) and a recent report from Ferrari's group described an increase in sexual excitability in dogs after α-MSH (Bertolini et al., 1969).

Purified MSH preparations have been reported to produce feelings of nervousness, anxiety and motor restlessness in three out of six human female subjects (Kastin et al., 1968). These symptoms were thought to resemble those found in extrapyramidal disease (Ayd, 1961) and Cotzias et al. (1967) noticed that large doses of MSH aggravated the tremor of Parkinson's disease. Cotzias et al. (1967) also implied that the extrapyramidal symptoms in some patients receiving tranquillizing drugs might result from changes in the secretion of MSH from the pituitary. Tranquillizers certainly stimulate MSH secretion in experimental mammals (see section 3.6.1) and chronic administration may result in small changes in MSH secretion in man (see section 5.4.2).

6.8.2 Learning behaviour

In a series of studies which started in 1965, DeWied and his colleagues have investigated the effects of ACTH and MSH peptides on learning behaviour. ACTH, MSH and analogues such as ACTH1-24, ACTH1-10, ACTH4-10 were found to delay the extinction of a conditioned avoidance response (DeWied, 1965, 1966, 1969; DeWied et al., 1972). ACTH11-24, on the other hand, was without effect and it would appear that ACTH4-10 is the shortest amino acid sequence capable of affecting the avoidance response.

It has been demonstrated that α-MSH also delays the extinction of a passive avoidance response (Sandman et al., 1971a; Dempsey et al., 1972) and an appetitive response (Sandman et al., 1969). Further experiments suggested that these effects of MSH were not due to the failure of the animals to inhibit a response (Sandman et al., 1971b, 1972) or an increase in general activity (Kastin et al., 1973a). Although an effect on memory cannot be completely ruled out (Sandman et al., 1971a; Stratton and Kastin, 1973) Kastin and his co-workers have favoured the idea that the behavioural effects of MSH are related to an increase in the emotional state of the animal (Sandman et al., 1971b; Stratton and Kastin, 1973, 1974; Kastin et al., 1973c). Rats injected with MSH may become more aroused and this could lead to an increased attention to certain sensory cues (Sandman et al., 1972; Stratton and Kastin, 1973). Thus rats receiving MSH may learn a simple task more readily and because of the delayed extinction show slower learning of a second task (Stratton and Kastin, 1973).

Synthetic α-MSH has been reported to affect attention in human beings. A significant improvement in the Benton visual retention test occurred after infusion of α-MSH, although no change in verbal retention was found (Kastin et al., 1971b).

6.8.3 Sexual behaviour

There have been several reports that injection of MSH and ACTH peptides into the CNS stimulate penile erection and ejaculation in a number of different mammals (Ferrari et al., 1963; Bertolini et al., 1969; Baldwin et al., 1974). This effect is particularly evident in the rabbit, becoming apparent 15–60 min after administration of the peptide and persisting for several hours (Bertolini et al., 1975). No effect is seen in castrated animals and it appears that testosterone is essential for the sexual response to the MSH and ACTH peptides (Bertolini *et al.*, 1975).

Numerous peptides, including α-MSH, β-MSH, β-LPH and various ACTH analogues, produce sexual excitement in the male and Bertolini *et al.* (1975) consider ACTH5-10 to be the essential sequence for this effect. Bohus *et al.* (1975) have, however, reported that testosterone-treated castrated rats are "sluggish" copulators after ACTH4-10, although this peptide tended to motivate male rats to seek contact with a female.

The MSH peptides also affect sexual behaviour in the female. A recent report describes two effects of α-MSH in oestrogen and progesterone primed female rats (Everard *et al.*, 1977). In rats showing poor receptivity a subcutaneous injection of α-MSH potentiated the effect of progesterone on lordosis, but in receptive rats α-MSH tended to inhibit the lordotic response. Preliminary findings suggest that ACTH1-39 and ACTH1-16 elicit similar effects (Everard, Wilson and Thody, unpublished observations). Intraventricular administration of ACTH1-24 has also been shown to stimulate lordosis and ovulation in the rabbit (Sawyer *et al.*, 1975). ACTH4-10, on the other hand, failed to induce ovulation and was much less effective in stimulating lordosis (Sawyer *et al.*, 1975). Similarly ACTH4-10 produced no effect on lordosis in the female rat (Meyerson and Bohus, 1976).

The lack of effect of ACTH4-10 on sexual behaviour in the female and its inhibitory effect in the male makes it unlikely that this moiety is responsible for the sexual excitation elicited by the MSH and ACTH peptides. Additional amino acid residues on the intact MSH and ACTH molecules are obviously necessary for the stimulation of sexual behaviour. Smaller peptides, such as ACTH4-10, might compete with the intact molecules and in so doing have an inhibitory effect on sexual behaviour.

6.8.4 *Possible mechanisms and sites of action*

The way in which MSH peptides affect neural processes is not understood. Kastin *et al.* (1968) considered that MSH might affect the CNS through its effect on serum calcium. These workers found that infusion of MSH produced a significant decrease in serum calcium in human subjects. Similar decreases in serum calcium after MSH have been found in rabbits (Friesen, 1964). Patients with hypocalcaemia seem to be more sensitive to extrapyramidal symptoms induced by tranquillizing drugs (Schaaf and Payne, 1966; Lichtigfeld and Simpson, 1967) and Kastin *et al.* (1968) offer the interesting concept that the decline in serum calcium after MSH is responsible for the increase in responsiveness of the CNS to MSH.

Indeed hypocalcaemia is generally thought to be the cause of the psychological and neurological changes that occur in hypoparathyroidism.

The fact that MSH peptides act on the spinal cord to facilitate synaptic transmission (Krivoy and Guillemin, 1961; Krivoy et al., 1963; Krivoy, 1969) suggests that these peptides may have a direct neural action. This action is preceded by a long latent period and this occurs whether the action is facilitation of the monosynaptic reflex in the spinal cord of cats (Krivoy and Guillemin, 1961) or the stretching effect observed in dogs by Ferrari et al. (1963). To explain this latency Krivoy (1969) has presented evidence which shows that β-MSH alters the recovery period of nerve cells causing them to remain in a hyperexcitable state for a longer period of time. With continuous input these phenomena will summate (Krivoy et al., 1963) and the latent period may thus allow sufficient summation to occur so that hyperexcitability becomes manifest.

Whether such mechanisms are involved in the behavioural effects of MSH peptides is not clear. Nevertheless, the effect of MSH on conditioned avoidance behaviour is thought to be through a direct action on the CNS rather than through an action on the thyroid or adrenal glands. The thyroid gland has been implicated in acquisition and retention of avoidance behaviour (see DeWied, 1969) and it is well known that MSH peptides can stimulate thyroid activity (see section 6.5.2). However, the inhibitory action of ACTH1-10 on the extinction of the avoidance response is unaffected by thyroidectomy (see DeWied, 1969). The adrenal gland is also involved in avoidance behaviour (see DeWied et al., 1972) but it is unlikely that the behavioural effects of MSH and ACTH peptides are mediated with the adrenal glands. In the first place MSH peptides have no action on the adrenal cortex (see section 6.5.1) and secondly glucocorticoids tend to facilitate rather than inhibit the extinction of the avoidance response (DeWied, 1969).

It is possible that the MSH peptides act on the autonomic nervous system. Sakamoto and Prasad (1968) noted similar effects in rats treated with β-MSH and noradrenaline and the effect of β-MSH was prevented by adrenergic blocking agents. However, the doses of MSH used by Sakamoto and Prasad (1968) did not produce behavioural effects (Bohus and DeWied, 1966).

There is much evidence suggesting a relationship between RNA synthesis in the brain and learning processes (see DeWied, 1969). This prompted the hypothesis that ACTH and MSH like peptides influence learning behaviour through an effect on RNA and protein metabolism in the brain (DeWied, 1969). The recent studies of Gispen and co-workers (Gispen and Schotman, 1970, 1973; Gispen et al., 1971, 1972; Schotman et al., 1972; Reith et al., 1974) would support this view.

Experiments have been performed in an attempt to localize the site of action of the MSH peptides on the CNS. Although bilateral lesions in the parafascicular nuclei had no effect on avoidance learning they did block the inhibitory effect of α-MSH on the avoidance response (Bohus and DeWied, 1967). Implantation of ACTH1-10 in the nucleus parafascicularis and adjacent areas also resulted in extinction of the avoidance response (Van Wimersma Greidanus and DeWied, 1971). It has therefore been concluded that this region of the thalamus may be important in the maintenance of conditioned avoidance behaviour (Van Wimersma Greidanus et al., 1972). Electrophysiological studies suggest that the mid-brain limbic system is also an important site of action of the MSH and ACTH peptides (Sandman et al., 1971b; Urban et al., 1974).

Very little is known of the way in which the MSH peptides affect sexual behaviour. An effect on brain amine metabolism is one possibility. Sexual behaviour is known to be influenced by changes in the catecholamine–serotonin balance and α-MSH has been shown to alter serotonin and dopamine turnover in the brain of the rat (Leonard et al., 1976).

7 Concluding remarks

7.1 MSH SECRETION

The one thing that is clear about MSH secretion is that it is under an inhibitory control by the hypothalamus. What is not clear, however, is how this control is mediated. Some workers consider that MSH secretion is controlled by hypothalamic peptides in the same way as other adenohypophysial hormones. However, the pars intermedia in most mammals is not connected to the hypothalamus by the hypophysial portal system and it is not known how hypothalamic peptides might be transported. One possibility is that these peptides are liberated from neurosecretory fibres that have been found in the pars intermedia. More information is required as to the nature and site of production of these hypothalamic peptides.

Hypothalamic catecholamines appear to have an important role in regulating MSH release. While catecholamines may act as neurotransmitters affecting MIF release from nerve endings in the hypothalamus (or the pars intermedia) there is evidence that they have a direct effect on MSH release at the pituitary levels. It is not known which of these two systems is the more important or whether both mechanisms play an integral part in the control of MSH.

Virtually all of our knowledge on the control of MSH secretion in the mammal has come from studies in the rat. Strictly speaking these studies have been concerned with the control of α-MSH secretion since this is

the major MSH in the rat. Rather less is known about the control of
β-MSH secretion. The β-MSHs are structurally different to α-MSH and
unlike the latter are not confined to the intermediate lobe of the pituitary.
Considering these differences it might not be surprising to find that the
control of these two hormones is different.

Attempts to study the control of β-MSH secretion have been made in
man. Initially β-MSH was thought to be the major MSH in man but
recent studies suggest that human β-MSH may only exist as part of the
larger LPH molecule (Bloomfield *et al.*, 1974; Scott and Lowry, 1974).
The LPHs cross-react with β-MSH in some radioimmunoassays (Gilkes
et al., 1975b) and thus the results obtained with such systems are more
relevant to β- or γ-LPH. This could explain why the control of β-MSH
secretion in man appears to be different from the control of MSH secretion
in other mammals.

7.2 SIGNIFICANCE OF MSH IN THE MAMMAL

Although MSH was discovered some fifty years ago its physiological
function in the mammal is still unknown. Its role as a pigmentary hormone
is well established in the lower vertebrates but with the evolution of hair
in the mammal the control of skin colour has little significance. The fact
that MSH does produce darkening of human skin in itself demonstrates
an effect, not a function, and it is unlikely that MSH has any physiological
role as a pigmentary hormone in man. Indeed the human pituitary having
no distinct intermediate lobe has apparently lost the ability to produce
MSH (see section 5). The lack of a potent pigmentary hormone in man
makes it difficult to explain the increased pigmentation that occurs in
certain conditions. In some conditions the LPHs may be involved. These
hormones have only slight melanocyte-stimulating activity but they may
have a melanogenic effect, together with ACTH, when secreted in large
amounts as in Addison's and Cushing's disease.

In some mammals the MSH peptides may have acquired new roles.
Numerous extrapigmentary effects have been described for the MSH
peptides and several of these have been mentioned in the present article.
With the development of hair one extrapigmentary effect of MSH that
could have special significance is its action on the sebaceous gland. Control
of sebaceous gland activity is clearly important in hairy mammals where
sebum is necessary for lubrication and waterproofing the hair. In other
mammals, such as the armadillo, elephant, pangolin, whale and man,
body hair is reduced or virtually absent and the need for a sebotrophic
hormone may well have been lost. This could explain the lack of a distinct
pars intermedia in these animals and it would be interesting to know if

these mammals have lost the ability to produce any of the MSH peptides. This may have happened in man (see sections 2 and 5) and it would seem unlikely that MSH peptides are responsible for the seborrhoea that is associated with certain clinical conditions, as was originally suggested (Burton *et al.*, 1973).

Nevertheless, an intermediate lobe is present in the human foetal pituitary and appears to be capable of producing α-MSH (Silman *et al.*, 1976). Thus while the absence of MSH in adult man rules out any possibility of its having an effect at that stage its presence in the foetus means that it could be important during early life. Through an action on foetal sebaceous glands MSH could be concerned with the production of the vernix that protect the foetus from the amniotic fluid.

Stimulation of the sebaceous glands by α-MSH during early life could also have a lasting effect on their activity. α-MSH has been shown to have such an effect in the rat and a similar conditioning effect in man could be important in disorders such as acne, hirsuties and cutaneous virilism where seborrhoea is a feature.

In some rodents sebaceous glands have become modified to take on specialized roles concerned with behaviour through the release of pheromones. The finding that α-MSH stimulates preputial gland activity is interesting since through its sebotrophic action MSH may have acquired a behavioural role controlling the production of pheromones. This possibility has received support from the recent finding that α-MSH stimulated the release of an aggression promoting pheromone from the preputial glands of male mice (Nowell and Wouters, 1975).

The preputial glands also produce sex pheromones (Gawienowski *et al.*, 1975, 1976), and α-MSH has been shown to stimulate their production in the female rat (Thody and Dijkstra, 1977). The interesting possibility arises that MSH is able to influence sexual behaviour in two ways: firstly through a direct action on the CNS and secondly through the release of pheromones from modified sebaceous glands.

The most studied extrapigmentary effect of the MSH peptides is their action on the CNS. The presence of MSH peptides in the brain supports the view that these peptides have a role in brain function and their influence on adaptive behaviour is now well documented. Adaptive responses are motivated by fear and hunger and it seems that the MSH peptides are able to facilitate adaptation to these and possibly other environmental stimuli through an effect on arousal or attention. Behaviour is, however, but one aspect of adaptation and MSH may also have "adaptive" value through various peripheral effects. Such a function of MSH in the mammal could be analogous to its role in the camouflage response of the lower vertebrates.

Thus, although MSH may have lost its pigmentary significance during the course of evolution, it may have retained an "adaptive" role.

Further studies are required to test the physiological significance of these extra-pigmentary effects and their relationship to changes in MSH secretion. Further information is also required as to the relative importance of the different MSH peptides. Although α-MSH and β-MSH have many biological activities in common they differ not only in structure but also in their distribution and it is likely that they have different physiological roles in the mammal.

References

Abe, K., Island, D. P., Liddle, G. W., Fleischer, N. and Nicholson, W. E. (1967a). *Journal of Clinical Endocrinology and Metabolism*, **27**, 46.

Abe, K., Nicholson, W. E., Liddle, G. W., Island, D. P. and Orth, D. N. (1967b), *Journal of Clinical Investigation*, **46**, 1609.

Abe, K., Nicholson, W. E., Liddle, G. W., Orth, D. N. and Island, D. P. (1969). *Journal of Clinical Investigation*, **48**, 1580.

Aldinger, E. E., Hawley, W. E., Schally, A. V. and Kastin, A. J. (1973). *Journal of Endocrinology*, **56**, 613.

Ances, I. G. and Pomerantz, S. H. (1974). *American Journal of Obstetrics and Gynaecology*, **119**, 1062.

Ayd, F. J. (1961). *Journal of the American Medical Association*, **175**, 1054.

Bagnara, J. T. and Hadley, M. E. (1973). "Chromatophores and Color Change". Prentice-Hall, Englewood Cliffs, New Jersey.

Baker, B. I. (1973) *Journal of Endocrinology*, **57**, 393.

Baker, B. L. and Drummond, T. (1972). *American Journal of Anatomy*, **134**, 395.

Bal, H. and Smelik, P. G. (1967). *Experientia*, **23**, 759.

Baldwin, D. M., Haun, C. K. and Sawyer, C. H. (1974). *Brain Research*, **80**, 291.

Barbarossa, C. and Pende, T. (1950). *Archivio e Maragliano di Patologia e Clinica*, **5**, 27.

Bargmann, W. and Knoop, A. (1960). *Zeitschrift für Zellforschung und mikroskopische anatomie*, **52**, 256.

Barrnett, R. J. and Greep, R. O. (1951). *Endocrinology*, **49**, 337.

Bertolini, A., Vergoni, W., Gessa, G. L. and Ferrari, W. (1969). *Nature (London)*, **221**, 667.

Bertolini, A., Gessa, G. L. and Ferrari, W. (1975). *In* "Sexual Behavior: Pharmacology and Biochemistry" (Eds M. Sandler and G. L. Gessa), p. 247. Raven Press, New York.

Bissonnette, T. H. and Baily, E. E. (1944). *Annals of the New York Academy of Sciences*, **45**, 221.

Bitensky, M. W. and Demopoulos, H. B. (1970). *Journal of Investigative Dermatology*, **54**, 83.

Björklund, A., Meurling, P., Nilsson, G. and Nobin, A. (1972). *Journal of Endocrinology*, **53**, 161.

Björklund, A., Moore, R. Y., Nobin, A. and Stenevi, U. (1973). *Brain Research*, **51**, 171.

Bloomfield, G. A., Scott, A. P., Lowry, P. T., Gilkes, J. J. H. and Rees, L. H. (1974). *Nature, (London)*, **252**, 492.

Bogdanove, E. M. and Halmi, N. S. (1953). *Endocrinology*, **53**, 274.

Bohus, B. (1974). *Progress in Brain Research*, **41**, 175.

Bohus, B. and DeWied, D. (1966). *Science*, **153**, 318.

Bohus, B. and DeWied, D. (1967). *Physiology and Behaviour*, **2**, 221.

Bohus, B., Hendrickx, H. H. L., van Kolfschoten, A. A. and Krediet, T. G. (1975). *In* "Sexual Behavior: Pharmacology and Biochemistry" (Eds M. Sandler and G. L. Gessa), p. 269. Raven Press, New York.

Bower, A., Hadley, M. E. and Hruby, V. J. (1971). *Biochemical and Biophysical Research Communications*, **45**, 1185.

Bower, A., Hadley, M. E. and Hruby, V. J. (1974). *Science*, **184**, 70.

Bowers, C. Y., Redding, T. W. and Schally, A. V. (1964). *Endocrinology*, **74**, 559.

Brooks, C. M. (1938). *American Journal of Physiology*, **121**, 157.

Burgers, A. C. J. (1963). *Annals of the New York Academy of Science*, **100**, 669.

Burton, J. L., Shuster, S., Cartlidge, M., Libman, L. J. and Martell, U. (1973). *Nature (London)*, **243**, 349.

Calne, D. B. (1970). "Parkinsonism: Physiology, Pharmacology and Treatment." Edward Arnold, London.

Cameron, E. and Foster, C. L. (1971). *Journal of Endocrinology*, **49**, 479.

Carrillo, A. J., Kastin, A. J., Dunn, J. D. and Schally, A. V. (1973). *Neuroendocrinology*, **12**, 120.

Cehovic, G. (1962). *Comptes Rendus hebdomadaire des séances de l'Académie des Sciences*, **254**, 1872.

Cehovic, G. (1965a). *Comptes Rendus de séances scientifiques de la société de Biologie*, **159**, 1491.

Cehovic, G. (1965b). *Comptes Rendus hebdomadaire des séances de l'Académie des Sciences*, **261**, 1405.

Celis, M. E. (1975). *Neuroendocrinology*, **18**, 256.

Celis, M. E. and Taleisnik (1973). *Life Sciences*, **13**, 493.

Celis, M. E. and Taleisnik, S. (1974). *Proceedings of the Society for Experimental Biology and Medicine*, **145**, 142.

Celis, M. E., Taleisnik, S. and Walter, R. (1971a). *Proceedings of the National Academy of Sciences*, **68**, 1428.

Celis, M. E., Taleisnik, S. and Walter, R. (1971b). *Biochemical and Biophysical Research Communications*, **45**, 564.

Celis, M. E., Hase, S. and Walter, R. (1972). *FEBS Letters*, **27**, 327.

Celis, M. E., Macagno, R. and Taleisnik, S. (1973). *Endocrinology*, **93**, 1229.

Chen, S., Tchen, T. T. and Taylor, J. (1973). *Pigment cell*, **1**, 1.

Chrétien, M. (1973). *In* "Methods in Investigative and Diagnostic Endocrinology: Peptide Hormones" (Eds S. A. Berson and R. S. Yalow), vol. 2A, part II, p. 617, 2. North Holland, Amsterdam and London; Elsevier, pub. co., New York.

Chrétien, M. and Li, C. H. (1967a). *Canadian Journal of Biochemistry*, **45**, 1163.

Chrétien, M. and Li, C. H. (1967b). *Canadian Medical Association Journal*, **96**, 342.

Clive, D. and Snell, R. S. (1967). *Journal of Investigative Dermatology*, **49**, 314.

Cooper, M. F., Thody, A. J. and Shuster, S. (1974). *Biochimica et Biophysica Acta*, **360**, 193.

Cooper, M. E., Bowden, P. E., Thody, A. J. and Shuster, S. (1975). *Journal of Endocrinology*, **64**, 63P.

Cotzias, G. C., Van Woert, M. H. and Schiffer, L. M. (1967). *New England Journal of Medicine*, **276**, 374.

Courrier, R. and Cehovic, G. (1960). *Comptes Rendus hebdomadaire des séances de l'Académie des Sciences*, **251**, 822.
Cseh, G., Gray, L. and Goth, E. (1968). *FEBS letters*, **2**, 42.
Dahlberg, B. C. G. (1961). *Acta Endocrinologica (Copenhagen)*, **38**, suppl. 60, 1.
Daniel, P. M. and Prichard, M. M. L. (1958). *American Journal of Pathology*, **34**, 433.
Davies, B. M. A. (1964). *Acta Endocrinologica (Copenhagen)*, **45**, 55.
Dempsey, G. L., Kastin, A. J. and Schally, A. V. (1972). *Hormones and Behaviour*, **3**, 333.
DeWied, D. (1965). *International Journal of Neuropharmacology*, **4**, 157.
DeWied, D. (1966). *Proceedings of the Society for Experimental Biology (New York)*, **122**, 28.
DeWied, D. (1969). *In* "Frontiers of Neuroendocrinology" (Eds W. F. Ganong and L. Martini), p. 97. Oxford University Press, London and New York.
DeWied, D., Van Delft, A. M. L., Gispen, W. H., Weijnen, J. A. W. M. and Van Wimersma Greidanus, T. B. (1972). *In* "Hormones and Behaviour" (Ed. S. Levine), p. 135. Academic Press, New York and London.
Dixon, H. B. F. (1960). *Biochimica et Biophysica Acta*, **37**, 38.
Dixon, H. B. F. and Stack-Dunne, M. P. (1955). *Biochemical Journal*, **61**, 483.
Dixon, J. S. (1960). *Biochimica et Biophysica Acta*, **37**, 38.
Dixon, J. S. and Li, C. H. (1960). *Journal of American Chemical Society*, **82**, 4568.
Dixon, J. S. and Li, C. H. (1961). *General and Comparative Endocrinology*, **1**, 161.
Donald, R. A. and Toth, A. (1973). *Journal of Clinical Endocrinology and Metabolism*, **36**, 925.
Dubois, M. P. (1972). *Zeitschrift für Zellforschung und mikroskopische anatomie*, **125**, 200.
Duchen, L. W. (1962). *Journal of Endocrinology*, **25**, 161.
Dyster-Aas, H. K. and Krakau, C. E. T. (1965). *Acta Endocrinologica (Copenhagen)*, **48**, 609.
Enemar, A. (1963). *Archives of Zoology*, **16**, 169.
Enemar, A. and Falck, B. (1965). *General and Comparative Endocrinology*, **5**, 577.
Everard, D., Wilson, C. A. and Thody, A. J. (1977). *Journal of Endocrinology*, **73**, 32P.
Ferrari, W., Gessa, G. L. and Vargiu, L. (1961). *Experientia*, **17**, 90.
Ferrari, W., Gessa, G. L. and Vargiu, L. (1963). *Annals of the New York Academy of Sciences*, **104**, 330.
Forgács, P. (1956). *Acta Endocrinologica (Copenhagen)*, **23**, 7.
Francis, M. G. and Peaslee, M. H. (1974). *Neuroendocrinology*, **16**, 1.
Friesen, H. (1964). *Endocrinology*, **75**, 692.
Fuxe, K. and Hokfelt, T. (1969). *In* "Frontiers in Neuroendocrinology" (Eds W. F. Ganong and L. Martini), p. 47. Oxford University Press, New York.
Gawienowski, A. M., Orsulak, P. J. Stacewicz-Sapientzakis, M. and Joseph, B. M. (1975). *Journal of Endocrinology*, **67**, 283.
Gawienowski, A. M., Orsulak, P. J. Stacewicz-Sapientzakis, M. and Pratt, J. J. (1976). *Psychoneuroendocrinology*, **1**, 411.
Geschwind, I. I. (1966). *In* "Symposium on Structure and Control of the Melanocyte", p. 28. Springer-Verlag, Berlin.
Geschwind, I. I. and Huseby, R. A. (1966). *Endocrinology*, **79**, 97.
Geschwind, I. I., Li, C. H. and Barnifi (1956). *Journal of American Chemical Society*, **78**, 4494.

Geschwind, I. I., Li, C. H. and Barnifi, L. (1957). *Journal of American Chemical Society*, **79**, 1003.

Gilkes, J. J. H., Eady, R. A. J., Rees, L. H., Munro, D. D. and Moorhead, J. F. (1975a). *British Medical Journal*, **1**, 656.

Gilkes, J. J. H., Bloomfield, G. A., Scott, A. P., Lowry, P. J., Ratcliffe, J. G., Landon, J. and Rees, L. H. (1975b). *Journal of Clinical Endocrinology and Metabolism*, **40**, 450.

Gispen, W. H. and Schotman, P. (1970). *Progress in Brain Research*, **32**, 236.

Gispen, W. H. and Schotman, P. (1973). *Progress in Brain Research*, **39**, 443.

Gispen, W. H., DeWied, D., Schotman, P. and Jensz, H. S. (1971). *Brain Research*, **31**, 341.

Gispen, W. H., Schotman, P. and De Kloet, E. R. (1972). *Neuroendocrinology*, **9**, 285.

Goodman, H. M. (1965). *Endocrinology*, **76**, 216.

Gosbee, J. L., Kraicer, J., Kastin, A. J. and Schally, A. V. (1970). *Endocrinology*, **86**, 560.

Graf, L., Cseh, G. and Schweizer, J. M. (1969). *Biochimica et Biophysica Acta*, **229**, 276.

Grant, N. H., Clark, D. E. and Rosanoff, E. I. (1973). *Biochemical and Biophysical Research Communications*, **51**, 100.

Greer, M. A. and Erwin, H. C. (1956). *Endocrinology*, **58**, 665.

Guillemin, R., Schally, A. V., Lipscomb, H. S., Anderson, R. N. and Long, J. M. (1962). *Endocrinology*, **70**, 471.

Hadley, M. E., Bower, A. and Hruby, V. J. (1973). *Yale Journal of Biology and Medicine*, **46**, 602.

Hamilton, J. M., Saluja, P. G. and Thody, A. (1976). *Senologia*, **1**, 79.

Harris, J. I. (1959). *Nature (London)*, **184**, 167.

Hess, R., Barratt, D. and Gelzer, J. (1968). *Experientia*, **24**, 584.

Hoekstra, A. and van der Wal, P. G. (1971). *Netherland Journal of Zoology*, **21**, 159.

Holmes, R. L. (1961). *Journal of Endocrinology*, **22**, 7.

Holmes, R. L. (1962). *Journal of Endocrinology*, **24**, 53.

Honnebier, W. J. and Swaab, D. F. (1974). *Journal of Obstetrics and Gynaecology of the British Commonwealth*, **81**, 439.

Howe, A. (1973). *Journal of Endocrinology*, **59**, 385.

Howe, A. and Maxwell, D. S. (1966). *Journal of Physiology (London)*, **183**, 70P.

Howe, A. and Maxwell, D. S. (1968). *General and Comparative Endocrinology*, **11**, 169.

Howe, A. and Thody, A. J. (1969a). *Journal of Physiology (London)*, **203**, 159.

Howe, A. and Thody, A. J. (1969b). *Nature (London)*, **222**, 781.

Howe, A. and Thody, A. J. (1970). *Journal of Endocrinology*, **46**, 201.

Howe, A. and Thody, A. J. (1971). *Journal of Physiology (London)*, **209**, 5P.

Hruby, V. J., Smith, C. W., Bower, A. and Hadley, M. E. (1972). *Science*, **175**, 1331.

Huntington, T. and Hadley, M. E. (1974). *Endocrinology*, **96**, 472.

Island, D. P., Shizume, N., Nicholson, W. E., Abe, K., Ogata, E. and Liddle, G. W. (1965). *Journal of Clinical Endocrinology and Metabolism*, **25**, 975.

Iturriza, F. C. (1969). *General and Comparative Endocrinology*, **12**, 417.

Ivy, H. K. and Albert, A. (1957). *Endocrinology*, **61**, 667.

Johnsson, S. and Högberg, B. (1952). *Nature (London)*, **169**, 286.

Karkun, J. N., and Sen, D. P. (1965). *Indian Journal of Medical Research*, **53**, 226.

Karkun, J. N., Kar, A. B. and Sen, D. P. (1963). *Annals of Biochemistry and Experimental Medicine*, **23**, 253.

Kase, N. (1967). *In* "Textbook of Medicine" (Eds P. B. Beeson and W. McDermott), p. 1336. W. B. Saunders, Philadelphia and London.

Kastin, A. J. and Barbeau, A. (1972). *Canadian Medical Association Journal*, **107**, 1079.

Kastin, A. J. and Ross, G. T. (1964). *Encrinodology*, **75**, 187.

Kastin, A. J. and Schally, A. V. (1966a). *General and Comparative Endocrinology*, **7**, 452.

Kastin, A. J. and Schally, A. V. (1966b). *Endocrinology*, **79**, 1018.

Kastin, A. J. and Schally, A. V. (1967a). *General and Comparative Endocrinology*, **8**, 344.

Kastin, A. J. and Schally, A. V. (1967b). *Nature (London)*, **213**, 1238.

Kastin, A. J. and Schally, A. V. (1970). *Proceedings of the Seventh Pan American Congress of Endocrinology*, São Paulo, Brazil. International Congress Series No. 238, p. 311. Excerpta Medica, Amsterdam.

Kastin, A. J. and Schally, A. V. (1972). *In* "Pigmentation: Its Genesis and Biologic Control" (Ed. V. Riley), p. 215. Appleton-Century-Crofts, New York.

Kastin, A. J., Schally, A. V., Viosca, S. Barrett, L. and Redding, T. W. (1967a). *Neuroendocrinology*, **2**, 257.

Kastin, A. J., Redding, T. W. and Schally, A. V. (1967b). *Proceedings of the Society of Experimental Biology and Medicine*, **124**, 1275.

Kastin, A. J., Arimura, A., Viosca, S., Barrett, L. and Schally, A. V. (1967c). *Neuroendocrinology*, **2**, 200.

Kastin, A. J., Kullander, S., Borglin, N. E., Dahlberg, B., Dyster-Aas, K., Krakau, C. E. T., Ingvar, D. H., Miller, M. C., Bowers, C. Y. and Schally, A. V. (1968). *Lancet*, **i**, 1007.

Kastin, A. J., Gennser, G., Arimura, A., Miller, M. C. and Schally, A. V. (1968). *Acta Endocrinologica (Copenhagen)*, **58**, 6.

Kastin, A. J., Schally, A. V., Viosca, S. and Miller, M. C. (1969). *Endocrinology*, **84**, 20.

Kastin, A. J., Arimura, A., Schally, A. V. and Miller, M. C. (1971a). *Nature New Biology*, **231**, 29.

Kastin, A. J., Miller, C. H., Gonzalez-Barcena, D., Hawley, D., Dyster-Aas, K., Schally, A. V., Parra, M. L. V. and Velasco, M. (1971b). *Physiology and Behaviour*, **7**, 893.

Kastin, A. J., Gual, C. and Schally, A. V. (1972a). *Recent Progress in Hormone Research*, **28**, 201.

Kastin, A. J., Zarate, A., Miller, M. C., Hernandez-Ayup, S., Dyster-Aas, K., Gual, C. and Schally, A. V. (1972b). *Journal of Reproduction and Fertility*, **28**, 185.

Kastin, A. J., Plotnikoff, N. P., Viosca, S., Anderson, M. S. and Schally, A. V. (1973a). *Yale Journal of Biology and Medicine*, **46**, 617.

Kastin, A. J., Beach, G. D., Hawley, W. D., Kendall, J. W., Edwards, M. S. and Schally, A. V. (1973b). *Journal of Clinical Endocrinology and Metabolism*, **36**, 770.

Kastin, A. J., Miller, C. H., Nockton, R., Sandman, C. A., Schally, A. V. and Stratton, L. (1973c). *Progress in Brain Research*, **39**, 461.

Kobayashi, Y. (1964). *In* "Gunma Symposia on Endocrinology", vol. 1, p. 173, University of Gunma, Maebashi, Japan.

Kobayashi, Y. (1965). *Zeitschrift fur Zellforschung und Mikroskopische anatomie*, **68**, 155.

Koneff, A. A., Simpson, M. E. and Evans, H. M. (1946). *Anatomical Record*, **94**, 169.

Kordon, C. and Bachrach, D. (1959). *Journal de Physiologie* (Paris), **51**, 500.

Krähenbühl, C. and Desaulles, P. A. (1969). *Experientia*, **25**, 1193.

Kraicer, J., Gosbee, J. L. and Bencosme, S. A. (1973). *Neuroendocrinology*, **11**, 156.

Krayer, O., Astwood, E. B., Wand, D. R. and Alper, M. H. (1961). *Proceedings of the National Academy of Sciences, U.S.A.* **47**, 1227.

Krivoy, W. A. (1969). *Psychopharmacology Bulletin*, **5**, 29.

Krivoy, W. A. and Guillemin, R. (1961). *Endocrinology*, **69**, 170.

Krivoy, W. A., Lane, M. and Droeger, D. C. (1963). *Annals of the New York Academy of Sciences*, **104**, 312.

Kurosumi, K., Matsuzawa, T. and Shibasaki, S. (1961). *General and Comparative Endocrinology*, **1**, 433.

Lee, T. H. and Lee, M. S. (1973). *Yale Journal of Biology and Medicine*, **46**, 493.

Lee, T. H., Lerner, A. B. and Buettner-Janusch, V. (1967). *Journal of Biological Chemistry*, **236**, 1390.

Lee, T. H., Lee, M. S. and Lu, M. Y. (1972). *Endocrinology*, **91**, 1180.

Legait, E. (1963). *In* "Cytologie de l'Adenohypophyse" (Eds J. Benoit and C. DaLage), p. 215. C.N.R.S., Paris.

Legait, H. and Legait, E. (1962). *In* "Neurosecretion" (Eds H. Heller, and R. B. Clark), p. 165. Academic Press, London and New York.

Leonard, B., Kafoe, W. F., Thody, A. J. and Shuster, S. (1976). *Journal of Neuroscience Research*, **2**, 39.

Lerner, A. B. (1961). *Archives of Dermatology*, **3**, 97.

Lerner, A. B. and Lee, T. H. (1955). *Journal of American Chemical Society*, **77**, 1066.

Lerner, A. B. and Lee, T. H. (1973). *In* "Methods in Investigative and Diagnostic Endocrinology: Peptide Hormones" (Eds S. A. Berson and R. S. Yalow), vol. 2A, part II, p. 405. North Holland, Amsterdam and London; Elsevier, New York.

Lerner, A. B. and McGuire, J. S. (1961). *Nature (London)*, **189**, 176.

Lerner, A. B. and Takahashi, Y. (1956). *Recent Progress in Hormone Research*, **12**, 303.

Lerner, A. B., Shizume, K. and Bunding, I. (1954). *Journal of Clinical Endocrinology and Metabolism*, **14**, 1463.

Lerner, A. B., Snell, R. S., Chanco-Turner, M. L. and McGuire, J. S. (1966). *Archives of Dermatology*, **94**, 269.

Levina, S. E. (1968). *General and Comparative Endocrinology*, **11**, 151.

Li, C. H. (1959). *Laboratory Investigation*, **8**, 574.

Li, C. H. (1964). *Nature (London)*, **201**, 924.

Li, C. H., Schnabel, E., Chung, D. and Lo, T. B. (1961). *Nature (London)*, **189**, 143.

Li, C. H., Barnifi, L., Chrétien, M. and Chung, D. (1965). *Nature (London)*, **208**, 1093.

Lichtigfeld, F. J. and Simpson, G. M. (1967). *New England Journal of Medicine*, **276**, 874.

Liddle, G. W. (1973). *In* "Methods in Investigative and Diagnostic Endocrinology: Peptide Hormones" (Eds S. A. Berson and R. S. Yalow), vol. 2A, part II, p. 421. North Holland, Amsterdam and London; Elsevier, New York.

Lohmar, P. and Li, C. H. (1967). *Biochimica and Biophysica Acta*, **147**, 381.

Long, J. M., Krivoy, W. A. and Guillemin, R. (1961). *Endocrinology*, **69**, 176.

Lowry, P. J. and Chadwick, A. (1970a). *Nature (London)*, **226**, 219.

Lowry, P. J. and Chadwick, A. (1970b). *Biochemical Journal*, **118**, 713.

Lowry, P. J. and McMartin, C. (1972). *Journal of Endocrinology*, **55**, xxxiii.

Marks, V. (1959). *Acta Endocrinologica (Copenhagen)*, **32**, 527.

May, R. M. and Stutinsky, F. (1947). *Archives d'anatomie microscopique et de morphologie experimentale*, **36**, 201.

McGuinness, B. W. (1963). *Annals of the New York Academy of Sciences*, **100**, 640.

Meyerson, B. J. and Bohus, B. (1976). *Pharmacology, Biochemistry and Behaviour*, **5**, 539.

Miahle-Voloss, C. (1958a) *Acta Endocrinologica (Copenhagen)* suppl. 35, 1.

Miahle-Voloss, C. (1958b). *Acta Endocrinologica (Copenhagen)*, **35**, 7.

Nair, R. M. G., Kastin, A. J. and Schally, A. V. (1971). *Biochemical and Biophysical Research Communications*, **43**, 1376.

Nair, R. M. G., Kastin, A. J. and Schally, A. V. (1972). *Biochemical and Biophysical Research Communications*, **47**, 1420.

Nelson, D. H., Meakin, T. W. and Thorn, G. W. (1960). *Annals of Internal Medicine*, **52**, 560.

Nobin, A., Björklund, A. and Stenevi, U. (1972). *Proceedings of the Fourth International Congress of Endocrinology*, Washington. International Congress Series No. 256, p. 50. Excerpta Medica, Amsterdam.

Norman, R. J., Weatherhead, B. and Vincent, D. S. (1972). *Journal of Endocrinology*, **55**, xxi.

Nowell, N. W. and Wouters, A. (1975). *Journal of Endocrinology*, **65**, 36P

Olivecrona, H. (1957). *Acta Physiologica Scandinavica*, **40**, suppl. 136, 1.

Oliver, C., Eskay, R. L. and Porter, J. C. (1976). 5th International Congress of Endocrinology, Hamburg, Germany, Abst. No. 593, p. 243.

Ooki, T., Kotsu, T., Kinutani, M. and Daikoku, S. (1973). *Neuroendocrinology*, **11**, 22.

Orías, R. and McCann, S. M. (1972). *Endocrinology*, **90**, 700.

Page, R. B., Boyd, J. E. and Mulrow, P. J. (1974). *Endocrine Research Communications*, **1**, 53.

Peaslee, M. H. and Einhellig, F. A. (1973). *Toxicology and Applied Pharmacology*, **25**, 507.

Peaslee, M. H. and Milburn, S. E. (1971). *Journal of Endocrinology*, **51**, 253.

Peaslee, M. H., Goldman, M. and Mulburn, S. E. (1972). *Comparative and General Pharmacology*, **3**, 191.

Penny, R. J. and Thody, A. J. (1976). *Journal of Endocrinoolgy*. **69**, 2P.

Phifer, R. F. and Spicer, S. S. (1970). *Laboratory Investigation*, **23**, 543.

Phifer, R. F., Orth, D. N. and Spicer, S. S. (1974). *Journal of Clinical Endocrinology and Metabolism*, **39**, 684.

Plummer, N. A. (1974). Ph.D. Thesis, University of Newcastle upon Tyne.

Plummer, N. A., Thody, A. J., Burton, J. L., Goolamali, S. K., Shuster, S., Cole, E. N. and Boyns, A. R. (1975). *Journal of Clinical Endocrinology and Metabolism*, **41**, 380.

Pomerantz, S. H. and Chuang, L. (1970). *Endocrinology*, **87**, 302.

Porath, J., Roos, P., Landgrebe, F. W. and Mitchell, G. M. (1955). *Biochimica et Biophysica Acta*, **17**, 598.

Privat de Garilhe, M., Gros, C., Porath, J. and Lindner, E. B. (1960). *Experientia*, **16**, 414.

Raben, M. S., Landolt, R., Smith, F. A., Hofman, K. and Yajima, H. (1961). *Nature (London)*, **189**, 681.

Racadot, J. (1958). *Comptes Rendus des Séances de la Société de Biologie et de ses filiales*, **152**, 135.

Reith, M. E. A., Schotman, P. and Gispen, W. H. (1974). *Brain Research*, **81**, 571.

Rochefort, G. J., Rosenberger, J. and Saffran, M. (1959). *Journal of Physiology (London)*, **146**, 105.

Roux, M. (1962). *Comptes Rendus des Séances de la Société de Biologie et de ses filiales*, **156**, 1664.

Rudman, D., Brown, S. J. and Malkin, M. F. (1963). *Endocrinology*, **72**, 527.

Rudman, D., Rio, E. D., Bixler, T. J. and Barnett, J. (1970). *Endocrinology*, **86**, 1410.

Rudman, D., Del Rio, A. E., Hollins, B. M., Houser, Keeling, M. E,. D. H., Sutin, J., Scott, J. W., Sears, R. A. and Rosenberg, M. Z. (1973). *Endocrinolgy*, **92**, 372.

Rust, C. C. (1965). *General and Comparative Endocrinology*, **5**, 222.

Rust, C. C. and Meyer, R. K. (1968). *Science*, **11**, 548.

Rust, C. C. and Meyer, R. K. (1969). *Science*, **165**, 921.

Sakamoto, A. (1966). *Nature (London)*, **211**, 1370.

Sakamoto, A. and Prasad, K. N. (1968). *In* "Protein and Polypeptide Hormones" (Ed. M. Margoulies), part 2, p. 503. *Excerpta Medica Foundation International Congress*, Series 161.

Sandman, C. A., Kastin, A. J. and Schally, A. V. (1969). *Experientia*, **25**, 1001.

Sandman, C. A., Denman, P. M., Miller, L. H., Schally, A. V. and Kastin, A. J. (1971). *Journal of Comparative and Physiological Psychology*, **76**, 103.

Sandman, C. A., Kastin, A. J. and Schally, A. V. (1971a). *Physiology and Behaviour*, **6**, 45.

Sandman, C. A., Miller, L. H., Kastin, A. J. and Schally, A. V. (1972). *Journal of Comparative Physiological Psychology*, **80**, 48.

Sawin, C. T., Abe, K. and Orth, D. N. (1970). *Archives of Internal Medicine*, **125**, 708.

Sawyer, C. H., Baldwin, I. M. and Haun, C. K. (1975). *In* "Sexual Behavior: Pharmacology and Biochemistry" (Eds M. Sandler and G. L. Gessa), p. 259. Raven Press, New York.

Schaaf, M. and Payne, C. A. (1966). *New England Journal of Medicine*, **275**, 991.

Schally, A. V. and Kastin, A. J. (1966). *Endocrinology*, **79**, 768.

Schally, A. V., Lipscomb, H. S., Long, J. M., Dear, W. E. and Guillemin, R. (1962). *Endocrinology*, **10**, 478.

Schotman, P., Gispen, W. H., Jansz, H. S. and DeWied, D. (1972). *Brain Research*, **46**, 349.

Scott, A. P. and Lowry, P. J. (1974). *Biochemical Journal*, **139**, 593.

Scott, A. P., Bennett, H. P. J., Lowry, P. J., McMartin, C. and Ratcliffe, J. G. (1972). *Journal of Endocrinology*, **55**, xxxvi.

Scott, A. P., Bennett, H. P. J., Lowry, P. J., McMartin, C. and Ratcliffe, J. G. (1973). *Journal of Endocrinology*, **58**, xv.

Scott, A. P., Lowry, P. J., Ratcliffe, J. G., Rees, L. H. and Landon, J. (1974). *Journal of Endocrinology*, **61**, 355.

Scott, G. T. and Stillings, W. A. (1972). *Endocrinology*, **90**, 545.

Seelig, S. and Sayers, G. (1971). *Federation Proceedings of the Federation of American Societies for Experimental Biology*, **30**, 316.

Selye, H. and Hall, C. E. (1943). *Anatomical Record*, **86**, 579.

Shapiro, M., Nicholson, W. E., Orth, D. N., Mitchell, W. M., Island, D. P. and Liddle, G. W. (1972). *Journal of Clinical Endocrinology and Metabolism*, **90**, 249.

Shizume, K. and Lerner, A. B. (1954). *Journal of Clinical Endocrinology and Metabolism,* **14,** 1491.

Shimizu, N., Ogata, E., Nicholson, W. E., Island, D. P., Ney, R. L. and Liddle, G. W. (1965). *Journal of Clinical Endocrinology and Metabolism,* **25,** 984.

Shuster, S. and Thody, A. J. (1974). *Journal of Investigative Dermatology,* **62,** 172.

Shuster, S., Burton, J. L., Thody, A. J., Plummer, N., Goolamali, S. K. and Bates, D. (1973). *Lancet,* **i,** 463.

Silman, R. E., Chard, T., Lowry, P. J., Smith, I. and Young, R. M. (1976). *Nature (London),* **260,** 716.

Siperstein, E. R. and Greer, M. A. (1956). *Journal of National Cancer Institute,* **17,** 569.

Smelik, P. G. (1966). *Acta Physiologica et Pharmacologica Néelandica,* **14,** 1.

Smith, A. G., Shuster, S., Comaish, J. S., Plummer, N. A., Thody, A. J., Alvarez-Ude, F. and Kerr, D. N. S. (1975). *British Medical Journal,* **1,** 658.

Smith, A. G., Shuster, S., Thody, A. J., Alvarez-Ude, F. and Kerr, D. N. S. (1976). *British Medical Journal,* **1,** 874.

Smith, A. G., Shuster, S., Thody, A. J. and Peberdy, M. (1977). *Journal of Investigative Dermatology,* **68,** 169.

Snell, R. S. (1962). *Journal of Endocrinology,* **25,** 249.

Snell, R. S. (1964). *Journal of Investigative Dermatology,* **42,** 337.

Snell, R. S. and Bischitz, P. G. (1960). *Journal of Investigative Dermatology,* **35** 73.

Snell, R. S. and Turner, R. (1966). *Journal of Investigative Dermatology,* **47,** 147.

Soboleva, E. L. (1964). *Bulletin of Experimental Biology and Medicine, USSR,* **55,** 577.

Steelman, S. L. and Guillemin, R. (1959). *Proceedings of the Society for Experimental Biology and Medicine,* **101,** 600.

Stefan, Y. and Dubois, M. P. (1972). *Zeitschrift für zellforschung und mikroskopische anatomie,* **133,** 353.

Stratton, L. O. and Kastin, A. J. (1973). *Physiology and Behaviour,* **10,** 689.

Stratton, L. O. and Kastin, A. J. (1974). *Hormones and Behaviour,* **5,** 149.

Strauch, G., Girault, D., Rifai, M. and Bricaire, H. (1973). *Journal of Clinical Endocrinology and Metabolism,* **37,** 990.

Stutinsky, F., Bonvallet, M. and Dell, P. (1950). *Annales d'endocrinologie,* **11,** 1.

Sulman, F. G. (1956). *Journal of Clinical Endocrinology and Metabolism,* **16,** 755.

Sulman, F. G. and Eviatar, A. (1956). *Acta Endocrinologica (Copenhagen),* **23,** 120.

Swaab, D. F. and Honnebier, W. J. (1974). *Progress in Brain Research.* **41,** 255.

Taleisnik, S. and Celis, M. E. (1972). *Proceedings of the Fourth International Congress of Endocrinology,* Washington. International Congress Series No. 273. Excerpta Medica, Amsterdam.

Taleisnik, S. and Orías, R. (1965). *American Journal of Physiology,* **208,** 293.

Taleisnik, S. and Tomatis, M. E. (1967a). *Endocrinology,* **81,** 819.

Taleisnik, S. and Tomatis, M. E. (1967b). *American Journal of Physiology,* **212,** 157.

Taleisnik, S. and Tomatis, M. E. (1968). *Neuroendocrinology,* **3,** 307.

Taleisnik, S. and Tomatis, M. E. (1969). *Neuroendocrinology,* **5,** 24.

Taleisnik, S. and Tomatis, M. E. (1970). *Neuroendocrinology,* **6,** 368.

Taleisnik, S., Orías, R. and Olmos de J. (1966). *Proceedings of the Society of Experimental Biology and Medicine,* **122,** 325.

Taleisnik, S., Olmos de J., Orías, R. and Tomatis, M. E. (1967). *Journal of Endocrinology,* **39,** 485.

Taleisnik, S., Tomatis, M. E. and Celis, M. E. (1972). *Neuroendocrinology*, **10**, 235.
Taleisnik, S., Celis, M. E. and Tomatis, M. E. (1974). *Neuroendocrinology*, **13**, 327.
Thody, A. J. (1969a). *General and Comparative Endocrinology*, **13**, 477.
Thody, A. J. (1969b). Ph.D. Thesis, University of London.
Thody, A. J. (1974). *Neuroendocrinology*, **16**, 323.
Thody, A. J. and Dijkstra, H. (1977). *Journal of Endocrinology*. To be published.
Thody, A. J. and Hinks, W. M. (1973). *Journal of Endocrinology*, **59**, 657.
Thody, A. J. and Plummer, N. A. (1973). *Journal of Endocrinology*, **58**, 263.
Thody, A. J. and Shuster, S. (1970). *Journal of Endocrinology*, **48**, 139.
Thody, A. J. and Shuster, S. (1971a). *Journal of Endocrinology*, **51**, vi.
Thody, A. J. and Shuster, S. (1971b). *Journal of Endocrinology*, **49**, 325.
Thody, A. J. and Shuster, S. (1971c). *Journal of Endocrinology*, **50**, 533.
Thody, A. J. and Shuster, S. (1972a). *Nature (London)*, **237**, 346.
Thody, A. J. and Shuster, S. (1972b). *Journal of Endocrinology*, **54**, 239.
Thody, A. J. and Shuster, S. (1972c). *Journal of Endocrinology*, **54**, 519.
Thody, A. J. and Shuster, S. (1973a). *Journal of Endocrinology*, **58**, xxxv.
Thody, A. J. and Shuster, S. (1973b). *Nature (London)*, **245**, 207.
Thody, A. J. and Shuster, S. (1975). *Journal of Endocrinology*, **64**, 503.
Thody, A. J., Plummer, N. A., Smith, A. G. and Shuster, S. (1974a). *European Journal of Clinical Investigation*, **4**, 363.
Thody, A. J., Plummer, N. A., Burton, J. L. and Hytten, F. F. (1974b). *Journal of Obstetrics and Gynaecology of the British Commonwealth*, **81**, 875.
Thody, A. J., Shuster, S., Plummer, N. A., Leigh, J., Goolamali, S. K. and Smith, A. G. (1974c). *Journal of Clinical Endocrinology and Metabolism*, **38**, 491.
Thody, A. J., Penny, R. J. and Clark, M. D. (1975a). *Journal of Endocrinology*, **64**, 62P.
Thody, A. J., Penny, R. J., Clark, D. and Taylor, C. (1975b). *Journal of Endocrinology*, **67**, 385.
Thody, A. J., Goolamali, S. K., Burton, J. L., Plummer, N. A. and Shuster, S. (1975c). *British Journal of Dermatology*, **92**, 43.
Thody, A. J., Cooper, M. F., Meddis, D., Bowden, P. E. and Shuster, S. (1975d). *Journal of Endocrinology*, **67**, 18P.
Thody, A. J., Cooper, M. F., Bowden, P. E., Meddis, D. and Shuster, S. (1976). *Journal of Endocrinology*. **71**, 279.
Thody, A. J., Meddis, D. and Shuster, S. (1977). *Journal of Endocrinology*. **72**, 28P.
Tilders, F. J. H. (1973). *Journal of Endocrinology*, **57**, xxxv.
Tilders, F. J. H. and Mulder, A. H. (1975). *Journal of Endocrinology*, **64**, 63P.
Tilders, F. J. H. and Smelik, P. G. (1975). *Neuroendocrinology* **17**, 296.
Tilders, F. J. H., Mulder, A. H. and Smelik, P. G. (1975). *Neuroendocrinology*, **18**, 125
Tomatis, M. E. and Taleisnik, S. (1968a). *Journal of Endocrinology*, **42**, 505.
Tomatis, M. E. and Taleisnik, S. (1968b). *Acta Physiologica Latino Americana*, **18**, 96.
Uotila, U. U. (1939). *Endocrinology*, **25**, 605.
Urban, I., Lopes de Silva, F. H., Storm van Leeuwen, W. and De Wied, D. (1974). *Brain Research*, **69**, 361
Van Wimersma Greidanus, T. B. and DeWied, D. (1971). *Neuroendocrinology*, **7**, 291.
Van Wimersma Greidanus, T. B., Bohus, B. and DeWied, D. (1972). *Proceedings of the Fourth International Congress of Endocrinology*, Washington. International Congress Series No. 273, p. 197. Excerpta Medica, Amsterdam.

Vasquez-Lopez, E. (1944). *Journal of Pathology and Bacteriology*, **56**, 1.

Vincent, D. S. (1969). *Journal of Endocrinology*, **43**, xiii.

Vincent, D. S. and Kumar, T. C. A. (1968). *Journal of Endocrinology*, **41**, xviii.

Vincent, D. S. and Kumar, T. C. A. (1969). *Zeitschrift für Zellforschung und mikroskopische anatomie*, **99**, 185.

Werner, R. (1959). *Comptes Rendus de l'Association des Anatomistes*, **45**, 783.

Werner, S. C., Tierney, J. and Tallberg, T. (1964). *Journal of Clinical Endocrinology and Metabolism*, **24**, 339.

Wilson, M. J. and Spaziani, E. (1973). *Zeitschrift für Zellforschung und mikroskopische anatomie*, **140**, 451.

Wingstrand, K. G. (1966). *In* "The Pituitary Gland" (Eds G. W. Harris and B. T. Donovan), vol. 3, pp. 1–27. Butterworths, London.

Wong, G. and Pawelek, J. (1973). *Nature New Biology*, **241**, 213.

Wong, G., Pawelek, J., Sansone, M. and Morowitz, J. (1974). *Nature (London)*, **248**, 351.

Yamazaki, E., Sakiz, E. and Guillemin, R. (1963). *Annales d'endocrinologie*, **24**, 795.

Ziegler, B. (1963). *Zeitschrift für Zellforschung und mikroskopische anatomie*, **59**, 486.

Zahnd, G. R. and Von Mulhendahl, K. E. (1971) quoted by Strauch *et al.* (1973).

The Pineal Gland:
A Review of the Biochemistry, Physiology and Pharmacological Potential of Melatonin and other Pineal Substances

KENNETH M. SHAW, MA, MRCP

Medical Unit, University College Hospital, London, England

1 Introduction

Throughout the centuries man has been continually intrigued by the pineal gland, a single, small, cone-shaped organ situated in the depth of the brain. Philosophers have claimed various properties. Herophilus believed that the mind was located within the ventricles of the brain, and that the pineal gland served as a sphincter to control the flow of thought. With remarkable foresight, Galen proposed that the pineal was likely to be glandular in nature. Little further was known until 1662 when Descartes with true romanticism claimed that the pineal was the seat of the soul, controlling bodily activities by "animal humours" which passed along threads connecting the eye and internal organs (Descartes, 1662). Thomas Gibson (1763), reviving Galen's idea of a gland, suggested that the pineal served to separate lymph from blood. Others believed it regulated the flow of spinal fluid, while some associated the tendency of the pineal to undergo progressive calcification with the development of mental illness.

It was not until 1898, when Heubner reported sexual precocity in a young boy with a pineal tumour, that endocrine activity was seriously considered (Heubner, 1898). In 1918 the Swedish anatomist, Holmgren, using the light microscope, observed a similarity between the frog pineal and the eye, and he believed that the pineal represented a third eye (Holmgren, 1918). Unable to find similar photoreceptor cells in the human pineal, he suggested that in man it was but a vestigial remnant of this primitive dorsal eye. Meanwhile, contemporary with Holmgren's observations in Sweden, McCord and Allen at John Hopkins University showed that extract of bovine pineal gland caused blanching of the skin of tadpoles (McCord and Allen, 1917), a remarkable chance finding as the extract was without effect in the cow itself, and a similar substance has yet to be found in the frog. It took another forty years to isolate the active principle, but after obtaining extract from over a quarter of a million bovine pineals, Lerner and his co-workers succeeded in isolating an indole, N-acetyl-5-methoxytryptamine subsequently known as melatonin (Lerner et al., 1958).

2 Human anatomy

In man the pineal gland is about 8 mm in diameter lying deep in between the cerebral hemispheres, and yet without any direct neural contact to the brain. Its site and anatomical relations are shown in Fig. 1. Further details of its innervation by sympathetic tracts originating in the superior cervical ganglion are discussed later.

3 Comparative studies

Much of our present knowledge concerning the anatomy of the pineal gland has resulted from the pioneering work of Dr Arien Kappers of the Netherlands Central Institute for Brain Research, Amsterdam. He has shown that the mammalian pineal gland (from studies mostly in the rat) has no direct connection with the brain itself, but is exclusively innervated

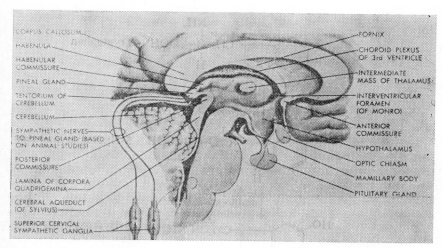

FIG. 1. Anatomy of human pineal gland (reproduced from Netter Medical Illustration by permission of Ciba Laboratories).

by the peripheral automomic system (see review articles: Kappers, 1971a, 1971b), mostly sympathetic postganglionic fibres from the superior cervical ganglia. These sympathetic fibres terminate in boutons with close contact to the pineal cell or pinealocyte. Although acetylcholine can be demonstrated within these nerve endings, it is probable that, like other sympathetic nerves elsewhere, noradrenaline is the active neurotransmitter. The mammalian pineal cell is essentially secretory in function, actively synthesizing, storing and secreting melatonin and other methoxyindoles. A rich capillary network is to be found in the parenchyma surrounding the pineal cells, and into this circulation pineal secretions are probably released. There has been some debate concerning the possibility of direct release into the cerebrospinal fluid as melatonin is more potent when administered experimentally by this route. But as yet, there is no evidence that this occurs.

When comparative studies of pineal structure and function are made, a fascinating phylogenetic evolution becomes evident. It would appear that the mammalian pineal gland originates from the primitive "third eye" of fishes and amphibia. From the basic light responsive function in these lower animals, a progressive loss of photoreceptor activity and a development of secretory function can be seen to evolve, when intermediate stages such as birds and reptiles are studied. The amniotic (fish, amphibia) pineal has a structure rather similar to the retina with cells which are derived from neuroepithelium and which are directly responsive to light

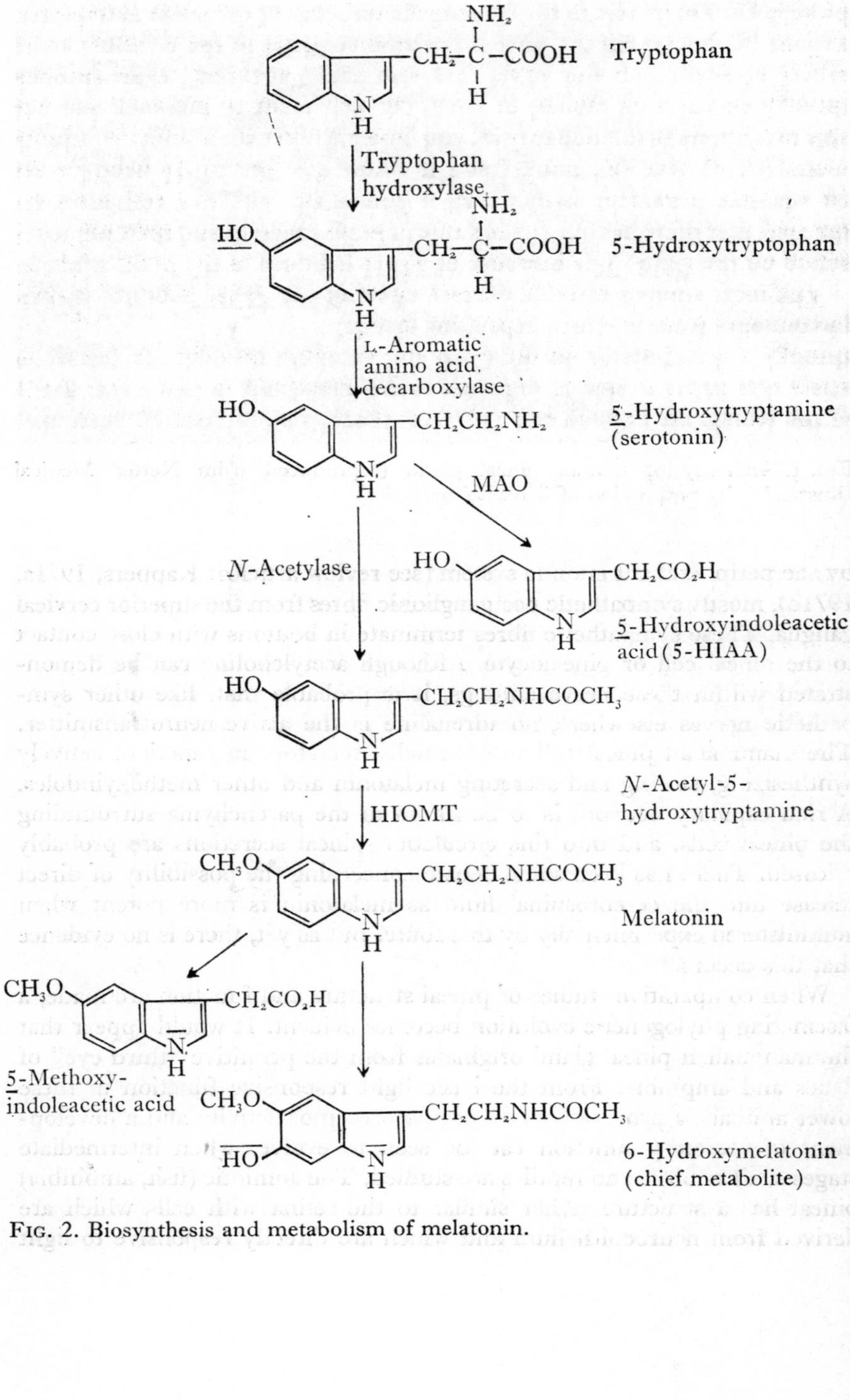

Tryptophan

Tryptophan hydroxylase

5-Hydroxytryptophan

L-Aromatic amino acid decarboxylase

5-Hydroxytryptamine (serotonin)

MAO

N-Acetylase

5-Hydroxyindoleacetic acid (5-HIAA)

N-Acetyl-5-hydroxytryptamine

HIOMT

Melatonin

5-Methoxyindoleacetic acid

6-Hydroxymelatonin (chief metabolite)

Fig. 2. Biosynthesis and metabolism of melatonin.

stimuli. These messages are then relayed to the brain. During phylogenetic development the pineal cell loses its capacity to receive photic stimuli directly, and neural contact with the brain is lost. Secretory function gradually develops, and at the same time complex autonomic innervation connecting the pineal gland to the retina is acquired. This neural pathway is discussed in detail later (see section 5.3), but it is appropriate to note here that the pineal cell can respond indirectly to external light changes via this autonomic innervation connecting the eye and the retina. Thus it can be seen that evolution has transformed a primitive photoreceptor organ into a highly developed neuroendocrine gland, capable of producing hormones, which in turn may be profoundly influenced by alterations in environmental lighting.

4 Biochemistry

4.1 PINEAL PRINCIPLES

Following the isolation of melatonin, Axelrod and co-workers conducted a series of experiments to identify the nature of the enzyme needed for the synthesis of melatonin. In view of the methoxy group it was clear that methylation was important, but no such enzyme was known. However, when N-acetylserotonin was incubated with (Me-^{14}C)S-adenosylmethionine (a methyl donor) in the presence of bovine pineal extract, ^{14}C-labelled melatonin was extracted (Axelroad and Weissbach, 1960). The melatonin-forming enzyme was subsequently isolated from the cow pineal gland and identified as hydroxyindole-O-methyl transferase (HIOMT). This enzyme, although virtually unique to the pineal, has also recently been found in the mammalian retina and harberian gland, but there is no evidence that melatonin is produced anywhere else than within the pineal gland. The properties of HIOMT have been studied by Axelrod and his colleagues (Axelrod and Weissbach, 1961). They showed that N-acetylserotonin is the best substrate, while serotonin has approximately one-tenth of the activity of N-acetylserotonin as a methyl acceptor. They concluded that melatonin was enzymatically formed from N-acetylserotonin and S-adenosylmethionine (Fig. 2).

Apart from melatonin, the pineal contains other biologically active substances, including serotonin, noradrenaline and histamine. Large amounts of serotonin have been demonstrated (Giarman and Day, 1959). When serotonin is incubated with A, S-adenosylmethionine and bovine pineal extract melatonin is produced, indicating that the pineal is capable of synthesizing melatonin from serotonin in stepwise fashion (Weissbach et al., 1960). Further studies (Wurtman et al., 1968a) showed that the pineal contains all the enzymes at the high concentrations necessary for the synthesis of melatonin from tryptophan (Fig. 2).

Tryptophan enters the pineal cell from the circulation, where it is first hydroxylated to 5-hydroxytryptophan and decarboxylated to serotonin. There is apparently a reciprocal relationship between the storage of noradrenaline and serotonin in the pineal gland such that when levels of noradrenaline are low, levels of serotonin are high.

4.2. METABOLISM

Melatonin is almost completely metabolized by the liver, where it is 6-hydroxylated and then excreted in the urine as a glucouronide or sulphate conjugate (Kopin et al., 1961).

The metabolic fate of exogenous ^{14}C-melatonin in rats and rabbits has been studied (Kveder and McIsaac, 1961). Within 30 minutes of administration a significant amount of activity in the brain was noted, and within 24 hours, 70 per cent and 20 per cent of the activity were excreted in the urine and faeces respectively. They confirmed that melatonin was largely metabolized to N-acetyl-6-hydroxy-5-methoxytryptamine; a trace of unchanged melatonin was excreted, 2 per cent was metabolized to 5-methoxyindoleacetic acid, and two other unidentified metabolites were detected.

Serotonin has two pathways of metabolism. Acetylation to N-acetyl-serotonin has been described as a necessary step in the biosynthesis of melatonin, but deamination by monoamine oxidase can also occur in the pineal. The deaminated products are then either oxidized to 5-hydroxy-indoleacetic acid or reduced to 5-hydroxytryptophol.

Much remains unknown about the biochemistry of the pineal. Other aspects of pineal metabolism have been discussed by Krass and colleagues (1971). There is an active hexose monophosphate pathway, known to be important in hormone synthesis providing further evidence of endocrine activity. A high turnover of ^{32}P in the carbohydrate fraction of the pineal has been noted with increased uptake during the hours of darkness consistent with a diurnal rhythm. Large amounts of cystathionine and taurine are present as free amino acids, possibly as precursors of 5-adenosylmethionine necessary for the synthesis of melatonin. A number of other biologically active polypeptides are known to be present in the pineal, but, apart from melatonin, their nature has yet to be determined. A peptide binding protein substance, epiphysin, similar to but differing in certain aspects to the posterior pituitary substance, neophysin, has been detected in appreciable amounts. Cholinergic activity can be demonstrated in the pineal but its role is uncertain.

5 Physiology

5.1 GENERAL

The vast majority of knowledge on the physiological actions of the pineal gland and melatonin is derived from studies in animals. Little is known of their importance in man; interest is great and speculation considerable, but evidence is accumulating that the pineal gland has important neuro-endocrine activity.

Early observations on the action of melatonin demonstrated its potent ability to contract the frog melanophore and thereby blanch its skin. This appears to be an adaptation to light and darkness. In fishes and amphibia the ability to change skin pigmentation in response to changing light conditions is lost when the pineal body is removed. Melatonin, when given to human volunteers causes no consistent change in skin pigmentation, largely because human skin lacks the melanophore cell responsive to melatonin.

Evidence of endocrine activity is obtained from studies based on classical ablation, substitution and transplantation experiments. Yet the pineal gland shows certain peculiarities (Martini, 1971). It is not a vital organ as animals can survive pinealectomy; nor does administration of pineal extract restore normal function after ablation—the neural connections are clearly an integral and necessary component.

5.2 RELATIONSHIP TO LIGHT AND GONADAL FUNCTION

The best documented aspects of pineal physiology are related to the inter-action of the pineal gland and the gonad, and their responses to light. Profound changes in gonadal function can be observed in most birds and animals when exposed to continuous light or darkness. Hamsters and rats develop delayed sexual maturation with atrophy of the gonads during continuous darkness, and these changes can be prevented by pinealectomy. In contrast, continuous light exposure in the rat leads to early onset of sexual development and increase in ovarian weight; these effects can be reduced by administration of bovine pineal extract.

It has been shown that these changes in gonadal function in response to light are probably mediated via the pineal gland. Fiske et al. (1960) showed that constant light caused a reduction in the size of the pineal gland. Later a reduction in HIOMT and melatonin synthesis were demonstrated under similar conditions (Wurtman et al., 1963a) and the reverse changes rapidly occur when the animal is moved into darkness. Subtle changes in pineal weight have been noted during the 24-hour day with the minimum weight at the end of the daylight hours followed by an increase in weight during darkness. Clearly the chemistry of the pineal gland can be affected by environmental lighting.

The inhibitory gonadal effect of the pineal and melatonin has been well established. Melatonin administration to rats leads to reduction in ovarian weight, delayed vaginal opening and a disturbance of the ovulatory cycle (Wurtman et al., 1963b). Melatonin also interferes with the increased oestrus produced by constant light exposure (Chu et al., 1964). It would appear that melatonin and other pineal principles produce some of these effects by altering the secretion of gonadotrophins from the anterior pituitary gland. In the adult male rat testicular weight is determined by the gonadotrophin follicle-stimulating hormone (FSH), and the weight of the prostate gland and seminal vesicles by luteinizing hormone (LH). Pinealectomy leads to increased weight of the testes (Fraschini and Martini, 1970), prostate and seminal vesicles (Motta et al., 1967). This would suggest that the pineal normally maintains the anterior pituitary gland under inhibitory control. When melatonin is administered to male rats by subcutaneous injection, pituitary and testicular weights are unaffected, whilst pronounced atrophy occurs in the prostate and seminal vesicles, indicating a selective effect of melatonin on LH but not FSH activity. Further evidence of differential effect has been obtained from experiments involving brain implants of melatonin and other pineal principles under stereotaxic control (Fraschini and Martini, 1970). Brain implants have the advantage of direct action and avoid the blood-brain barrier. A series of elegant studies involving the implantation of various pineal substances into the median eminence of the hypothalamus in castrated male rats has shown the following: serotonin and 5-methoxytryptophol reduce pituitary FSH levels and do not affect LH, while melatonin and 5-hydroxytryptophol reduce pituitary LH levels and not FSH. These results are not obtained when implantation is made directly into the anterior pituitary itself. Melatonin also leads to reduced pituitary and plasma LH levels following mid-brain implantation and intraventricular injection. Further information on these effects is required.

5.3   NEURAL CONTROL

How does the pineal gland respond to light? In the lower animals— amphibia, reptiles and possibly birds—the pineal is directly photoreceptive, but in mammals, where light would have to pentrate thick cranial bone, dura mater and brain to reach the pineal, this is unlikely, although studies with photoelectric cells implanted in the temporal lobe show that a surprisingly large amount of light can penetrate deep into the brain. In higher animals the neural connections, particularly sympathetic innervation, become increasingly important; when these connections are severed the pineal response to light and darkness is lost. Bilateral enucleation of the eye or cervical sympathetic ganglionectomy abolish the effects of environmental lighting on HIOMT activity. By a series of experiments in the rat, making discrete neural transections at various stages, it has been established that light reaches the pineal by the following pathway:

Retina → inferior accessory optic tract (the primary optic nerve is not involved) → medial fore-brain bundle → preganglionic sympathetic nerves → superior cervical ganglion → postganglionic sympathetic nerves → pineal gland (see Fig. 3).

A similar pathway probably occurs in all mammals. In birds, blinding or ganglionectomy does not prevent the pineal light response, and an alternative mechanism must be present, possibly a direct pineal response to external light, particularly long wavelengths.

In mammals action spectrum studies have shown that inhibition of HIOMT activity is most effective in the green band, which fits well with the known action spectrum of the retinal pigment, rhodopsin. Light

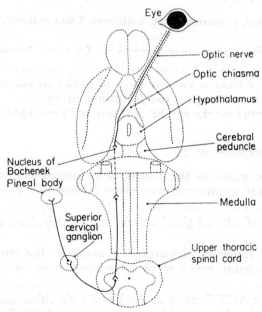

FIG. 3. Neuro-optic pathway connecting the pineal gland to the eye in the rat. (Wurtman *et al.*, 1968b).

messages are transmitted from the retina to the pineal gland via the sympathetic nerves. Organ culture studies involving the ability of pineal tissue to take up ^{14}C-labelled tryptophan and synthesize ^{14}C-melatonin have shown that noradrenalin stimulates melatonin synthesis, probably via cyclic AMP. This action can be inhibited by β-adrenergic blocking drugs. It has, therefore, been proposed that in response to information received from the retina, the sympathetic nerves release noradrenaline, which then acts at β-adrenergic receptor sites in the pineal gland to activate the adenyl cyclase system which in turn triggers HIOMT activity.

5.4   PINEAL AND BRAIN ACTIVITY

There is good evidence that much of pineal action is mediated via receptors in the brain. It is not known whether the pineal gland releases melatonin into the circulation or into the CSF, although injection of ^{3}H-labelled melatonin into the cerebral ventricles leads to a 100-fold greater retention of the administered dose compared with systemic injection (Anton-Tay and Wurtman, 1969). Both routes lead to a selective concentration in the hypo-thalamus and mid-brain, known to be important sites of melatonin activity.

Pinealectomy leads to increased motor and EEG activity (Reiss et al., 1963; Nir et al., 1969), whilst melatonin administration reduces spontaneous motor activity, promotes sleep with slow EEG activity, and prolongs barbiturate induced sleep (Fraschini and Martini, 1970). Melatonin probably modifies central neurotransmitter function. Increased levels of γ-aminobutyric acid (GABA) and serotonin have been noted (Anton-Tay, 1971), probably mediated via activation of pyridoxal kinase (Anton-Tay et al., 1970) which catalyses the formation of pyridoxal phosphate, a co-enzyme essential for the synthesis of serotonin and GABA.

5.5   OTHER ENDOCRINE EFFECTS

The role of the pineal in the control of adrenocorticotrophin (ACTH) secretion from the anterior pituitary gland is uncertain. Pinealectomy can lead to reduced adrenal ascorbic acid levels (Asagoe and Mamamoto, 1959), an index of adrenal gland activity and increased secretion of corti-costerone (Kinson and Singer, 1967), suggesting that the pineal gland inhibits adrenal function. However, the effects on the pituitary–adrenal axis following administration of pineal substances are conflicting. Some workers (Barchas et al., 1969) have been unable to detect any change in corticosterone or ACTH levels in the blood with either acute or chronic administration of melatonin. Others (Fraschini et al., 1968) have reported decreased adrenal weight following intrahypothalamic implantation of melatonin, whilst Gromova *et al.* (1967) have shown that acute administration of melatonin can actually increase corticosterone production. These confusing results prompted Motta and co-workers (1971) to make further studies of the effects of pineal indoles and methoxy-indoles on the pituitary-adrenal axis in rats. Pineal substances were injected directly into the cerebrospinal fluid of the lateral ventricle via an indwelling cannula under resting conditions. One hour after the injection of a large dose of melatonin, plasma corticosterone levels were significantly depressed. A similar reduction was also achieved following injection of 5-hydroxytryptophol, 5-methoxytryptophol, noradrenaline and dopamine. Further experiments showed that both melatonin and dopamine suppressed stress-induced (intravenous histamine) corticosterone production. However, when the animals were pretreated with reserpine, a depletor of central catecholamines, the corticosterone response to histamine was much greater and unaffected by melatonin administration. These findings support the hypothesis (Giuliani *et al.*, 1966) that ACTH secretion is under inhibitory control by a central adrenergic mechanism. It is suggested that melatonin acts via this inhibitory mechanism and that this is abolished with reserpine.

In the rat, blood corticosterone levels are highest in the afternoon and it is tempting to suggest that light has suppressed pineal activity and melatonin synthesis which in turn has released ACTH secretion from inhibitory control. However it is unlikely that such a simple scheme will entirely explain diurnal variation of corticosteroid production. Little is known about such changes in man. Indeed, ACTH release in man occurs, in contrast, in the early hours of the morning towards the end of the dark period. Oral melatonin administration in man is without effect on the HPA axis (personal observations).

Disordered pineal function may have implications in diabetes mellitus, as the pineal gland clearly plays a part in carbohydrate metabolism (Milcu *et al.*, 1971). Following pinealectomy in rats, there is diminution in glucose tolerance after a glucose load, hyperglycaemia and a rise in plasma insulin levels. Administration of pineal extract leads to increased glucose tolerance and hypoglycaemia. Milcu *et al.* have suggested that these changes are due to an alteration in adrenocorticosteroid production, but a direct action on the pancreas, possibly mediated via serotonergic mechanisms within the pancreas, has yet to be excluded. The association of impaired glucose tolerance and elevated plasma insulin levels is a well-established finding in maturity onset diabetes in man.

Melatonin injection into the rat cerebral ventricle stimulates release of prolactin (Kamberi *et al.*, 1971), an effect not obtained when melatonin is directly injected into the anterior pituitary, suggesting that melatonin may have suppressed the release of prolactin inhibitory hormone from the hypothalamus. The importance of prolactin in man is only now becoming evident as modern specific immunoassay techniques are developed.

Although pinealectomy or continuous light in rats lead to raised melanocyte-stimulating hormone (MSH) levels, and melatonin adminis-tration suppresses MSH levels (Kastin *et al.*, 1967a, 1967b), the signi-ficance is uncertain. A depressant effect of melatonin on thyroid function (Baschieri *et al.*, 1963) has been reported, but alleged effect on aldosterone production has not been confirmed.

Of considerable interest is an association of pineal hyperplasia with insulin-resistant diabetes that has been recently reported (West, 1972; West *et al.*, 1974). Bizarre features, including an unusual facies, dental abnormalities and thickened nails were noted in a young girl of five who developed diabetes with raised serum insulin levels. Despite treatment with large doses of insulin, chlorpropamide and metformin, the patient's condition progressively deteriorated and she died of uncontrollable diabetic ketoacidosis at the age of eight years. Pineal hyperplasia was discovered at autopsy. Since her death her younger brother has also presented with diabetes and similar clinical features, suggesting a familial syndrome. Although the presence of a pineal tumour has not been established, a trial of oral melatonin therapy was carried out. Marked sedation occurred but there was no improvement in the hyperglycaemia or reduction in the raised serum insulin levels.

5.6 CIRCADIAN RHYTHM

One of the most fascinating aspects of pineal physiology is the circadian rhythmicity. Many such rhythms are known to occur in mammals, but the pineal, with its close relationship to external lighting conditions, provides a possible clue as to the way these mechanisms might be mediated. Could the pineal be the long sought after "biological clock"? HIOMT activity follows a 12-hour light/12-hour darkness response pattern, with greatest activity during darkness. This pattern can be altered by artificial changes in light. *N*-acetyltransferase, another pineal enzyme, has a ten-fold increase in activity during darkness, synchronous with HIOMT and rising just after the onset of darkness. Comparable diurnal changes in urinary melatonin excretion have been demonstrated in man.

Pineal serotonin has also marked diurnal changes with highest levels during the daylight falling rapidly with darkness (Quay, 1963). However, this rhythm is preserved with continuous darkness or blinding (Snyder *et al.*, 1965) but abolished when the postganglionic sympathetic nerves are severed. Reversal of external lighting conditions alters the rhythm (Snyder *et al.*, 1967). These observations suggest that pineal serotonergic rhythmicity is endogenous, although dependant on the sympathetic neural input and subject to modification by external lighting conditions.

Pineal noradrenaline also has a diurnal rhythm (Wurtman *et al.*, 1967) with high levels at night and low levels during the day. In contrast to serotonin, this rhythm is not endogenous and is readily abolished by continuous light or darkness.

In an attempt to correlate pineal activity with circadian rhythms outside the pineal, Nir and colleagues (Nir, 1971) studied the 24-hour rhythm of urinary 17-ketosteroid excretion in female rats. A definite rhythm was established with twice the excretion in the hours of darkness. Pinealectomy was without effect on this rhythm in adult rats, but when immature rats were subjected to pinealectomy the rhythm commenced at a much earlier stage of maturation. This is tentative work and it awaits to be seen to what extent the pineal gland is an overall controller of biological rhythms.

6 Pineal pathology

6.1 PINEAL TUMOURS

Very little information concerning the role of the pineal in man is available. Pineal tumours provide an opportunity to study the pathology of the pineal, but their occurrence is rare, and caution must be exercised when interpreting the effects of disease processes in terms of normal physiological activity. In 1954 Kitay and Altschule reviewed the case reports of 473 pineal tumours. Over half were under twenty years of age with a three-fold predilection for males. Although a high incidence (26 per cent) of precocious puberty occurred in these patients, a smaller fraction was associated with hypogonadism and delayed pubescence. It is possible to distinguish between true pinealomas, where enhanced pineal function would be anticipated, and nonparenchymatous tumours where effects comparable to pinealectomy might be observed. Nonparenchymatous tumours, essentially destructive in nature, are associated with precocious puberty, whilst the true parenchymatous tumour is associated with depressed gonadal function. The latter, true pinealoma, has a typical histology. Two cell types occur: large spheroidal cells and small darkly staining cells. Teratomata account for a small proportion (10–15 per cent) and these are often malignant.

Pineal tumours produce their effects in two ways. Firstly, there may be features of a space occupying mass within the brain, i.e. cranial nerve palsies, obstructive hydrocephalus. Secondly, a disturbance of pineal endocrine function can lead to altered gonadal activity as just described.

Ectopic pineal tumours are occasionally reported, particularly sited in the hypothalamus, where local pressure effects can lead to signs of optic chiasma compression and hypopituitarism. Hypernatraemia, diabetes insipidus and loss of thirst perception have also been reported (Christie and Ross, 1968).

6.2 PINEAL CALCIFICATION

It is a well-known observation that the pineal gland undergoes progressive calcification with age, but apart from acting as an important landmark for the neuroradiologist, calcification appears to serve little function. Calcification does not interfere with the endocrine activity of the pineal and it is not possible to interpret the commencement of sexual maturation, as once believed, in terms of the onset of pineal calcification.

7 Clinical aspects of melatonin administration

7.1 NORMAL VOLUNTEERS

Anton-Tay and colleagues studied the effects of melatonin administration in 11 healthy student volunteers (Anton-Tay et al., 1971). The students were placed under resting conditions in a soundproof darkened cubicle and then asked to perform certain tasks to determine response and speed of reaction. At the same time brain activity was monitored by electroencephalogram (EEG). Melatonin in 1 per cent ethanol was given intravenously as a single injection, while ethanol only was used in control experiments. A rapid induction of sleep associated with vivid dreams occurred with melatonin. On awakening there was no significant impairment of reaction time; certain EEG changes were observed, but apart from a mild euphoriant effect, no adverse reaction or behavioural change was encountered. Personal experience of oral melatonin in single does up to 500 mg confirms sedative activity, which begins about 30 minutes after ingestion and lasts for an interval of 30 to 60 minutes. One colleague noticed an exacerbation of his migraine.

7.2 PARKINSONISM

Recent advances in determining the neurochemical pathogenesis of the disease parkinsonism has led to study of a large number of centrally active substances, including melatonin. Parkinsonism is a disorder of the extrapyramidal motor system classically leading to the clinical features of tremor, rigidity and poverty of movement (bradykinesia). It is a progressive illness which can cause marked disability and immobility in the severely afflicted. The epidemic of encephalitis lethargica in the 1920s gave rise to a particularly distressing form of parkinsonism, while more recently drug-induced parkinsonism is increasingly recognized following the administration of drugs such as phenothiazines, butyrophenones (dopamine-blocking agents) and reserpine (depletes cerebral catecholamines). But the majority of parkinsonian cases are due to a degeneration of the basal ganglia in the brain, particularly involving the substantia nigra and corpus striatum. The substantia nigra, as the name implies, is normally pigmented, and loss of this pigmentation is characteristic of parkinsonism. Following the acceptance of dopamine as a neurotransmitter in its own right as well as a precursor of noradrenaline (Blaschko, 1957), Carlsson and colleagues showed that dopamine was particularly concentrated in the corpus striatum, and a central role for dopamine was proposed (Carlsson et al., 1958; Carlsson, 1959). Then, in 1960, Ehringer and Hornykiewiez discovered that the brains of patients dying from parkinsonism contained much reduced dopamine concentrations. This observation naturally led to attempts at repleting dopamine stores in parkinsonian patients. Dopamine itself failed to cross the blood-brain barrier and it was necessary to give the immediate precursor dopa (3,4-dihydroxyphenylalanine) which crosses the blood-brain barrier, and is then decarboxylated to dopamine. Initial studies of dopa in parkinsonism were discouraging (Birkmayer and Hornykiewicz, 1961; Barbeau et al., 1962), and the value of dopa in parkinsonism was not fully recognized until Cotzias and his colleagues reported striking benefit in 8 of 16 patients treated with large doses of ($\pm$) dopa (Cotzias et al., 1969). This renewed interest in dopa evolved from attempts at increasing brain melanin concentration in parkinsonism by injecting the pituitary hormone β-melanocyte stimulating hormone (β-MSH). β-MSH in fact worsened tremor and led to a darkening of the skin. Based on the speculative hypothesis that β-MSH could be diverting melanin precursers from the brain to the skin, a search for active precursors was carried out, dopa was reinvestigated and this time its beneficial role established. Many subsequent trials have confirmed the undoubted value of levodopa as the treatment of choice in parkinsonism, and more recently its combination with a decarboxylase inhibitor to prevent peripheral breakdown, thereby freeing a much larger amount for central action, has reduced many of the adverse reactions of levodopa alone.

It was these same observations that β-MSH worsened tremor which suggested the use of melatonin, known to antagonize the skin darkening effect of β-MSH. In a maximum daily dose of 1·35 g melatonin for fifty-one days, diminution of tremor was seen in one patient, but excess sedation deterred further study at that time (Cotzias et al., 1971a).

However, Anton-Tay and colleagues, studying the effects of melatonin administration to humans included observations on two parkinsonian patients (Anton-Tay *et al.*, 1971). Both patients were severely disabled and had had the disease for several years. 1·2 g melatonin as an elixir was administered daily for four weeks. Striking improvement in all symptoms and signs was recorded by the second week, and one patient, previously chairbound, was able to walk again. There was a general feeling of well-being and the performance of daily tasks was improved. Placebo substitution led to overall deterioration.

At the same time Cotzias and colleagues reported that adventitious movements induced by levodopa in mice could be blocked by melatonin (Cotzias *et al.*, 1971b). Involuntary movements are the commonest dose-limiting side-effect of levodopa therapy in man, and clearly such effects of melatonin in mice raise therapeutic implications in the treatment of parkinsonism. Prompted by these observations, and by the striking results of Anton-Tay, Cotzias *et al.* conducted a single blind study of the effects of melatonin in a further eleven parkinsonians (Papavasiliou *et al.*, 1972). Melatonin, in capsules of 50 mg or 100 mg, was administered by gradual increments to a maximum daily dose ranging from 3·0 g to 6·6 g. Sedation and somnolence were again encountered and episodes of flushing, diarrhoea, migrainous headaches and abdominal cramps occurred, rather akin to symptoms of carcinoid disease, suggesting serotonergic activity. Increased excretion of urinary hydroxylindole acetic acid in these patients gives further support to this view. However, no change in parkinsonism was observed. In those patients in whom levodopa was continued, no reversal of benefit or amelioration of dopa-induced dyskinesia was seen.

Our own studies of melatonin administration in parkinsonism in the Department of Neurology, University College Hospital, have been reported (Shaw *et al.*, 1973a, 1973b). Formulation of melatonin (obtained from Kochlight Labs, Colnbrook, Bucks.) was undertaken by Mr A. R. Williams, Group Chief Pharmacist. Supplies of melatonin being limited, a full pharmaceutical study was not possible. Preliminary tests indicated a proneness to oxidation, and it was thought advisable to avoid introducing any substance that might catalyse such a reaction (metallic ions, etc.) or to use a moist granulation process. The tablet ingredients, melatonin, dextrose and microcrystalline cellulose, were therefore compressed dry. No obvious abnormality of particle size was evident macroscopically, and it was considered that normal disintegration would occur during passage through the alimentary tract. Tablets containing 50 mg and 100 mg of melatonin were processed with 50 per cent of the tablets' gross weight consisting of soluble material. The 50 mg tablets disintegrated in 3 minutes (in the British Pharmacopœia test for disintegration) and the 100 mg tablets in 10 minutes using a guided disc. It was therefore anticipated that following oral ingestion there would be a somewhat slow release of melatonin which would then be rapidly absorbed into the circulation (see section 4.2). The best means of administering melatonin has yet to be fully determined. A suspension of melatonin with polyethylene glycol 400 may be a suitable alternative.

As melatonin supplies were limited, administration was restricted to four parkinsonian patients (three men, one woman, aged fifty-six to sixty-eight years, average sixty-two years) with moderately severe disease considered suitable for trial therapy. Although all continued to take anti-cholinergic drugs, none received levodopa during the study. Melatonin, commencing with 100 mg daily, was gradually increased to a maximum of 1·0 g daily in divided doses and continued for four weeks, after which time placebo substitution (lactose tablets) was made. Weekly assessment, using a standard 4-point scale of functional disabilities and physical signs and a computerized motor performance tracking device, were employed to assess change. However, there was no alteration in parkinsonian disabilities; nor was there any change following switch to placebo. All four patients noted a transitory sedation shortly after taking the tablets, suggesting central activity and therefore evidence of absorption. No other side-effects were noted.

In collaboration with Professor M. Sandler and Dr K. Blau of the Bernhard Baron Memorial Research Laboratories, Queen Charlotte's Hospital, London, urine collections were made during melatonin administration. Metabolites related to melatonin have been detected, but further analysis, including specific melatonin assay, is in process, and details will be reported elsewhere.

Hypothalamo-pituitary-adrenal function tests were carried out on admission before treatment was begun and after four weeks of treatment with melatonin. Cortisols were measured for diurnal variation and response to tetracosactrin stimulation: 24-hour urinary ketogenic steroids were measured before and after metyrapone suppression and a single insulin hypoglycaemic stress test was performed in three patients while on treatment only. Melatonin did not interfere with either the cortisol (Mattingly fluorometric method) or ketogenic steroid estimations. Normal diurnal rhythm of control was preserved, and a normal cortisol response after tetracosactrin stimulation was maintained. Urinary ketogenic steroid excretion was unaltered, and the metyrapone suppression test was not impaired. Normal insulin stress response was observed in three patients on melatonin.

7.3 EPILEPSY

Anton-Tay's studies (Anton-Tay, 1971) also included observations on melatonin administration to three epileptic patients, all of whom had had long-standing Grand Mal epilepsy associated with temporal lobe seizures. Electroencephalographic readings following melatonin administration showed a reduction in the electrical activity over the temporal lobe, depression of paroxysmal activity and increase in rapid eye movements (REM) during sleep. It would appear that melatonin raises the convulsive threshold, and may therefore provide potential therapy for epilepsy. Further studies of melatonin administration in epilepsy are needed.

8 Conclusion

In their preface to *The Pineal Gland* (Wolstenholme and Knight, 1971) the editors suggest that "the pineal gland may well be about to attract the same limelight as the adrenal cortex some twenty years ago, with an equal impact on the better understanding of human functioning and behaviour, in health and disease". It is only over the last decade that evidence of neuroendocrine activity has accumulated. The vast majority of knowledge is naturally derived from animal studies, and little information concerning pineal physiology in man is available, although intriguing glimpses and important clues of endocrine activity are provided in the rare cases of pineal tumour. It is likely that the main site of action of melatonin is the brain itself, and it is of interest that selective concentration of melatonin following administration occurs in the hypothalamus, where important neuroendocrine regulatory mechanisms are now well established. Hypothalamic hormones, e.g. thyroid-releasing hormone (TRH), luteinizing hormone releasing factor (LHRF) have been identified. TRH has been shown to play an essential role in maintaining normal thyroid activity. Its intravenous administration is helpful in distinguishing between various thyroid disorders. More recently, prospects of medical treatment of acromegaly have been raised by the discovery of a growth hormone inhibitory peptide (somatostatin). This substance may have further therapeutic value in brittle diabetics, by suppressing glucagon production, which may be contributing to the poor control of the hyperglycaemia. There are many other hypothalamo-pituitary hormones, e.g. prolactin, whose importance is increasingly recognized. In turn it is likely that the hypothalamus is controlled by yet higher centres. For instance, corticotrophin releasing factor (CRF) and ACTH are known to be under at least three regulatory mechanisms: stress or emotion, negative feedback control and the circadian or nyctohymeral rhythm. Centres such as the hippocampus and amygdaloid nucleus are probably involved in emotional control and on present evidence, discussed in this chapter, it is not unreasonable to postulate that the pineal gland is responsible for the circadian control. A hypothetical "biological clock" has long been advocated to explain the diurnal variations in hormonal patterns, and the pineal gland would fit this role. Its ability to adjust its enzyme activity and thereby its secretory response to external light conditions, and the apparent endocrine properties of melatonin are strong pointers in favour of this suggestion. It looks as though melatonin endocrine activity largely acts at the hypothalamic level, although direct effects on the thyroid and gonad may yet be found.

Accepting the thesis that the pineal gland is an endocrine gland in its own right, then, by analogy with other endocrine glands, it is likely that disease states will occur. Pineal tumours produce gross, crude changes, but what of more subtle disorders? Do underactive and overactive states exist? What are the effects of pineal deficiency and of pineal hyperactivity? These questions are open to conjecture, but it is not unreasonable to suggest that such states may have important implications when considering other endocrine disorders. Pineal dysfunction may play a part in the pathogenesis of such diseases as diabetes mellitus, thyroid disease and gonadal disorders. If deficiency states exist then there would be a possible need for replacement therapy. If over-activity occurs then drugs might be required to suppress pineal activity. Time and research will tell, but there are exciting future possibilities to be explored.

Apart from endocrine activity, melatonin undoubtedly possesses potent effects on the central nervous system. Although the studies in parkinsonism proved disappointing, attention was drawn to the powerful sedative and hypnotic properties, which need to be further explored. Certainly brain catecholamines may be altered by melatonin, for serotonin levels are elevated by melatonin administration. Such changes may have psychopharmacological potential. Certain psychiatric illnesses may be associated with brain catecholamine imbalance, e.g. manic-depression. It is not inconceivable that pineal dysfunction could be related and that melatonin therapy could be beneficial. Again further studies are needed.

The preliminary observations in epilepsy need confirming. Epilepsy is a disorder which can be refractory to all known therapies with consequent instability of control. Further rational drug development is restricted by ignorance of underlying mechanisms leading to the development of an epileptic fit, but in melatonin there is a substance with marked effects on brain activity—as judged by the electroencephalogram—and with possible ability to raise the convulsive threshold and thereby reduce the risk of an epileptic fit in a predisposed patient.

The report that melatonin reduces the incidence of levodopa-induced involuntary movements in mice (Cotzias *et al.*, 1971b) suggests that it may have therapeutic potential in the treatment of other involuntary movement disorders in man, e.g. spasmodic torticollis, chorea, tardive dyskinesia. All are singularly difficult to treat and rarely is satisfactory relief of symptoms obtained. The neuropharmacological actions of melatonin need to be elucidated.

But melatonin is not the only pineal product. Other biologically active substances are known to occur. What of their significance? It is likely that they too will have important physiological and metabolic activities, but as yet, sophisticated methods for their study in man are unavailable.

In summary, the human pineal body can be seen as an important neuroendocrine gland which has directly evolved from the photoreceptor organ of the lower vertebrates. It lies within the brain and yet is anatomically distinct. It produces hormones unique to itself and this activity is profoundly influenced by external environmental conditions, mostly by light and darkness, but also by other factors such as cold and stress. It is likely that the pineal plays an important part in regulatory control of hormonal homeostasis in the body. A vast amount of additional study is needed, and many workers are now actively engaged in this field. These unique pineal substances have potent biological properties and thereby potential pharmacological activity. Once these actions are elucidated and their role in man determined, it is likely that the pineal will turn a full circle, and, if not the actual seat of the soul, it will nevertheless be the centre of considerable interest, research, and hopefully pharmacological therapeutic potential.

References

Anton-Tay, F. (1971). *In* "The Pineal Gland", Ciba Foundation Symposium (Eds G. E. W. Wolstenholme and J. Knight), p. 213. Churchill Livingstone, London.

Anton-Tay, F. and Wurtman, R. J. (1969). *Nature (London)*, **221**, 474.

Anton-Tay, F., Sepulveda, J. and Gonzalez, S. (1970). *Life Sciences*, **9**, 1283.

Anton-Tay, F., Diaz, J. L. and Fernandez-Guardiola, A. (1971). *Life Sciences*, **10**, 841.

Assagoe, Y. and Hamamoto, A. (1959). *Yonago Acta Medica*, **3**, 192.

Axelrod, J. and Weissbach, H. (1960). *Science*, **131**, 1312.

Axelrod, J. and Weissbach, H. (1961). *Journal of Biological Chemistry*, **236**, 211.

Barbeau, A., Sourkes, T. L. and Murphy, G. F. (1962). *In* "Symposium sur les Monoamines et Système Nerveux Centrale" (Ed. J. de Ajuriageurra), p. 247. George et Cie, Geneva.

Barchas, J., Conner, R., Levine, S. and Vernikos-Danellis, J. (1969). *Experientia*, **25**, 413.

Baschieri, L., De Luca, F., Cramarossa, L., de Martino, C., Oliverio, A. and Negae, M. (1963). *Experientia*, **19**, 15.

Birkmayer, W. and Hornykiewicz, O. (1961). *Wiener Klinische Wochenschrift*, **73**, 757.

Blaschko, H. (1957). *Experientia*, **13**, 9.

Carlsson, A. (1959). *Pharmacological Reviews*, **11**, 490.

Carlsson, A., Lindquist, M., Magnussen, T. and Waldeck, B. (1958). *Science*, **127**, 471.

Christie, S. B. M. and Ross, E. J. (1968). *British Medical Journal*, **ii**, 669.

Chu, E. W., Wurtman, R. J. and Axelrod, J. (1964). *Endocrinology*, **75**, 238.

Cotzias, G. C., Papavasiliou, P. S. and Gellene, R. (1969). *New England Journal of Medicine*, **280**, 337.

Cotzias, G. C., Tang, L. C., Miller, S. T. and Ginos, J. Z. (1971a). *Science*, **173**, 450.

Cotzias, G. C., Papavasiliou, P. S., Ginos, J., Steck, A. and Duby, S. (1971b). *Annual Review of Medicine*, **22**, 305.

Descartes, R. (1662). *In* "De Homine".

Ehringer, L. H. and Hornykiewicz, O. (1960). *Weiner Klinische Wochenschrift*, **38**, 1236.

Fiske, V., Bryant, M. and Putnam, J. (1960). *Journal of Endocrinology*, **66**, 489.

Fraschini, F. and Martini, L. (1970). *In* "Hypothalamus" (Eds L. Martini, M. Motta and F. Fraschini), p. 529. Academic Press, New York and London.

Fraschini, F., Mess, B. and Martini, L. (1968). *Endocrinology*, **82**, 919.

Giarman, N. J. and Day, M. (1959). *Pharmacology*, **1**, 235.

Giuliani, G., Motta, M. and Martini, L. (1966). *Acta Endocrinologica*, **51**, 203.

Gromova, E. A., Kraus, M. and Krecek, J. (1967). *Journal of Endocrinology*, **39**, 345.

Heubner, O. (1898). *Deutsche Medischine Wochenschrift* (Vereins Beilag, No. 29), **24**, 214.

Holmgren, N. (1918). *Arkiv für Zoologi*, **11**, 1.

Kamberi, I. A., Mical, R. S. and Porter, J. C. (1971). *Endocrinology*, **88**, 1288.

Kappers, J. A. (1971a). *In* "The Pineal Gland", Ciba Foundation Symposium (Eds G. E. W. Wolstenholme and J. Knight), p. 3. Churchill Livingstone, London.

Kappers, J. A. (1971b). *Memoirs of the Society for Endocrinology*, **19**, 27.

Kastin, A. J. and Schally, A. V. (1967). *Nature (London)*, **213**, 1238.

Kastin, A. J. *et al.* (1967). *Neuroendocrinology*, **2**, 257.

Kinson, G. and Singer, B. (1967). *Journal of Endocrinology*, **37**, 37.

Kitay, J. I. and Altschule, M. D. (1954). *In* "The Pineal Gland". Harvard University Press, Cambridge, Massachusetts.

Kopin, I. J., Pare, C. M. B., Axelrod, J. and Weissbach, H. (1961). *Journal of Biological Chemistry*, **236**, 3072.

Krass, M. E., Labella, F. S., Shin, S. H. and Minnich, J. (1971). *Memoirs of the Society for Endocrinology*, **19**, 49.

Kveder, S. and McIsaac, W. (1961). *Journal of Biological Chemistry*, **236**, 3214.

Lerner, A. B., Case, J. D., Takahashi, Y., Lee, T. H. and Mori, W. (1958). *Journal of the American Chemical Society*, **80**, 2587.

McCord, C. P. and Allen, F. P. (1917). *Journal of Experimental Zoology*, **23**, 207.

Martini, L. (1971). *In* "The Pineal Gland", Ciba Foundation Symposium (Eds G. E. W. Wolstenholme and J. Knight), p. 1. Churchill Livingstone, London.

Milcu, S. M., Nanu-Ionescu, L. and Milcu, I. (1971). *In* "The Pineal Gland", Ciba Foundation Symposium (Eds G. E. W. Wolstenholme and J. Knight), pp. 345–60. Churchill Livingstone, London.

Motta, M., Fraschini, F. and Martini, M. (1967). *Proceedings of the Society for Experimental Biology and Medicine*, **126**, 431.

Motta, M., Schiaffini, O., Piva, F. and Martini, L. (1971). *In* "The Pineal Gland", Ciba Foundation Symposium (Eds G. E. W. Wolstenholme and J. Knight), p. 279. Churchill Livingstone, London.

Nir, I. (1971). *In* "The Pineal Gland", Ciba Foundation Symposium (Eds G. E. W. Wolstenholme and J. Knight), p. 373. Churchill Livingstone, London.

Nir, I., Behroozi, K., Assael, M., Ivriani, I. and Sulman, F. G. (1969). *Neuroendocrinology*, **4**, 122.

Papavasiliou, P. S., Cotzias, G. C., Duby, S. E., Steck, A. J., Bell, M. and Lawrence, W. H. (1972). *Journal of the American Medical Association*, **222**, 88.

Quay, W. B. (1963). *General Comparative Endocrinology*, **3**, 473.

Reiss, M., Davis, R. H., Sideman, M. B. and Plichta, E. S. (1963), *Journal of Endocrinology*, **28**, 127.

Shaw, K. M., Stern, G. M. and Sandler, M. (1973a). *Lancet*, **i**, 271.

Shaw, K. M., Stern, G. M. and Sandler, M. (1973b). *In* "Advances in Neurology" (Ed. D. Calne), vol. 3 p. 115. Raven Press, New York.

Snyder, S. H., Axelrod, J. Zweig, M. and Fischer, J. E. (1965). *Proceedings of the National Academy of Sciences, USA*, **53**, 301.

Snyder, S. H., Axelrod, J. and Zweig, M. (1967). *Journal of Pharmacology and Experimental Therapeutics*, **158**, 206.

Weissbach, H., Redfield, B. G. and Axelrod, J. (1960). *Biochimica et Biophysica Acta*, **43**, 352.

West, R. J. (1972). *Archives of Disease in Childhood*, **47**, 153.

West, R. J., Lloyd, J. K. and Turner, W. (1974). *In* "Abstracts Medical and Scientific Section British Diabetic Association".

Wolstenholme, G. E. W. and Knight, J. (1971). *In* "The Pineal Gland", Ciba Foundation Symposium (Eds G. E. W. Wolstenholme and J. Knight), p. ix. Churchill Livingstone, London.

Wurtman, R. J., Axelrod, J. and Phillips, L. S. (1963a). *Science*, **142**, 1071.

Wurtman, R. J., Axelrod, J. and Chu, E. W. (1963b). *Science*, **141**, 277.

Wurtman, R. J., Axelrod, J., Sedvall, G. and Moore, R. Y. (1967). *Journal of Pharmacology and Experimental Therapeutics*, **157**, 487.

Wurtman, R. J., Larin, F., Axelrod, J., Stein, H. M. and Rosasco, K. (1968a). *Nature (London)*, **217**, 953.

Wurtman, R. J., Axelrod, J. and Kelly, D. E. (1968b). "The Pineal". Academic Press, New York and London.

Potential Therapeutic Agents Derived from the Cannabinoid Nucleus

HARRY G. PARS, PhD, RAJ K. RAZDAN, PhD,
and JOHN F. HOWES, BPharm, PhD

SISA Incorporated, Concord Avenue, Cambridge, Massachusetts, USA

1   Introduction

1.1   HISTORICAL INTEREST IN DRUGS FROM CANNABIS

For centuries man has used various preparations of *Cannabis sativa* (Cannabinaceae) for their psychotomimetic and supposed medicinal effects. Since the pioneering studies of the earliest recorded pharmacologist in this field, Emperor Shen Nung of China, 2737 BC, the natural product has been investigated in various parts of the world for its potentially useful stimulant and depressant effects. The world literature abounds with folklore accounts of its use in medicine. The Indian Hemp Drug Commission Reports (1893–1894) cites *Cannabis indica* as one of the most important drugs of Indian Materia Medica. In Europe and America extracts of the plant were used for a variety of somatic and psychiatric illnesses, including migraine, depression, rheumatism and epilepsy. Tincture of Cannabis was listed in the US Pharmacopeia (USP) and in the National Formulary and could legally be prescribed by physicians for these and other ailments.

By 1940, totally synthetic isomers and homologs of the active principle of the plant were also being investigated in the US and a review of this period is in the La Guardia Report (1939–1944). However, the use of, and investigations with, cannabis and synthetic compounds began to decline by the late 1930s, and by 1942 neither cannabis nor any of its synthetically derived drugs were any longer listed in the USP. Its listing in the Merck Index (1950) also disappeared beginning with the 8th edition of this drug compendium. The demise of cannabis as a drug was perhaps due to the resinous, intractable nature of this natural product, but more probably because of a general lack of specific therapeutic activity, equivocal therapeutic results to date in man, clinically unacceptable subjective effects, and to the increasing availability of other drugs for the same indications.

1.2 BASIS FOR THE PURSUIT OF NEW DRUGS FROM CANNABIS

Bergel (1965) stated: ". . . it is regrettable that neither hashish nor one of its major constituents has an honest nitrogen from which one could make a soluble salt. . . ." In 1946 Anker and Cook succeeded in synthesizing a nitrogen-containing cannabinoid, which they reported to be inactive as an analgesic agent. Following this work Pars *et al.* (1966) reported the synthesis of a pharmacologically active series of nitrogen-containing analogs of the cannabinoids. Although the initial nitrogen-containing substances were not water-soluble, soluble ester salts were subsequently synthesized and investigated (Zitko *et al.*, 1972; Razdan *et al.* 1976c).

The basis for pursuing these and other analogs of the cannabinoids as potential therapeutic agents was stimulated by the following:

1. Cannabinoids have pharmacological profiles of action in laboratory animals which make them unique among (known) therapeutic agents.
2. There is no known physical-dependence liability associated with cannabis despite centuries of use.
3. Cannabinoids show extraordinary low toxicity in laboratory animals, including low lethality and little or no respiratory depression.
4. There are centuries of folklore suggesting pain relief, sedation, and other potentially useful therapeutic indications.

1.3 SCOPE AND PERSPECTIVE

The principal emphasis of this review is to direct the reader's attention to "the other side of marihuana research" (Pars, 1973). It is only relatively recently that the therapeutic potential of this field has been rediscovered. Reports are once again appearing in the literature which summarize new results and point to the therapeutic potential of cannabinoids (Archer, 1974; Cohen and Stillman, 1976). Included in these are the latest US Government studies in this field (Marihuana and Health Report, 1974).

It is the purpose of this review to summarize the current status of the chemistry and pharmacology of the active constituents of cannabis, Δ^9-tetrahydrocannabinol (I) and Δ^8-tetrahydrocannabinol (II), and carbocyclic (CHO) and heterocyclic (CHNO, CHOS) analogs, with respect to their therapeutic potential. It is beyond the scope of this review to document all the research currently in progress in this field. The chemistry of cannabinoids has been well reviewed by Mechoulam *et al.* (1976), Razdan (1973) and Neumeyer (1971). The biochemistry and pharmacology of cannabis and cannabinoids as psychotomimetics has also been reviewed in this series (Brimblecombe, 1973).

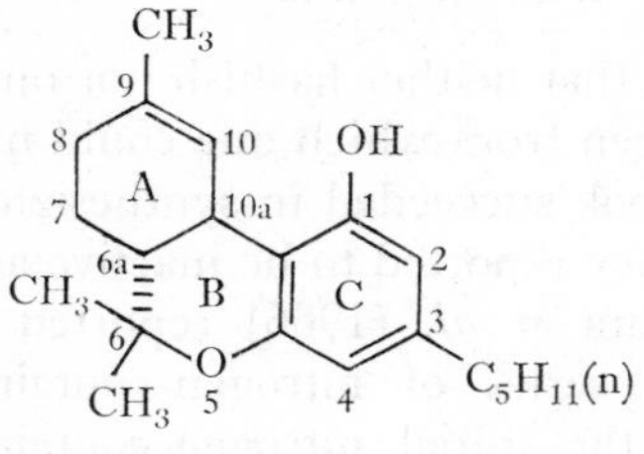

(I) Δ^9-THC 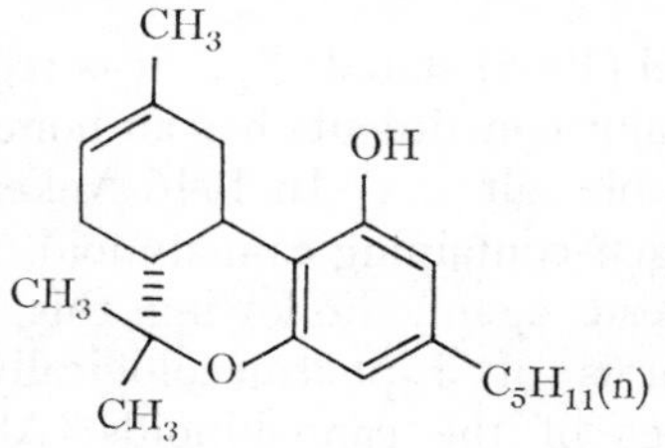   (II) Δ^8-THC

With the current availability of pure synthetic cannabinoids, water-soluble crystalline derivatives and nitrogen and sulfur analogs, and also with the availability today of more precise methods of pharmacologic study in animals and man, the earlier problems of identifying and discovering specific therapeutic effects will no doubt be overcome. Like morphine, lysergic acid diethylamide and cocaine which now have structurally related analgesics, oxytoxics, and local anesthetics respectively, similarly the socially abused cannabinoids may now be on the verge of generating a family of safer and more useful therapeutic agents.

2   Structure–activity relationships: carbocyclic (C, H, O) analogs

Δ^9-Tetrahydrocannabinol (THC) is the principal active cannabinoid of marijuana, hashish, charas etc. (see for example Mechoulam, 1973, and Razdan, 1973). The other cannabinoid of interest is Δ^8-THC which, in contrast to Δ^9-THC, is found only in a few varieties of the plant *Cannabis sativa*. There is yet a third type of cannabinoid of pharmacological interest which is synthetic, $\Delta^{6a,10a}$-THC (**III**). It was discovered by Roger Adams and his collaborators (1949) following the classical studies of the resinous cannabinoid fraction of the plant by Todd (1943), Cahn (1933) and their respective collaborators. It differs from the natural THC (**I**) in the relative position of the double bond in ring A and shows typical marijuana-like activity in rodents and in the dog ataxia test. Todd and particularly Adams carried out extensive structure–activity relationship (SAR) studies in the synthetic THCs and concluded that the marijuana activity varied with the alkyl substituent in the benzene ring. Adams found the 1,2-dimethylheptyl analog (C_9H_{19}) (**IIIb**), known as dimethylheptyl-pyran DMHP, to be the most potent compound, approximately 500 times more active than **IIIa**. He also showed that the natural THC (**I**, Δ^9-THC) was several-fold more active than the synthetic isomer **IIIa**. In various animals, Δ^9-THC and synthetic derivatives such as **IIIb** showed predominantly CNS depression and ataxia lasting from several hours to days depending upon the dose administered. The characteristic effect of THCs,

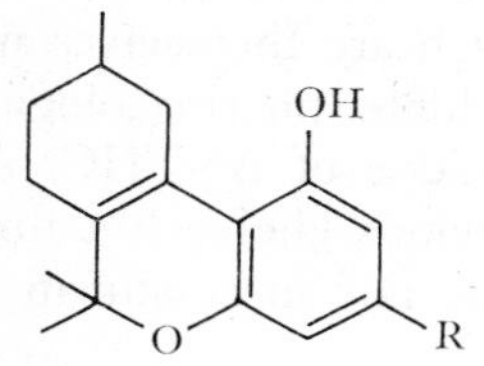

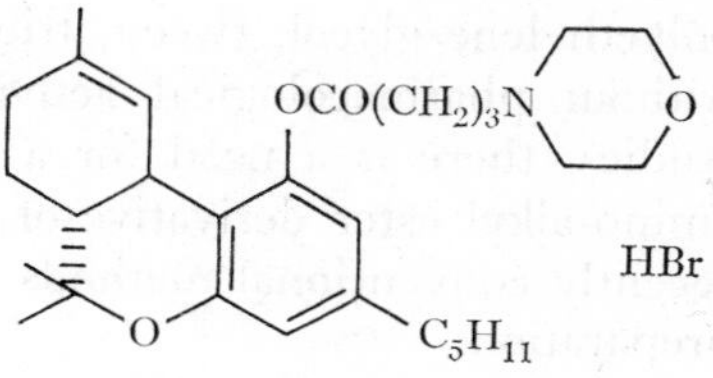

(III) a, $R = C_5H_{11}$
　　b, $R = CH(CH_3)CH(CH_3)(CH_2)_4CH_3$ (DMHP)
　　c, $R = C_6H_{13}$ (synhexyl)
　　d, $R = CH(CH_3)(CH_2)_3$—⟨⟩—F

(IV)

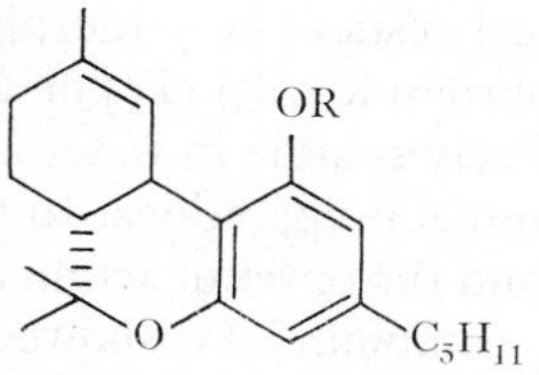

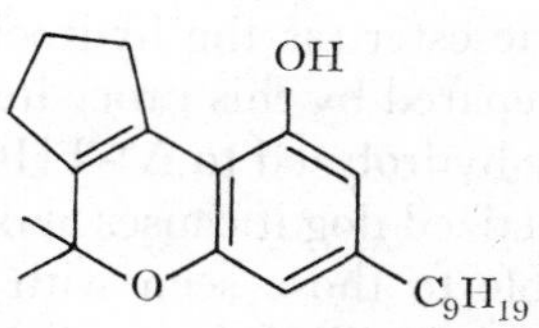

(V) a, $R = CO(CH_2)_3N(C_2H_5)_2 \cdot HCl$
　　b, $R = CH_2CH_2N(C_2H_5)_2$

(VI)

which distinguishes them from all other psychoactive drugs, is a postural arrest phenomenon with relaxed staring and associated with hypersensitivity to external stimuli. (For a detailed description of the gross behavioral effects of THCs in laboratory animals see Domino, 1971.) For example when Δ^9-THC is given at a dose of 0·2–0·5 mg kg^{-1} (iv) to dogs they stand in a trance-like state, weave from side to side, pitch forward and backward and overreact to a swinging object. When aroused, ataxia is evident for at least 3 or 4 hours after the injection. It is characteristic for the dogs to urinate and defecate soon after receiving the drug and sleep a great deal for the next 24 hours.

The phenolic hydroxyl group in the 1-position of Δ^9-THC is very important for eliciting activity in THCs. This has been demonstrated earlier and confirmed more recently by Razdan and co-workers (Uliss *et al.*, 1975). They therefore prepared ethers (Razdan *et al.*, 1970) and various straight-chain and hindered esters of the phenolic hydroxyl group in THCs (Zitko *et al.*, 1972; Razdan *et al.*, 1976c) which were expected to hydrolyze at different rates *in vivo* to the parent compound and hopefully selectively enhance the activity of THCs. Furthermore, THCs, being resinous materials insoluble in water, are administered in various solvents such as polyethylene glycol, tween, triton and alcohol which are themselves not without pharmacological activity. Hence, to facilitate pharmacological studies, there is a need for a water-soluble derivative of Δ^9-THC. An amino-alkyl ester derivative of Δ^9-THC is the obvious choice but until recently conventional methods of esterification were not successful in its preparation.

2.1 BASIC ESTER AND ETHER DERIVATIVES OF Δ^9-TETRAHYDROCANNABINOL

It was recently reported that water-soluble esters of Δ^9-THC type **IV**, can easily be prepared with carbodiimide as the condensing agent. This discovery led Razdan and co-workers (Razdan *et al.*, 1970, 1976c; Zitko *et al.*, 1972) to prepare numerous esters of THCs and synthetic analogs and to study their activity in selected pharmacological tests. The γ-morpholinobutyric ester (as the hydrochloride or hydrobromide salt) (**IV**) of Δ^9-THC, prepared by this procedure, is a solid, is freely soluble in water and is quickly hydrolyzed to Δ^9-THC by liver microsomal preparations. In the unanesthetized dog it causes ataxia and the dose and the onset of action are comparable to those seen with Δ^9-THC. Also, compound **IV** showed a similarity to Δ^9-THC in a number of other test procedures (see section 4). On the other hand, although the γ-diethylamino derivative (**Va**) (Razdan *et al.*, 1970) was similar to **IV** in pharmacological profile and in production of ataxia in unanesthetized dogs, the onset of action was considerably delayed and the effective dosage was five to ten times higher. In contrast to the activity of **IV** and **Va**, the diethylaminoethyl ether (**Vb**) of Δ^9-THC was quite different (Razdan *et al.*, 1970) and did not show the pharmacological profile of Δ^9-THC.

2.2 BASIC ESTERS OF DIMETHYLHEPTYLPYRAN (DMHP) AND ITS CYCLO-PENTENO ANALOG **VI**

The various basic esters of other carbocyclic analogs, such as DMHP (**IIIb**) and another potent analog **VI** (Razdan *et al.*, US Patent 1972) are listed in Tables 1 and 2 respectively. Some structure–activity relationships (SAR) based on animal studies in the two series (Razdan *et al.*, 1976c) are as follows:

In the case of DMHP (**IIIb**) derivatives (Table 1) the parent phenol is moderately active in tests for analgesia whereas the γ-morpholinobutyrate ester compound 2 in Table 1 is extremely active and is more potent than codeine. All the compounds except the thiomorpholino derivative (compound **4**) show potent anticonvulsant activity (audiogenic seizure). One of these derivatives (compound **3**) is of particular interest as an anticonvulsant since it is active in a variety of anticonvulsant tests (supramaximal electroshock, metrazol and psychomotor electroshock) and has the potency of diphenylhydantoin.

The derivatives of the carbocyclic analog (**VI**) (Table 2) show that the masking of the phenol as a basic ester markedly reduces or eliminates the effects on the rat motor activity as it does for compounds in Table 1. The analgesic activity is slightly enhanced only in the morpholino and homopiperidino derivatives and decreases in the pyrrolo derivatives or where the dimethylheptyl, C_9H_{19}, side chain is replaced by n-C_5H_{11} (compounds **7** and **9**). The tranquillizing activity is decreased except in the piperidino and morpholino compounds. In contrast to the DMHP derivatives (Table 1) these compounds have much less anticonvulsant activity and, surprisingly, the homopiperidino analog is inactive (compare **3** with **8**).

2.3 ANALOGS OF $\Delta^{6a, 10a}$-TETRAHYDROCANNABINOL

As indicated earlier Adams and Todd (1949 and 1943) had carried out extensive SAR studies in the synthetic THCs based on the dog ataxia and rabbit areflexia tests. These and the carbocyclic analogs synthesized up to 1972 have been reviewed by Mechoulam (1973). Recently Loev *et al.* (1973) reported a re-examination of SAR of $\Delta^{6a, 10a}$-THCs (**IIIa**) in the rat and found significant differences from those originally reported by Adams and Todd in the dog and the rabbit. In addition these authors prepared new analogs (see Table 3) and compared their relative CNS potencies against synhexyl in the rat. The 1,1-dimethylheptyl compound (**13**) was found to be the most potent compound in the rat, twice as active as DMHP (**IIIb**). This is in sharp contrast with the results of Adams who reported that compound **13** had only 1/20th the potency of DMHP (**IIIb**) in the dog. The present authors concluded from their studies that in general it appears that the length of the side chain from its attachment to the ring is more important than the total number of carbon atoms in the side chain in influencing potency, but the branching pattern of the side chain appears to influence the type of activity.

TABLE 1

Basic esters of dimethylheptylpyran, DMHP (IIIb)

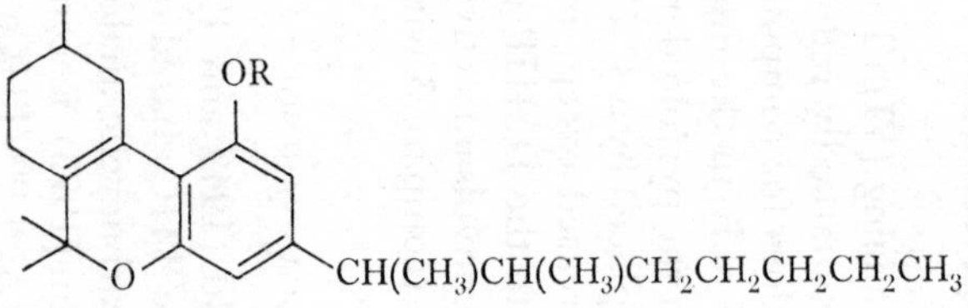

	DOPA[a] potentiation, mouse	Audiogenic seizure ED_{50} mg kg^{-1}	Mouse[b] fighting	Motor[b] activity rat	Analgesia[d] ED_{50} mg kg^{-1}	Ataxia[c] dog
IIIb H (DMHP)	+	2·9	+++(10)	+++(5)	19·6 (W)	++(1)
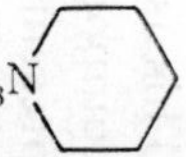 1 CO(CH₂)₃N⟨piperidine⟩ HCl	+	2·8	++(10)	++(5)	25·9 (W)	++(1)

No.	Structure	Salt						
2	CO(CH₂)₃N (morpholine, O) 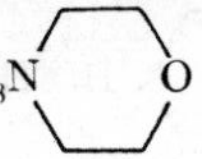	HBr	++	2·4	++(10)	+++(5)	2·34(W) 4·2 (RTF) 0·5 (HP)	+(0·05) ++(1·0)
3	CO(CH₂)₃N (azepane) 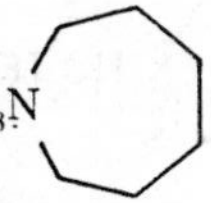	HCl	+	1·1	++(5)	++(1)		++(1·0)
4	CO(CH₂)₃N (thiomorpholine, S) 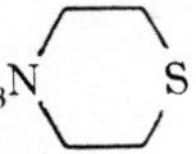	HCl	+	>100·0		++(2)		

---

[a] +, slight; ++, marked; +++, marked potentiation of the effect of levodopa (5 mg kg⁻¹), oral.

[b] +, 1–33 per cent; ++, 33–66 per cent; +++, 66–100 per cent reduction. Oral dose, mg kg⁻¹, in parentheses.

[c] +, decreased activity; ++, decreased activity and ataxia. Oral dose, mg kg⁻¹, in parentheses.

[d] W, writhing test in mice; RTF, rat tail flick test; HP, hot plate test in mice.

From Razdan et al. (1976c).

TABLE 2

Basic esters of the cyclopenteno analog (VI)[a]

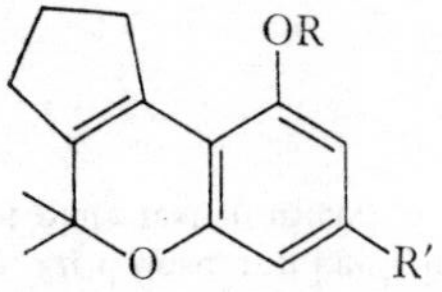

R		R'	DOPA	Audiogenic seizure ED$_{50}$ mg kg^{-1}	Mouse fighting	Motor activity	Analgesia	Ataxia dog
VI	H	C$_9$H$_{19}$	++	35·3	++(5)	+++(5)	25·3(W) 45·1(HP)	++(10)
5	COCH$_2$CH$_2$CH$_2$N⟨piperidine⟩ · HCl	C$_9$H$_{19}$	+	182·7	++(5) ++(10)	IA(5)	46·8(W) 30·2(HP)	+(1) ++(10)
6	COCH$_2$CH$_2$CH$_2$N⟨pyrrolidine⟩ · HCl	C$_9$H$_{19}$	++	50·7	+(10)	+(5)	>40(W)	+(1) ++(10)

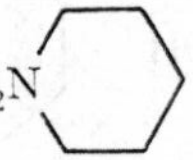

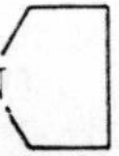

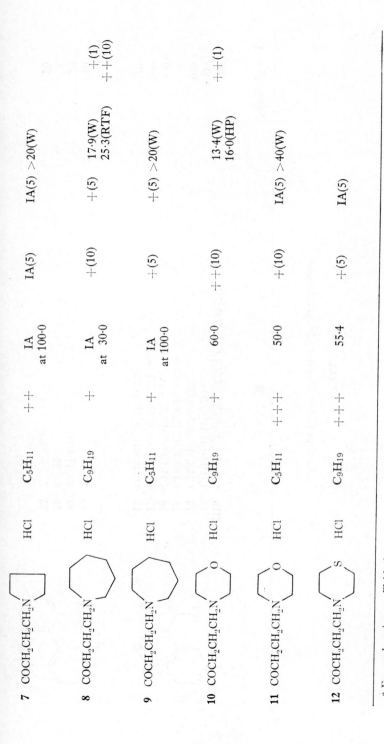

^{a} For explanation see Table 1.
IA, inactive. C_9H_{19}, 1,2-dimethylheptyl. C_5H_{11}, n-pentyl.
From Razdan et al. (1976c).

TABLE 3.

Analogs of $\Delta^{6a,10a}$-tetrahydrocannabinols[a]

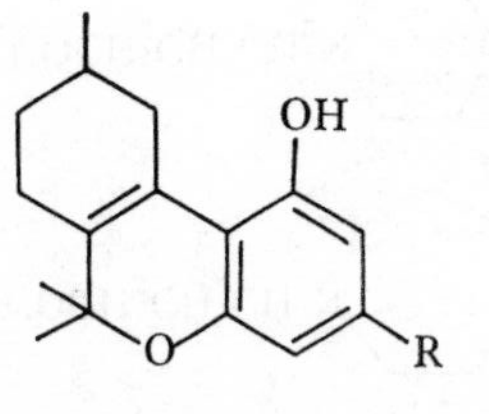

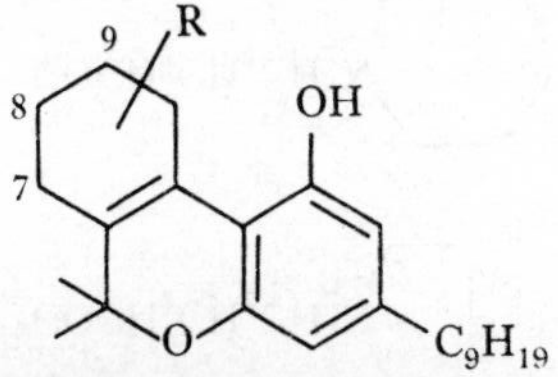

	R	Synhexyl = 1
IIIb	$CH(CH_3)CH(CH_3)(CH_2)_4CH_3$ (DMHP)	500
13	$C(CH_3)_2(CH_2)_5CH_3$	1000
14	$CH(C_2H_5)(CH_2)_5CH_3$	100
15	$CH_2CH(CH_3)(CH_2)_4CH_3$	2
16	$CH(CH_3)CH_2CH_2CH_3$	<0·6
17	$C(CH_3)=C(CH_3)(CH_2)_4CH_3$	500
18	$OCH(CH_3)(CH_2)_4CH_3$	10
19	H	10
20	9-CH_2CH_3	20
21	8-CH_3	1
22	7, 9-$(CH_3)_2$	50

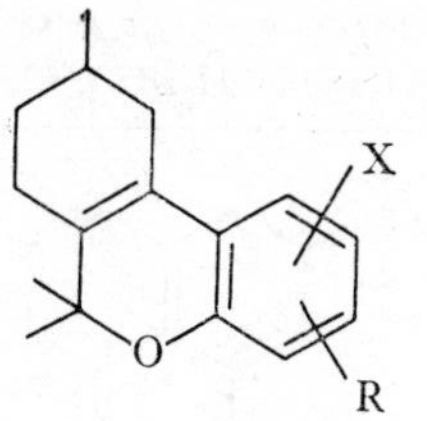

	R	X	
23	3-C$_9$H$_{19}$	1-OAc	>20
24	3-C$_9$H$_{19}$	1-OCH$_3$	<0.4
25	3-C$_9$H$_{19}$	H	1
26	2-C$_9$H$_{19}$	3-OH	10
27	3-C$_9$H$_{19}$	1-OH, 2-CH$_2$N(CH$_3$)$_2$	1
28	3-CH((CH$_2$)$_3$CH$_3$)$_2$	1-OH, 2-CH$_2$N(CH$_3$)$_2$ HCl	<0.4

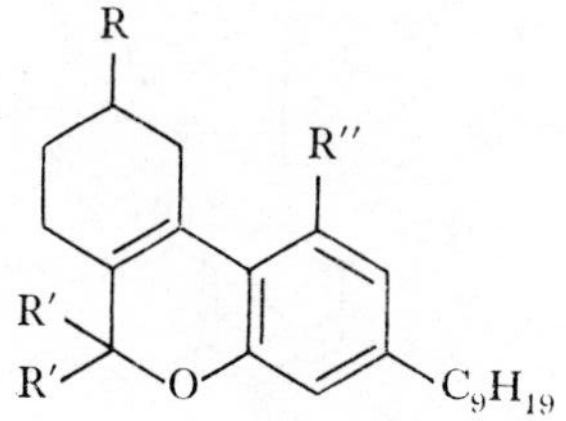

	R	R′	R″	
29	H	CH$_3$	OAc	>2
30	CH$_3$	CH$_2$CH$_3$	OH	2
31	CH$_3$	CH$_2$CH$_3$	OAc	0.5
32	CH$_3$	H	OH	5

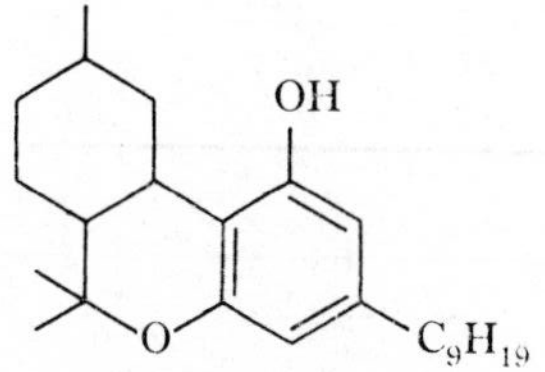

33	**IIIb** *cis*-dihydro	1
34	**IIIb** *trans*-dihydro	20

TABLE 3—*continued*

Analogs of $\Delta^{6a, 10a}$-tetrahydrocannabinols[a]

R	Synhexyl = 1
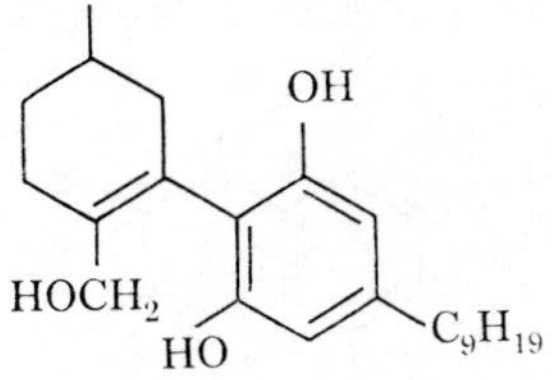 **35**	<1
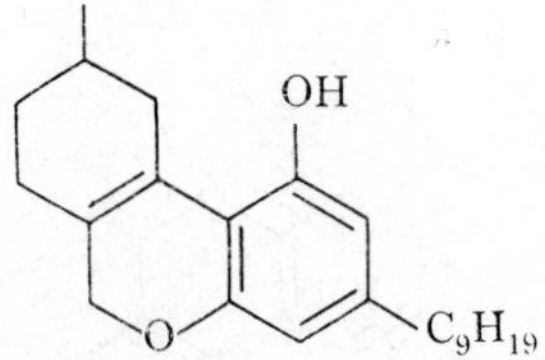 **36**	5

C_9H_{19}, $CH(CH_3)CH(CH_3)(CH_2)_4CH_3$

[a] Loev *et al.* (1973, 1974).

The effect of side-chain variation in $\Delta^{6a, 10a}$-tetrahydrocannabinols was studied extensively by Adams and co-workers. However, the changes in the side chain were confined to the length and the substitution pattern in the alkyl series only. Some cycloalkylalkyl derivatives were also studied (see for example, Todd *et al.*, 1943; Adams *et al.*, 1949; Loev *et al.*, 1973; and the review by Mechoulam, 1973). More recently the effect of an arylalkyl side chain in the $\Delta^{6a, 10a}$-THC series was reported by Winn *et al.* (1976). These authors have shown that biological activity is retained if the alkyl side chain is replaced by a phenylalkyl or a pyridylalkyl group. The former was active in the dog at 1 mg kg^{-1} and on this basis was considered to be equi-active with Adams' DMHP (**IIIb**). The most active compound in this series was the *p*-fluoro derivative **IIId** which was twice as active as DMHP in the dog (0·5 mg kg^{-1}). Basic esters, for example the γ-piperidino butyrate and the γ-morpholinobutyrate esters of **IIId**, were prepared as in the case of DMHP. These esters are more active than the parent phenol **IIId** in analgesic tests (Winn *et al.*, 1976). These results are very similar to those found in the DMHP series where the basic ester derivatives were more potent as analgesics than DMHP (Razdan *et al.*, 1976c).

2.4 COMPOUNDS RELATED TO Δ^9-TETRAHYDROCANNABINOL

The activity of Δ^9-THC related compounds is given in Table 4. The biological activity of Δ^9- and Δ^8-THCs decreases dramatically when the position of the n-C$_5$H$_{11}$ side chain and the phenolic hydroxyl group is interchanged (Uliss *et al.*, 1975) (compounds 37 and 38). These compounds arose as by-products from a new one-step synthesis (Razdan *et al.*, 1974a) of Δ^9-THC from *p*-mentha-2,8-dien-1-ol and olivetol. *cis*-Δ^9-THC (40) shows a similar profile to Δ^9-THC but is much less potent (Uliss *et al.*, 1975). This is consistent with its reported inactivity in monkeys (Mechoulam, 1973). Like the *trans* compounds, the positional *cis*-isomer 41 is much less active than 40 (Uliss *et al.*, 1975).

Compound 43 represents the first example of a Δ^9-THC derivative with a function in the geminal methyl position. It was prepared by Uliss *et al.* (1974) from the epoxide of (−)-cannabidiol diacetate utilizing a stereo-specific intramolecular epoxide cleavage by phenolate anion, and was found to be equiactive with Δ^9-THC. The same synthetic procedure also provided the first stereochemically unambiguous synthesis of cannabielsoin (42) and a novel cannabinoid (44) (containing a tetrahydrobenzoxepin ring system; Table 5) (Uliss *et al.*, 1974).

The interesting compound, 9-nor-Δ^8-THC (43a) was found to be equi-active with Δ^9- and Δ^8-THCs and was prepared from 9-nor-9-keto-THC by borohydride reduction followed by dehydration. The activity of

TABLE 4

Activity of the Δ⁸-THC derivatives in mice

	Dose (mg kg⁻¹)	Activity	Reference
37 C₅H₁₁ ... OH (−)-isomer	75·0 (iv)	—	Uliss et al. (1975)
39 C₅H₁₁ ... OH (−)-isomer	50·0 (iv)	Ataxia	Uliss et al. (1975)
38 C₅H₁₁ ... OH (−)-isomer	30·0 (iv)	—	Uliss et al. (1975)

40 (±)	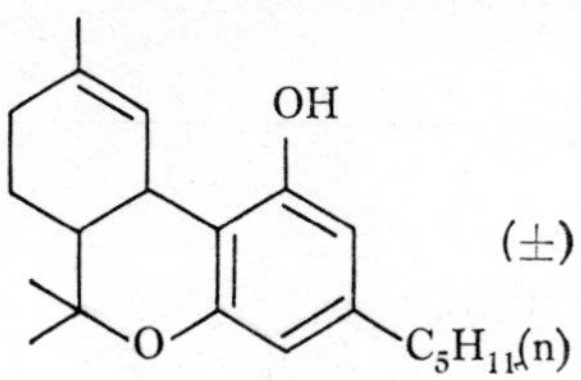 10·0 (iv)	Ataxia weak depressant	Uliss *et al.* (1975)
41 (±)	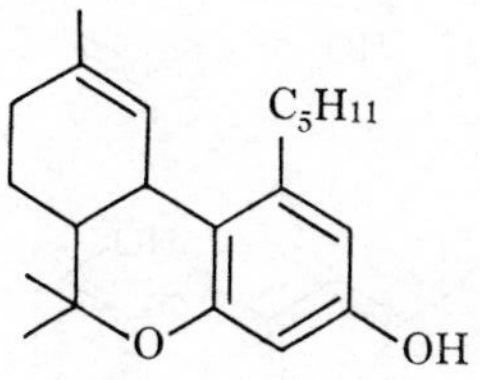 50·0 (iv)	Ataxia	Uliss *et al.* (1975)
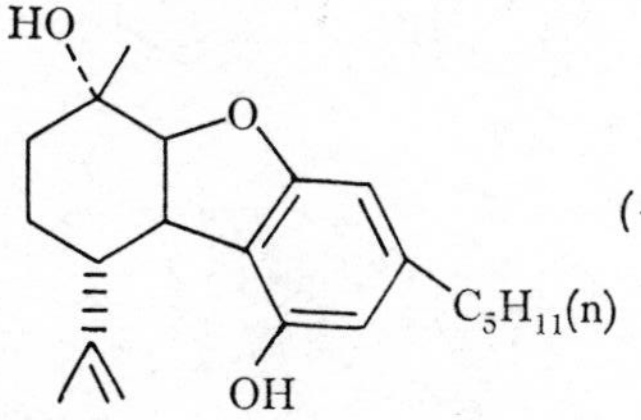 **42** (−)-isomer	10·0 (iv)	—	Uliss *et al.* (1974)

TABLE 4 —*continued*

Activity of the Δ⁹-THC derivatives in mice

	Dose (mg kg⁻¹)	Activity	Reference
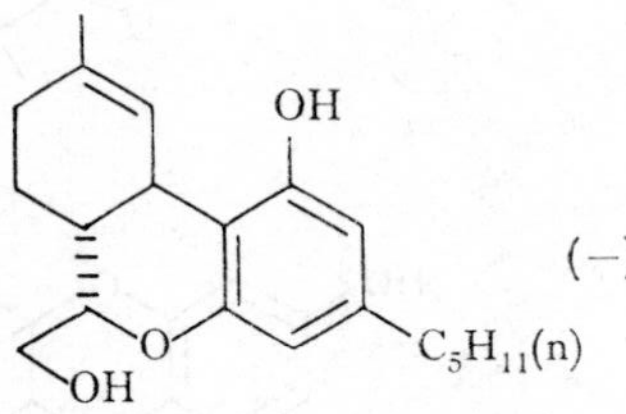 (−)-isomer 43	1·0 (iv)	Ataxia similar to Δ⁹-THC	Uliss et al. (1974) see also Razdan et al. (1976d)
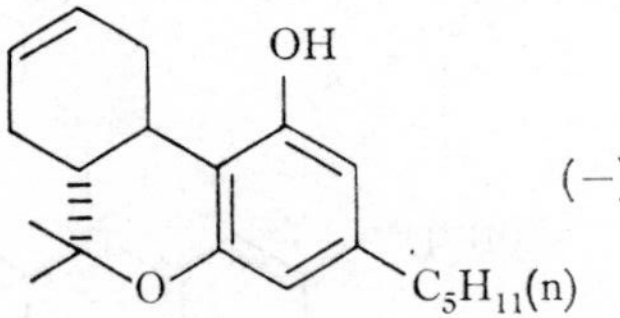 (−)-isomer 43a	0·2–0·4 (iv, dog)	Ataxia similar to Δ⁹-THC	Wilson (1974)

compound **43a** clearly supports the view that Δ^9- and Δ^8-THCs are active structures and their activity is not due to their 11-hydroxy metabolites (Wilson and May, 1974).

The compounds in Table 4 suggest the following structure–activity relationship: (a) the phenolic hydroxyl group in the C-1 position is extremely important for eliciting activity in THCs; (b) substitution of one of the geminal methyls by a hydroxymethyl in Δ^9-THC does not remove activity **(43)**; (c) metabolism to the 11-hydroxymethyl is not a prerequisite for activity of THCs.

2.5 MISCELLANEOUS

In Table 5 the novel benzoxocins **(45 to 55)** were synthesized by the condensation of carvone and olivetol in the presence of phosphorus oxychloride whereas the benzoxonins **(56, 57)** were similarly prepared from α-pinene or limonene (Houry *et al.*, 1974). These compounds are CNS-active and the authors conclude that the presence of a 1,2-dimethylheptyl side chain does not always give the most potent compound since the corresponding n-amyl substituted derivatives are equi or more potent. They also state that since the benzoxocins and benzoxonins are not planar, the flatness of the molecule is not a requirement for activity.

The lithium–ammonia reduction (Razdan *et al.*, 1974b) of **IIIb** (DMHP) gives the pyran ring-opened compound **58** (Table 5) which is very active (0·1 mg kg^{-1}, iv) in mice. This is in contrast to the very weak activity of cannabidiol. Another novel structure which has been synthesized (Cardillo *et al.*, 1973) is shown below but no biological data are reported.

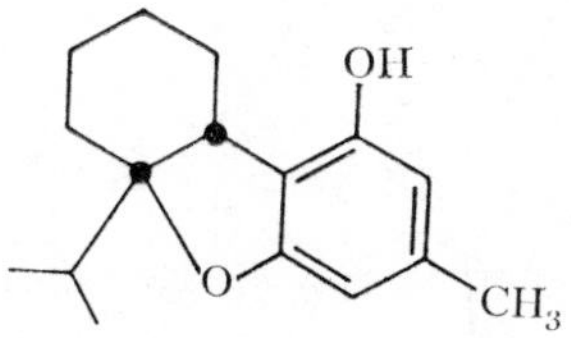

3 Structure–activity relationships: nitrogen and sulfur analogs

3.1 DESIGN CONSIDERATIONS

Interest in preparing nitrogen analogs was stimulated by the observation that THC is one of the very few potent drugs which act on the central nervous system yet has no nitrogen in its structure. In designing nitrogen

TABLE 5

Miscellaneous carbocyclic analogs

	Dose (mg kg^{-1})	Activity	Reference
44	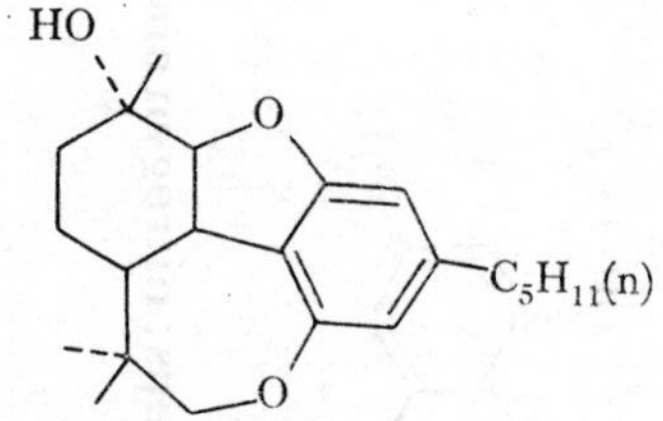 10·0 (iv, mice)	—	Uliss et al. (1974)
45 R=n-C$_5$H$_{11}$, R'=H, R''=CH$_3$	100–200 (po, rat)	Decreased motor activity ptosis, catalepsy, etc.	Houry et al. (1974)
46 R=C$_9$H$_{19}$[a], R'=H, R''=CH$_3$	10–25 (po, rat)		
47 R=n-C$_5$H$_{11}$, R'=CH$_3$, R''=H	100–200 (po, rat)		
48 R=C$_9$H$_{19}$[a], R'=CH$_3$, R''=H	10–25 (po, rat)		

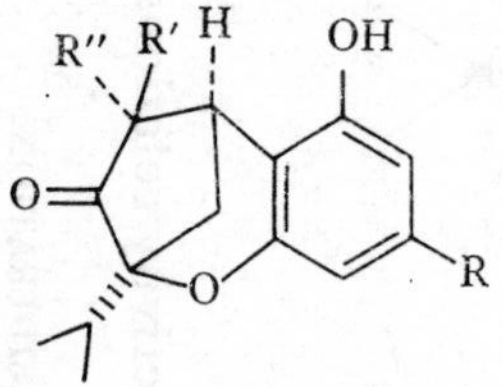

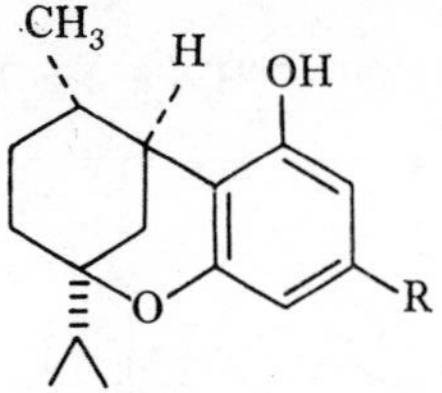

49   R=n—C_5H_{11}
50   R=$C_9H_{19}{}^{a}$

51   R=n—C_5H_{11}, R′=CH_3, R″=H
52   R=$C_9H_{19}{}^{a}$, R′=CH_3, R″=H
53   R=n—C_5H_{11}, R′=H, R″=CH_3
54   R=$C_9H_{19}{}^{a}$, R′=H, R″=CH_3

55

1–10 (po, rat)	Decreased motor activity ptosis, catalepsy, etc.	} Houry et al. (1974)
1–10 (po, rat)		
1–10 (po, rat)	Decreased motor activity ptosis, catalepsy, etc.	} Houry et al. (1974)
10–25 (po, rat)		
50 (po, rat)		
1–10 (po, rat)	Decreased motor activity ptosis, catalepsy etc.	Houry et al. (1974)
50 (po, rat)	Decreased motor activity ptosis, catalepsy, etc.	Houry et al. (1974)

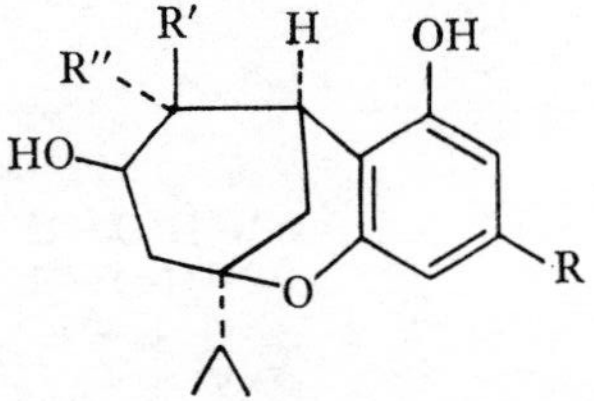

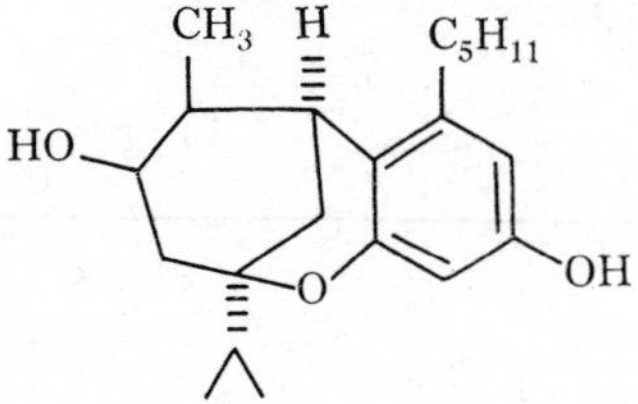

TABLE 5 —continued

Miscellaneous carbocyclic analogs

	Dose (mg kg^{-1})	Activity	Reference
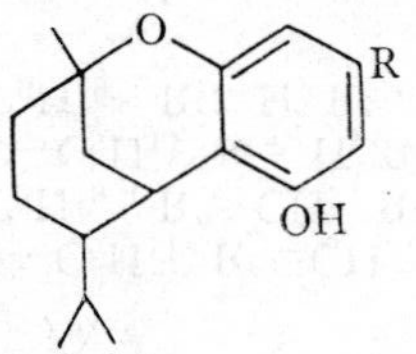 **56** R = C$_5$H$_{11}$(n) **57** R = C$_9$H$_{19}$[a]	10–25 (po, rat) 10–25 (po, rat)	Decreased motor activity ptosis, catalepsy, etc.	Houry et al. (1974, 1975)
58 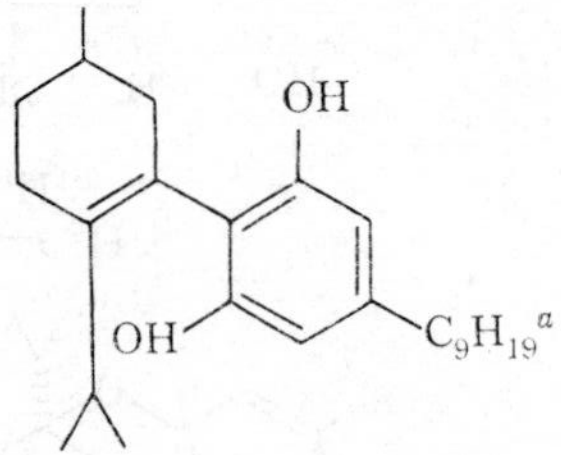	0·1 (iv, mouse)	Similar to DMHP LD50 >10·0	Razdan et al. (1974b)

[a] C$_9$H$_{19}$, CH(CH$_3$)CH(CH$_3$)(CH$_2$)$_4$CH$_3$.

analogs Pars and Razdan (1971, 1976) considered the following groups of moieties which are present in many agents active in the CNS:

(a) phenethylamine as found in many morphine and many morphine-like analgesics (e.g. phenethylamines, morphine, indoles, indolylethylamines);

(b) aryltetrahydropyridine moiety, which is found in particular in certain psychotomimetic agents (e.g. LSD, yohimbine); and

(c) arylpiperdine moiety as in pethidine and other strong analgesics.

There are other points of similarity in the structure of morphine, THC and LSD:

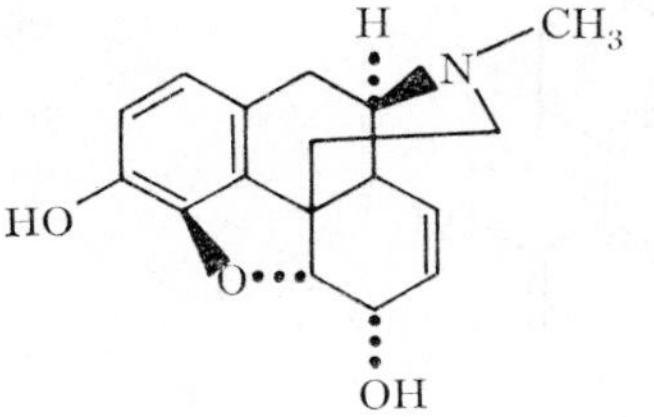

Morphine   Δ⁹-THC

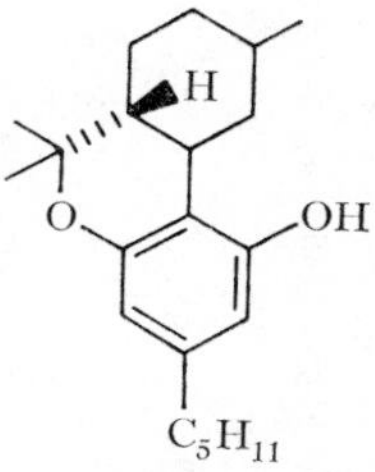

All have a planar ring (benzene in the case of morphine and Δ^9-THC, and indole in LSD) joined to a β-hydrogen atom two carbon atoms away.

Other points of striking structural similarity between the nitrogen-containing THC-analog **VII** and LSD, and another nitrogen-containing analog **VIII** and morphine are shown below (Razdan and Pars, 1970).

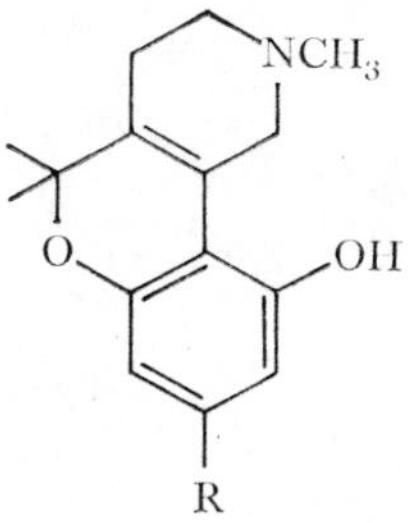

(VII) 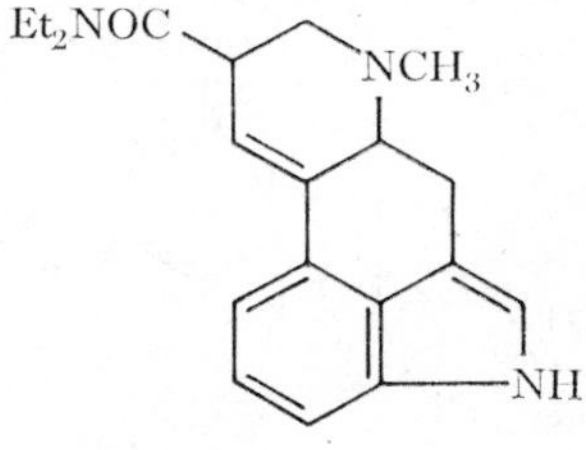   LSD

3.2 CHEMISTRY

As noted earlier, Anker and Cook (1946) synthesized compound **VII** ($R=n\text{-}C_5H_{11}$) and its dihydro derivative and found them to be without

analgesic activity. Other types of CNS activity were not mentioned in their
report.

Since 1966 various nitrogen analogs **VII** to **XIII** (Pars *et al.*, 1966, 1976;
Pars and Razdan 1971; Razdan and Pars 1970) and sulfur analogs **XIV** to
XVIII (Dewey *et al.*, 1970; Razdan *et al.*, 1976b) were synthesized, all of
which showed varying amounts of CNS activity in laboratory animals (see
section 8).

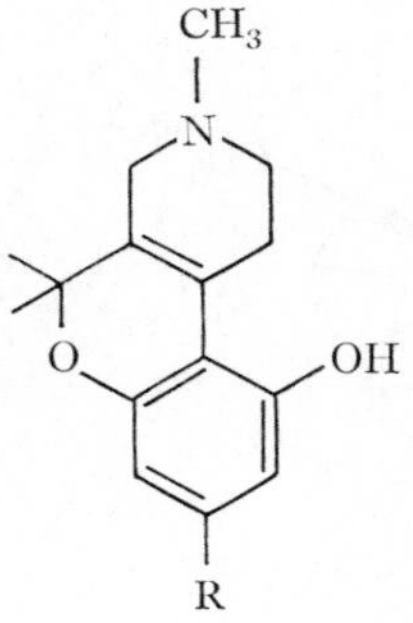

(**VIII**)

All the pyrans (**VII** to **XVIII**) except **XVI** were prepared according to the
general Scheme 1. The appropriate resorcinol and the keto-ester were
allowed to react under Pechmann conditions to give the pyrones which on
Grignard reaction with methyl magnesium iodide or bromide followed

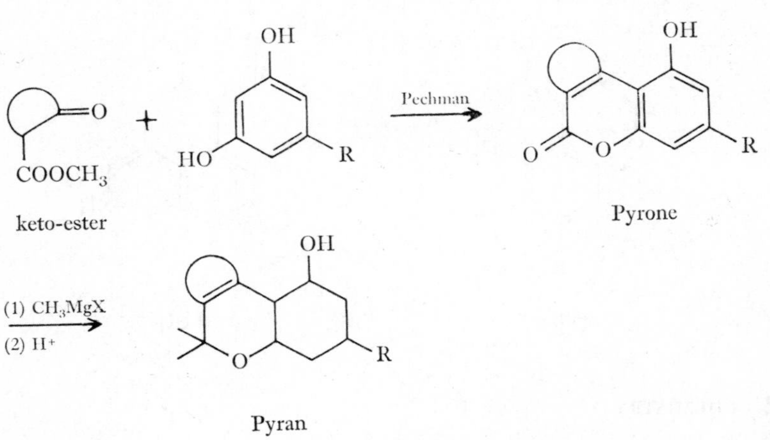

SCHEME 1

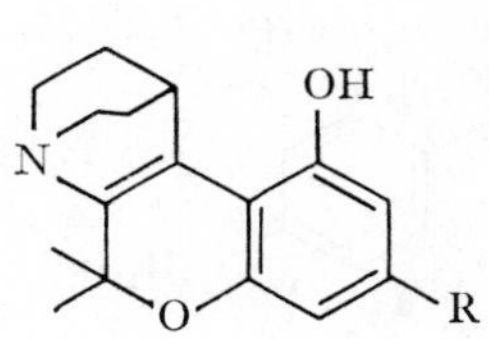

(IX)

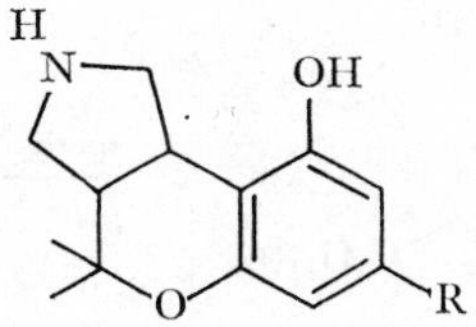

(X)

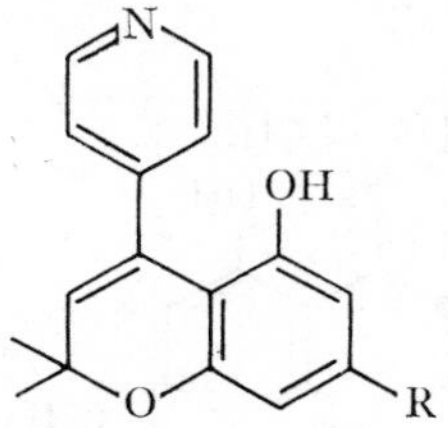

(XI)

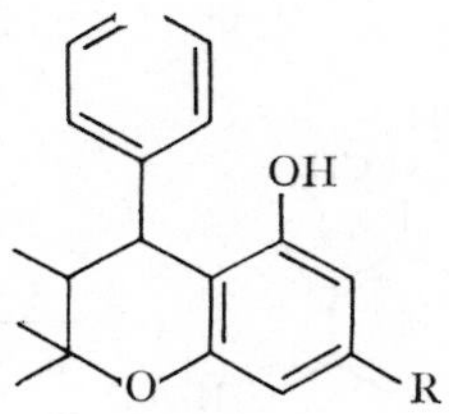

(XII)

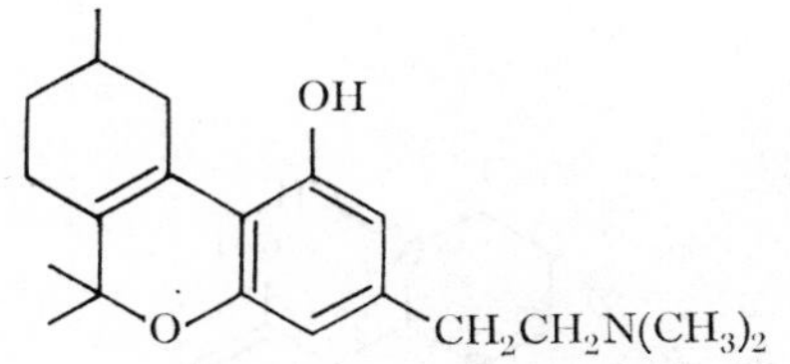

(XIII)

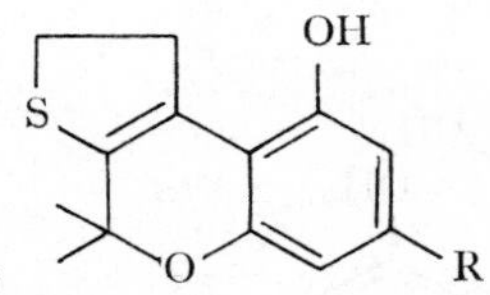

(XIV)

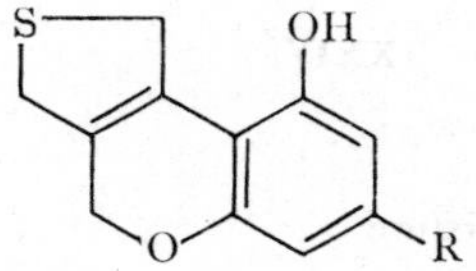

(XV)

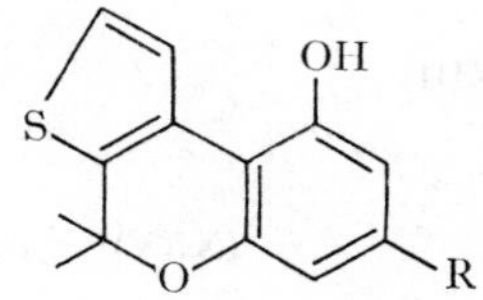

(XVI)

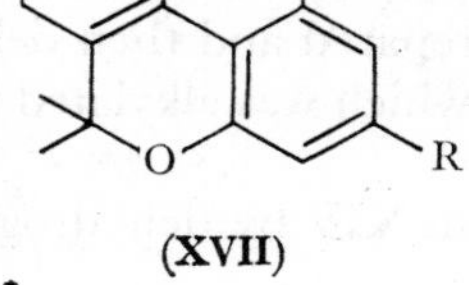

(XVII)

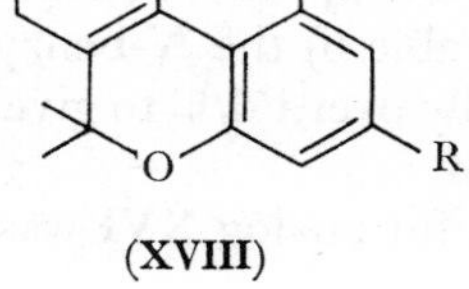

(XVIII)

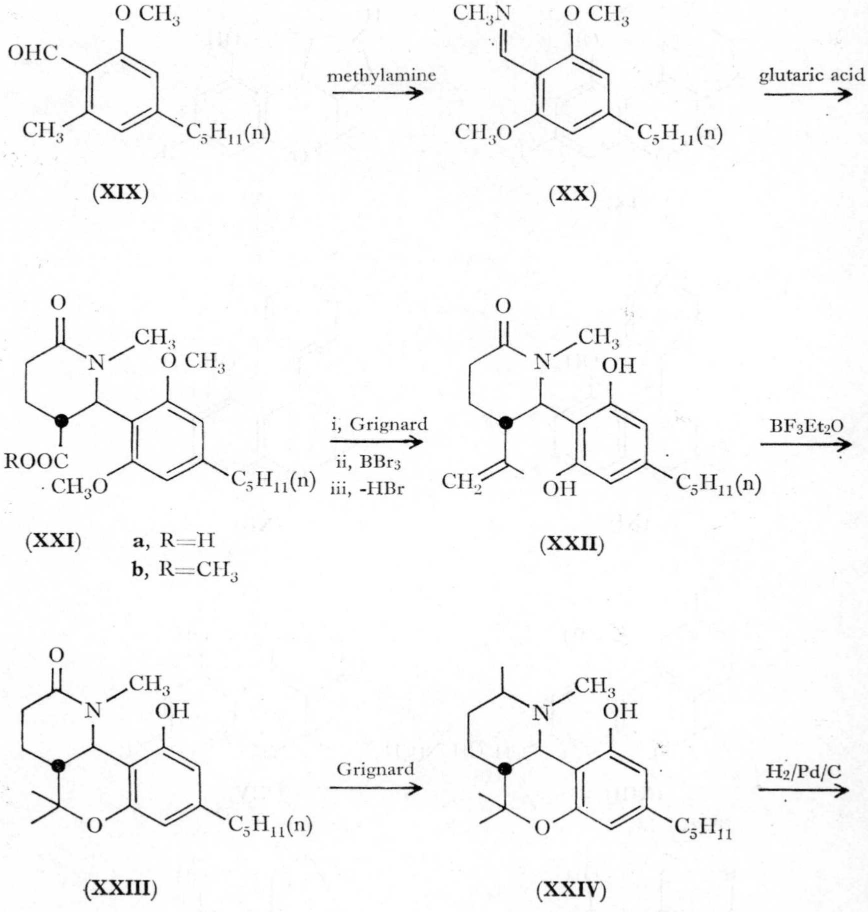

(XXV) diastereomeric mixture

SCHEME 2

by acid work-up afforded the pyrans. To prepare various *N*-substituted pyrans (Table 6) the *N*-benzylpyran was prepared and then debenzylated catalytically over Pd/C to give the nor-base which was alkylated to the final compound.

The sulfur analog **XVI** was prepared from **XIV** by dehydrogenation.

More recently Cushman and Castagnoli (1974) reported the synthesis (Scheme 2) of biologically active nitrogen analogs **XXV** having a *trans* ring fusion similar to that found in the natural THCs **I** and **II**. Their novel approach to the synthesis of these analogs utilizes the condensation of the Schiff base **XX** with glutaric anhydride to give predominantly the *trans*-piperidone **XXIa**. The ester **XXI** on Grignard treatment followed by de-methylation with borontribromide and subsequent dehydrohalogenation, afforded the olefin **XXII**. After ring closure with BF_3Et_2O compound

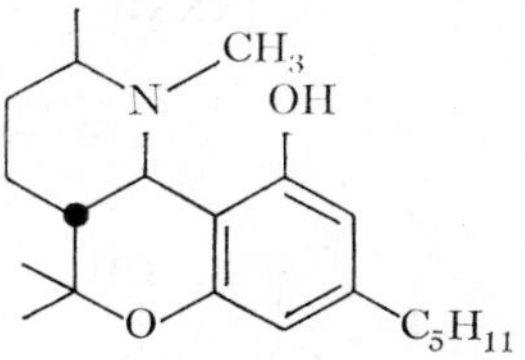

(**XXV**)

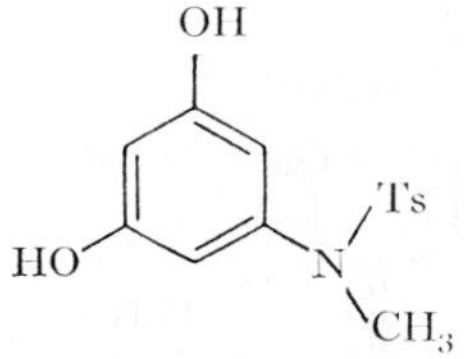

(**XXX**)

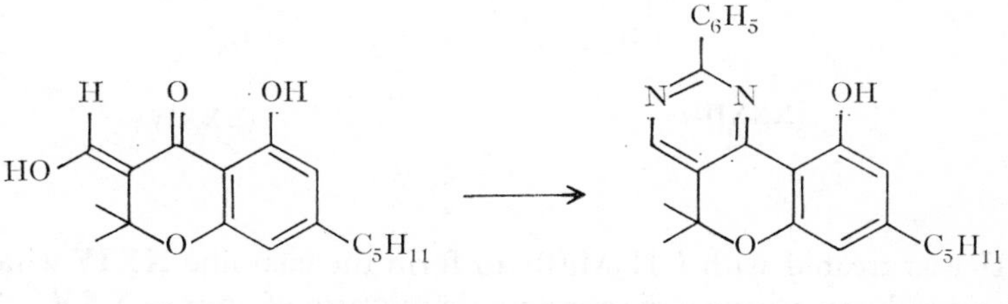

(**XXVII**)

(**XXVI**)

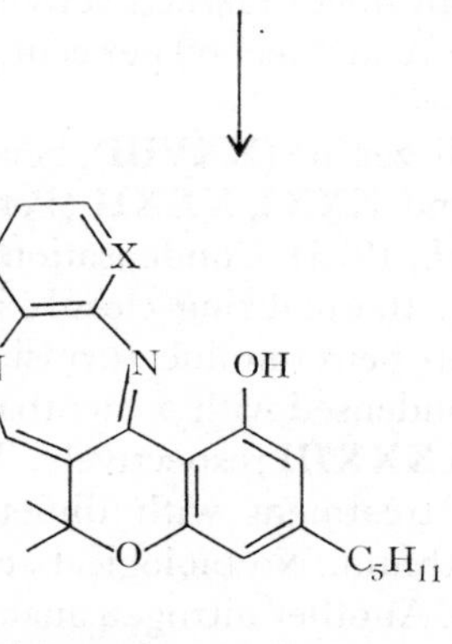

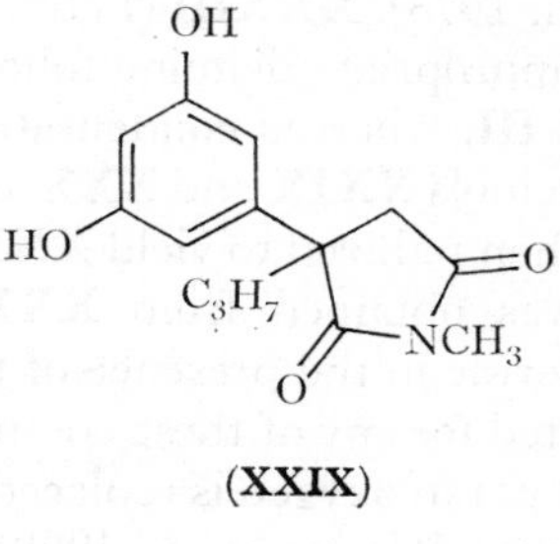

(**XXVIII**) a, X=CH

b, X=N

(**XXIX**)

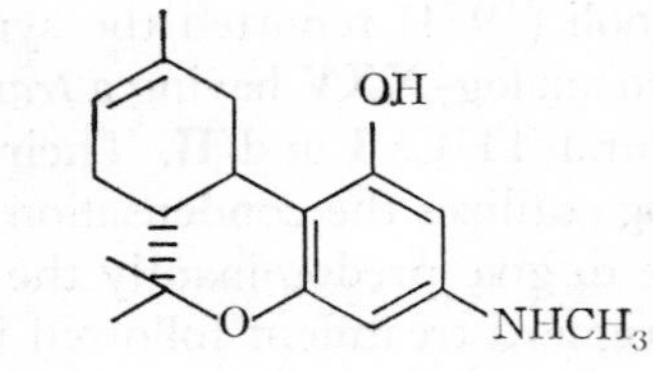

(XXXI)

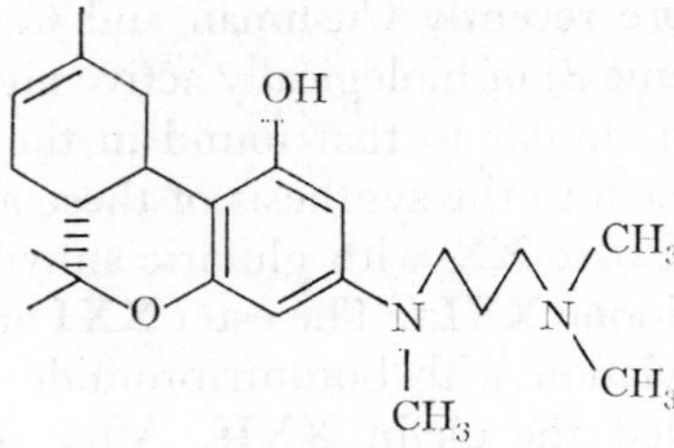

(XXXII)

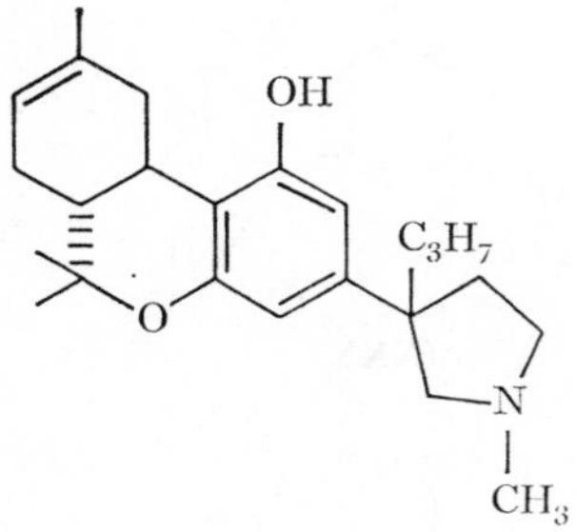

(XXXIII)

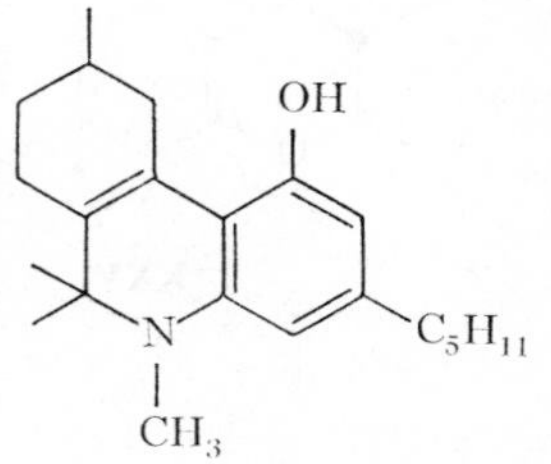

(XXXIV)

XXIII was treated with CH_3MgBr to form the enamine **XXIV** which on catalytic reduction gave a diastereomeric mixture of amines **XXV**.

Preliminary pharmacological results showed the mixture to possess both antidepressant (modified dopa test in mice; marked activity at 5 mg kg^{-1}) and anticonvulsant (audiogenic seizure in mice; 60 per cent protection at 30 mg kg^{-1}) activity.

Other nitrogen analogs include benzodiazepine (**XXVIII**), benzopyrano-pyrimidine (**XXVI**) (Greb et al., 1972), and **XXXI, XXXII** (Petrzilka and Lusuarndi, 1973), **XXXIII** (Petrzilka et al., 1973). Condensation of **XXVII** with the appropriate diamine followed by thermal ring-closure in vacuum gave **XXVIII**, whereas condensation with benzamidine furnished **XXVI**. The resorcinols **XXIX** and **XXX** were condensed with p-mentha-2,8-dien-1-ol and then reduced to yield **XXXI** and **XXXIII** respectively. The analog **XXXII** was obtained from **XXXI** on treatment with dimethylamino-propylchloride in the presence of butyllithium. No biological activity data was reported for any of these compounds. Another nitrogen analog **XXXIV** where the pyran oxygen is replaced by NCH_3 was synthesized and reported to be inactive (Hoops et al., 1968).

3.3 NITROGEN ANALOGS

SAR is discussed of various nitrogen analogs listed in Table 6 (Pars *et al.*, 1976) which includes analogs of type **VII**, the levo and dextro forms of *threo* and *erythro* isomers of compound **84**, which was the most potent of the series, analogs of type **VIII, IX, X, XI, XII, XIII** and other miscellaneous analogs.

All compounds were evaluated in a general pharmacology screen in mice. The procedure used was a modification of the Irwin mouse screen (see Irwin, 1964). Minimum effective doses (MED_{50} and LD_{50}) were determined. These nitrogen analogs were, like the cannabinoids, insoluble in aqueous media. They were solubilized in polyethylene glycol 200 and administered intravenously. The overt drug effects seen were qualitatively similar for all compounds tested. Most prominent effects were decreased locomotor activity, increased sensitivity to stimuli, depression and, at high doses, neuromuscular impairment.

Adams' most potent carbocyclic compound, DMHP (**IIIb**), had an MED_{50} of 0·075 mg kg^{-1} in these tests. Compound **64**, in Table 6, the nitrogen analog of DMHP, was less potent with an MED_{50} of 1 mg kg^{-1}. Altering the side chain (R′) of compound **64** further reduced potency (compounds **59** to **63**). Acetylation of the phenolic OH of compound **64** had little effect on its potency (compound **65**). Shifting the position in the ring of the nitrogen of compound **64** had no effect on potency (compound **90**). Changing the substituent on the nitrogen of compound **64** sometimes increased potency slightly and sometimes reduced potency (see for example compounds **66, 68, 70, 71–77, 80–81, 86**). A propargyl substituent (compound **84**) substantially increased potency as do other three-carbon substituents (**77, 79–81**). *N*-Propargyl compounds with long n-alkyl side chains were also potent in this test. Compound **84** was equipotent with DMHP. Resolution of compound **84** into its four stereoisomers showed the *erythro* isomers (**84a, 84b**) to be more potent than the *threo* isomers (**84c, 84d**). Compound **84** and its *erythro* isomers were the most potent nitrogen analogs tested. Alteration of the structure of compound **84** in the side chain (R′), by acetylation of the phenolic OH, slightly reduced potency (compound **85**). Shifting the position in the ring of the nitrogen or quarternization of the nitrogen significantly reduced its potency (compounds **95, 98, 99**).

3.4 BASIC ESTERS OF A NITROGEN ANALOG

A comparison of various basic esters, "water-soluble derivatives", of compound **84** and related compounds in selected pharmacological tests is given in Table 7 (Razdan *et al.*, 1976c). Formation of the basic esters of **84**

TABLE 6A

Comparative activity of analogs of compound VII in mice[a]

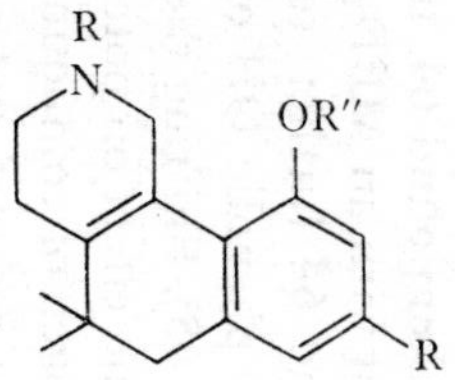

Compound number	R	R'	R''	Mouse data, mg kg⁻¹ (iv)	
				MED$_{50}$	LD$_{50}$
59	CH$_3$	CH$_3$	H	5·6	> 32·0[b]
60	CH$_3$	n-C$_5$H$_{11}$	H	18·0	> 32·0[b]
61	CH$_3$	CH(CH$_3$)C$_5$H$_{11}$	H	> 10·0[b]	> 10·0[b]
62	CH$_3$	CH(CH$_3$)C$_6$H$_{11}$	H	> 10·0[b]	> 10·0[b]
63	CH$_3$	CH(CH$_3$)C$_{12}$H$_{25}$	H	> 10·0[b]	> 10·0[b]
64	CH$_3$	C$_9$H$_{19}$	H	1·0	22·4
65	CH$_3$	C$_9$H$_{19}$	COCH$_3$	3·2	32·0
66	CH$_2$C$_6$H$_5$	C$_9$H$_{19}$	H	10·0	> 32·0[b]
67	H	C$_9$H$_{19}$	H	1·8	18·0
68	COCH$_3$	C$_9$H$_{19}$	H	5·6	> 32·0[b]
69	COCH$_3$	C$_9$H$_{19}$	COCH$_3$	1·8	> 32·0[b]
70	C$_2$H$_5$	C$_9$H$_{19}$	H	5·6	> 10·0[b]
71	n-C$_3$H$_7$	C$_9$H$_{19}$	H	0·42	3·2[b]

72	COC$_3$H$_5$	C$_9$H$_{19}$	H	10·0	> 32·0[b]
73	CH$_2$C$_3$H$_5$	C$_9$H$_{19}$	H	1·8	> 10·0
74	n-C$_5$H$_{11}$	C$_9$H$_{19}$	H	1·8	> 10·0[b]
75	CH$_2$C$_4$H$_7$	C$_9$H$_{19}$	H	0·56	25·0
76	CH$_2$CH$_2$C$_6$H$_5$	C$_9$H$_{19}$	H	3·2	> 10·0[b]
77	CH$_2$CH=CH$_2$	C$_9$H$_{19}$	H	0·75	> 10·0[b]
78	CH$_2$CH=CH$_2$	C$_9$H$_{19}$	COCH$_3$	0·42	32·0
79	CH$_2$CH=CHCl	C$_9$H$_{19}$	H	0·42	> 32·0[b]
80	CH$_2$CH=CHCl (cis)	C$_9$H$_{19}$	H	0·42	> 10·0[b]
81	CH$_2$CH=CHCl (trans)	C$_9$H$_{19}$	H	0·24	> 10·0[b]
82	CH$_2$CH=CHC$_6$H$_5$	C$_9$H$_{19}$	H	> 10·0	> 10·0[b]
83	CH$_2$CH=C(CH$_3$)$_2$	C$_9$H$_{19}$	H	3·2	> 10·0[b]
84	CH$_2$C≡CH	C$_9$H$_{19}$	H	0·042	40·0
85	CH$_2$C≡CH	C$_9$H$_{19}$	COCH$_3$	0·18	> 100·0[b]
86	CH$_2$C≡C—CH$_3$	C$_9$H$_{19}$	H	1·0	32·0
87	CH$_2$C≡CH	n-C$_7$H$_{15}$	H	0·13	> 32·0[b]
88	CH$_2$C≡CH	n-C$_9$H$_{19}$	H	0·32	> 20·0[b]

TABLE 6B

Comparative activity of isomers of compound **8**

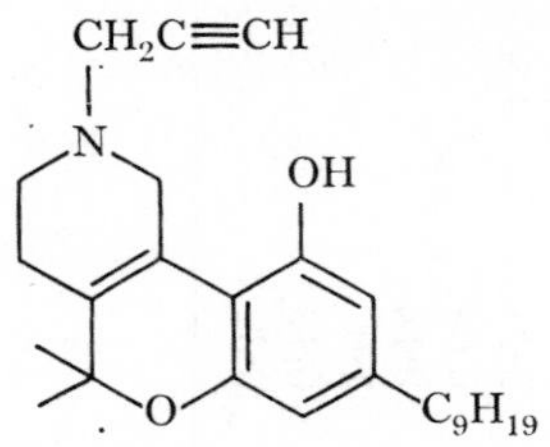

Compound number	Isomer	Mouse, data, mg kg^{-1} (iv)	
		MED$_{50}$	LD$_{50}$
84a	(+) *erythro*	0·013	> 10·0
84b	(−) *erythro*	0·056	> 10·0
84c	(+) *threo*	0·13	> 10·0
84d	(−) *threo*	0·13	> 10·0

TABLE 6C

Comparative activity of analogs of compound **VIII**

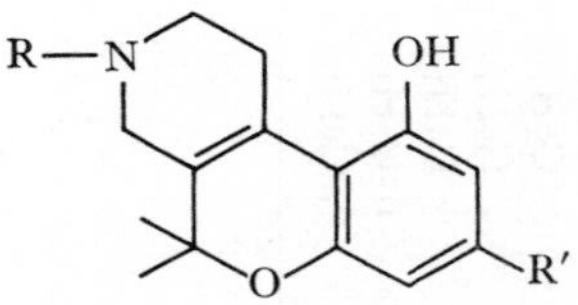

Compound number	R	R′	Mouse data, mg kg^{-1} (iv)	
			MED$_{50}$	LD$_{50}$
89	CH$_2$C$_6$H$_5$	CH$_3$	18·0	> 32·0[b]
90	CH$_3$	C$_9$H$_{19}$	1·8	> 32·0[b]
91	CH$_3$	C$_9$H$_{19}$	10·0	> 32·0[b]
92	H	C$_9$H$_{19}$	> 10·0[b]	> 10·0[b]
93	CH$_2$CH=CH$_2$	C$_9$H$_{19}$	> 32·0[b]	> 32·0[b]
94	*trans-*CH$_2$CH=CHCl	C$_9$H$_{19}$	> 32·0[b]	> 32·0[b]
95	CH$_2$C≡CH	C$_9$H$_{19}$	18·0	> 32·0[b]

TABLE 6—*continued*

Other analogs

Compound number		Mouse data, mg kg^{-1} (iv)	
		MED$_{50}$	LD$_{50}$
96 (IX)	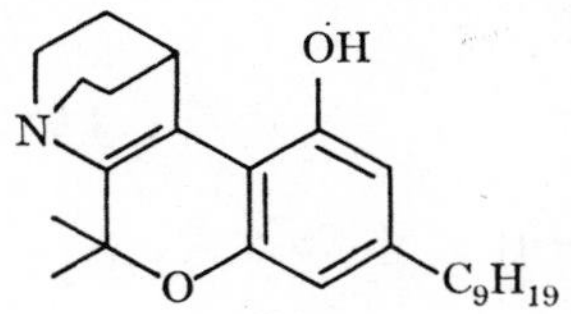	0·32	> 32·0^b
97	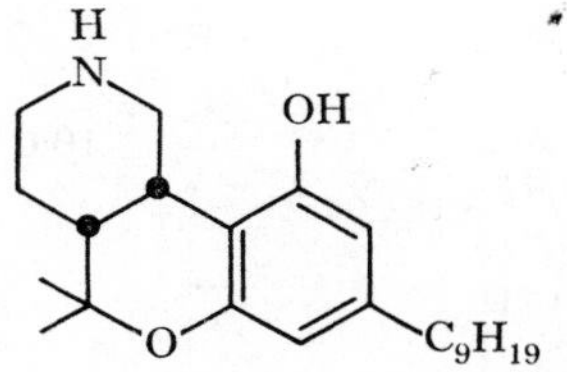	1·8	18·0
98	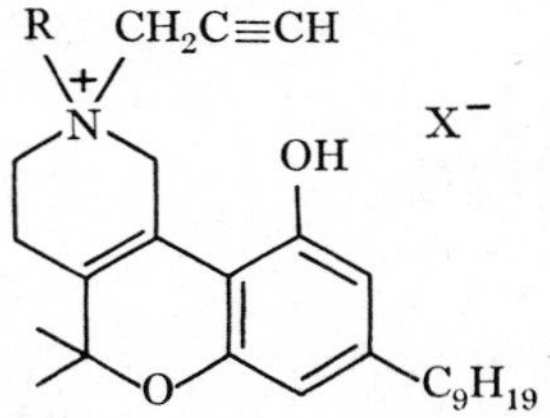 R=CH$_3$, X=I	5·6	5·6
99	R=CH$_2$C≡CH; X=Br	5·6	18·0
100 (X)	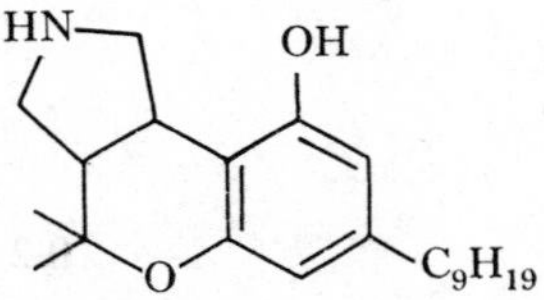	10·0	56·0
101 (XIII)	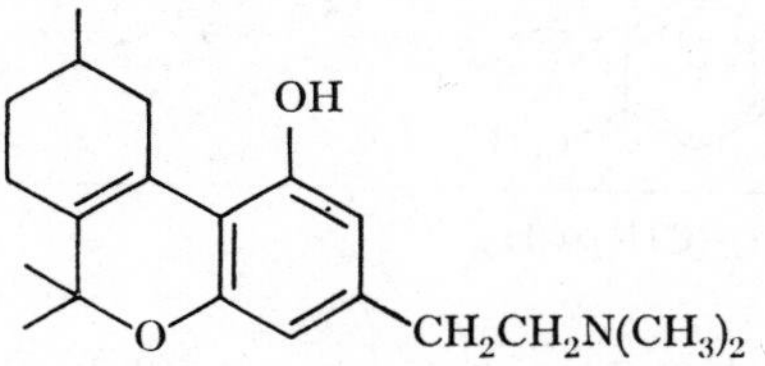	10·0	> 32·0^b

TABLE 6—*continued*

Other analogs—continued

Compound number	Mouse data, mg kg^{-1} (iv)	
	MED$_{50}$	LD$_{50}$
102	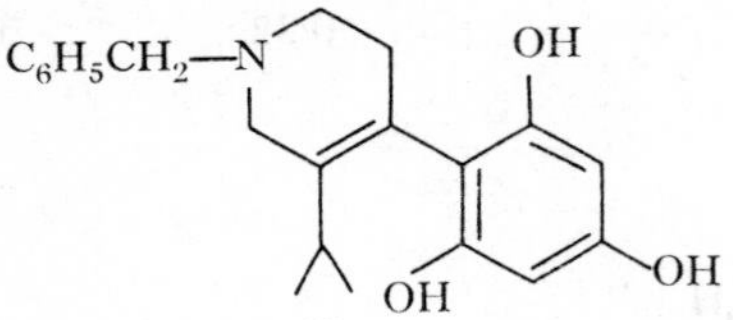 $> 1 \cdot 0^b$	$> 1 \cdot 0^b$
103	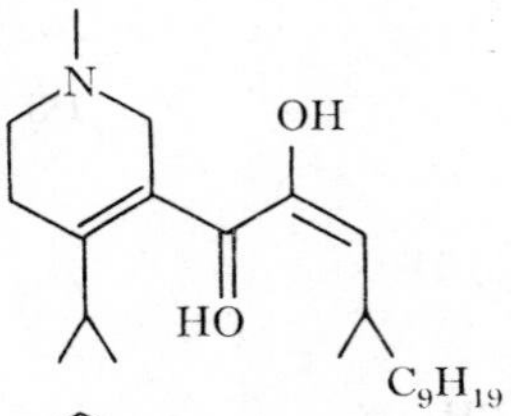 $10 \cdot 0$	$> 32 \cdot 0^b$
104	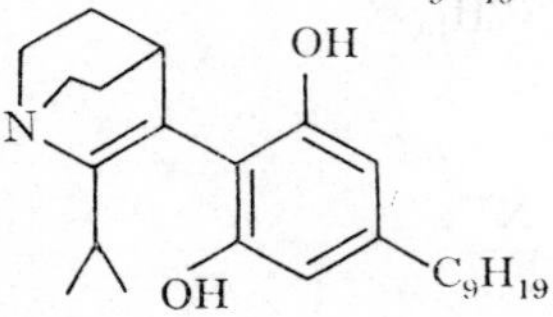 $5 \cdot 6$	$10 \cdot 0$
105^c (**XI**)	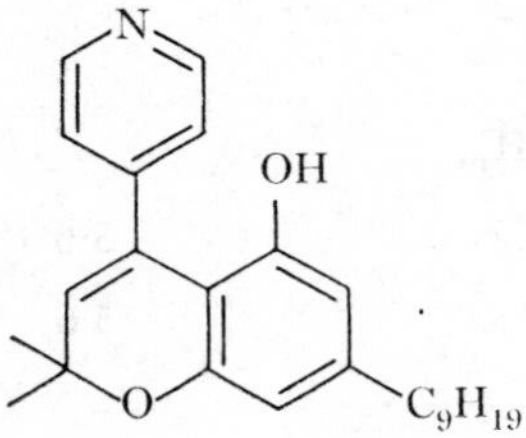 $0 \cdot 1$	$50 \cdot 0$
106^c (**XII**)	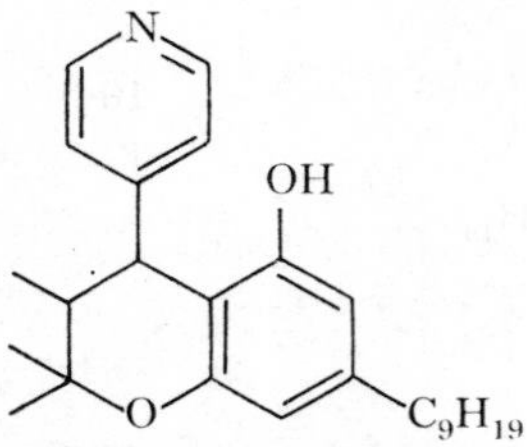 $0 \cdot 2$	$55 \cdot 0$

$C_9H_{19} = CH(CH_3)CH(CH)_3(CH_2)_4CH_3$.

^{a} Pars *et al.* (1976).

^{b} Higher doses not tested.

^{c} Presented at a symposium in Paris, 1967; Harris *et al.* (1967).

reduces the activity in the Dopa test and the rat motor activity of the parent phenol. A similar effect is also observed in their tranquillizing activity (mouse fighting) with the reduction being more pronounced in the case of hindered esters like α-methyl or α,α-dimethyl derivatives (compare **108** or **109** with **107**; **112** with **111**; **117** with **116**). The effect on analgesia varies with the nature of the substituent R. Thus compounds substituted by ω-piperdine and morpholine groups have analgetic activity, and α-methyl substitution in both cases has little or no effect, but α,α-dimethyl substitution decreased activity. Methyl substitution in the 2-position of the piperidine ring (**111** and **112**) retains activity and varying the length of the chain also has little effect. Replacement of piperidine or morpholine by pyrrolidine eliminates and diethylamine reduces analgetic activity. Similarly, quarternization of the basic nitrogen (**119**) or replacement of the aromatic side chain C_9H_{19} by n-C_5H_{11} (**115**) eliminates activity. The limited sedative-hypnotic studies show that this activity can be retained but is somewhat decreased by making a very hindered (α,α-dimethyl) ester. An interesting fact which emerges from these studies is the selectivity of action (analgesia and sedative hypnotic) in the ester derivatives compared to the parent phenol (compare **84** with **107, 108,** and **112**).

3.5   SULFUR ANALOGS AND THEIR BASIC ESTERS

Sulfur analogs including their basic esters are listed in Table 8 (Razdan *et al.*, 1976b). Only the five-membered-ring compounds (**120** and **123**) gave significant activity in the dopa test, and the activity was reduced when the five-membered ring was aromatized (compound **128**). Basic esters (**121** and **122**) of the parent phenol **120** showed reduced activity in this test. A similar SAR was found in the nitrogen analogs (Table 7). In the mouse fighting and rat motor-activity tests, no SAR were obvious. Interesting analgetic activity was found only in the parent phenol **124**, and this activity was reduced in the ester derivatives **125** and **126**. This change is in contrast to the nitrogen (Table 7) and carbocyclic analogs (Tables 1 and 2), in which esterification with the piperidino and morpholino acids retained analgetic activity.

In sedative-hypnotic activity tests in cats, compound **120** showed marginal activity and compounds **124** and **126** were inactive. These results differ from those found with the nitrogen (Table 7) and carbocyclic analogs, some of which showed potent sedative-hypnotic activity.

It appears that the sulfur atom should be adjacent to the double bond in order to elicit interesting activity in sulfur analogs and the ring size has no influence. However, a planar ring (as in compound **128**) eliminates activity.

TABLE 7

Basic esters of compound 84 and related compounds; comparative profiles[a,b]

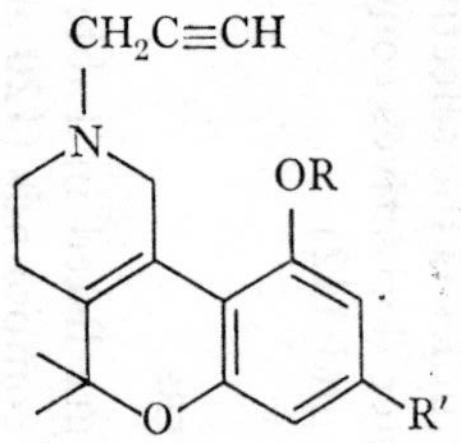

R	R'	DOPA	Mouse fighting	Motor activity	Analgesia ED$_{50}$ (mg kg^{-1})	Dog ataxia	Sedative hypnotic mg kg^{-1} (TST)
84 H	C$_9$H$_{19}$	+++	++(1) ++(5)	+++(1)	W(4·3) RTF(13·8) HP(7·7)	++(1)	0·1(+100) 0·25(+56) 0·5(+44)
107 COCH$_2$CH$_2$CH$_2$N⟨ ⟩ · HCl	C$_9$H$_{19}$	+	+(1) ++(5)	++(1)	W(12·0) RTF(12·5) HP(4·2)	++(1)	0·1(+38) 0·25(+33) 0·5(+48)
108 COCH(CH$_3$)CH$_2$CH$_2$N⟨ ⟩ · 2HCl	C$_9$H$_{19}$	+	IA(10)	++(10)	W(12-21) RTF(9·8)	+(1)	0·25(+58) 0·5(+45)

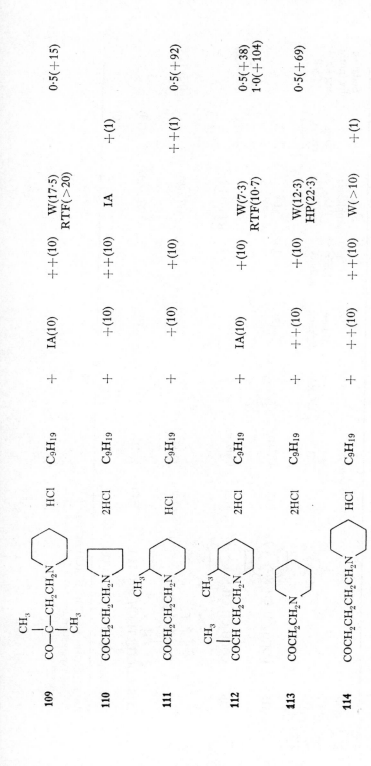

No.								
109	HCl	C$_9$H$_{19}$	+	IA(10)	++(10)	W(17·5) RTF(>20)		0·5(+15)
110	2HCl	C$_9$H$_{19}$	+	+(10)	++(10)	IA	+(1)	
111	HCl	C$_9$H$_{19}$	+	+(10)	+(10)		++(1)	0·5(+92)
112	2HCl	C$_9$H$_{19}$	+	IA(10)	+(10)	W(7·3) RTF(10·7)		0·5(+38) 1·0(+104)
113	2HCl	C$_9$H$_{19}$	+	++(10)	+(10)	W(12·3) HP(22·3)		0·5(+69)
114	HCl	C$_9$H$_{19}$	+	++(10)	++(10)	W(>10)	+(1)	

TABLE 7—continued

Basic esters of compound **84** and related compounds; comparative profiles[a,b]

	R		R'	DOPA	Mouse fighting	Motor activity	Analgesia ED_{50} (mg kg^{-1})	Dog ataxia	Sedative hypnotic mg kg^{-1} (TST)
115	$COCH_2CH_2CH_2N$(piperidino) 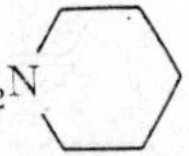	HCl	C_5H_{11}	+	+(5)	+(10)	IA		
116	$COCH_2CH_2CH_2N$(morpholino) 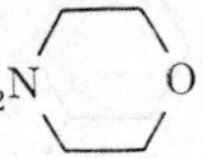	2HCl	C_9H_{19}	+	++(5)	+(10)	W(9·5) RTF(14·4)	++(1)	1·0(+30)
117	$COCH(CH_3)CH_2CH_2N$(morpholino) 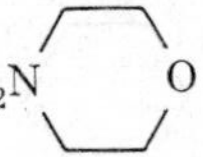	2HCl	C_9H_{19}	+	+(10)	++(10)	W(>10)		0·5(+36)
118	$COCH_2CH_2CH_2N(C_2H_5)_2$	HCl	C_9H_{19}	+	++(10)		W(>40)	++(10)	
119	Diquarternary Salt (2CH$_3$I) of **114**			+	++(10)	+	IA	+(10)	

C_9H_{19}, $CH(CH_3)CH(CH_3)(CH_2)_4CH_3$.

[a] For explanation see Table 1.

[b] Razdan et al. (1976c).

3.6 EFFECT OF ALKYL SUBSTITUENTS

The effects of alkyl substitution in the alicyclic ring of selected sulfur and carbocyclic analogs have been studied. These are summarized in Table 9 (Razdan *et al.*, 1976a).

Substitution at the C-1 position in the five-membered sulfur and carbocyclic series (compounds **129** and **132**) produced the most pronounced changes in the pharmacological activity. Thus a dramatic increase in potency in the analgesic and sedative-hypnotic tests was noted in the sulfur series (compare **129** with **120**). On the other hand, in the five-membered carbocyclic analogs, the potency in the audiogenic seizure test (anticonvulsant activity) increased the most, but the change in analgesic activity was moderate and there was no change in the sedative or hypnotic activity (compare **132** with compound **VI**). In both series, however, the potency was increased in the dog ataxia test, as compounds **129** and **132** were more active than **120** and compound **VI**.

In contrast to the marked pharmacological changes caused in the five-membered series, moving the methyl group to the C-10 position in the six-membered carbocyclic series, compound **135**, affected the activity only slightly, similar to the findings of Adams (1949) and Todd (1943). Our results for compound **135** compared to **IIIb** (DMHP) show that the anticonvulsant activity was decreased only slightly, the analgesic activity was increased (slightly), and the dog ataxia test results were unchanged.

It appears that methyl substitution in the close proximity of the phenolic hydroxyl group is very important in influencing the activity of some cannabinoids, particularly of those which have a planar five-membered alicyclic ring rather than a six-membered ring.

4 Pharmacology of Δ^9-tetrahydrocannabinol (THC) and other cannabis constituents: animal studies

The advances made during the past decade on the chemistry of cannabinoids has now made available pure Δ^9-THC, some of its metabolites, and other constituents of cannabis. A wide variety of biological investigations have been carried out with these substances and a number of reviews (see Mechoulam, 1973; Marihuana and Health, 1974; and Paton and Pertwee, 1973) have appeared which give extensive coverage to the pharmacology of these active constituents. Our intention in this section is to focus attention on that aspect of the pharmacological profile of Δ^9-THC as it pertains to potential therapeutic activity. For earlier reviews of such activity see Archer (1974) and Cohen and Stillman (1976).

TABLE 8

Sulfur analogs and their basic esters[a,b,c,d]

	DOPA	Mouse fighting	Motor activity	Analgesia ED_{50} (mg kg^{-1})	Dog ataxia
120 (XIV) R=H	+++	+(5) ++(10)	+(5)	W(71·8) HP(12·1)	+(0·1)
121 R=CO(CH$_2$)$_3$N⟩piperidine·HCl 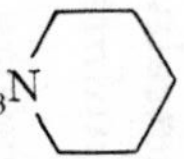	+	++(10)	+(5)	W(24)	IA(1)
122 R=CO(CH$_2$)$_3$N⟩morpholine·HCl 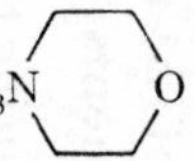	++	+(5) ++(10)	+(5)	HP(>50)	IA(1) ++(10)
123 (XV)	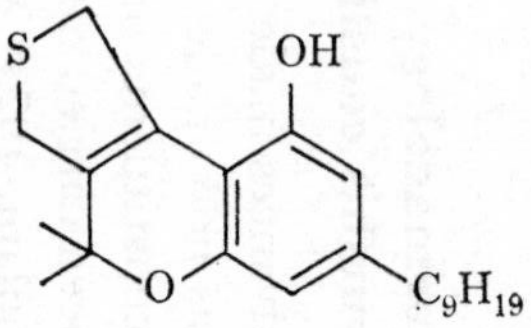 +++	++(10)	+(5)	W(51·7) HP(>120)	

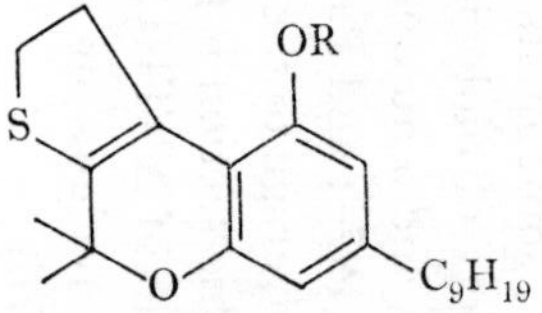

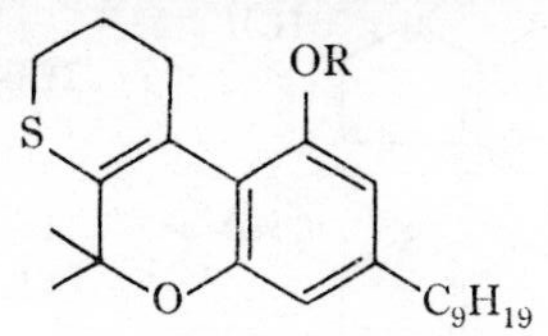

Compound					
124 (XVII) R=H	+	++(10)	+(5)	W(8·6) HP(5·7) RTF(2·7)	++(1)
125 R=CO(CH₂)₃N(piperidine) HCl	+	+(5)	+++(5)[b]	W(14·7)	
126 R=COCH(CH₃)CH₂CH₂N(piperidine) HCl	+	+++(10)	+(5)	W(22·6)	
127 (XVIII)	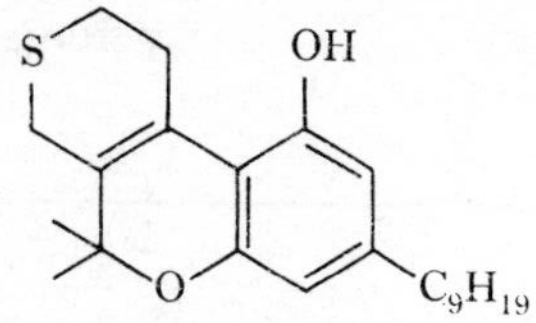 ++	+(5)	+(10)	W(>40) HP(>40)	++(10)
128 (XVI)	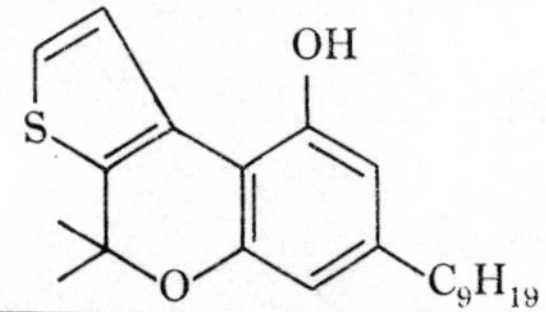 +	+(10)	+(5)	W(>10)	

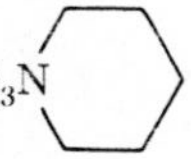

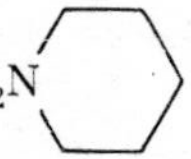

(Structures depict the chromeno-thiopyran ring systems with OR / OH and C_9H_{19} substituents for compounds 124, 127 and 128.)

[a] For explanation see Table 1.
[b] Inconsistent data.
[c] Razdan et al. (1976b).
[d] C_9H_{19}, $CH(CH_3)CH(CH_3)CH(CH_3)(CH_2)_4CH_3$.

TABLE 9

Alkyl substituted analogs—comparative profile[a,b,c]

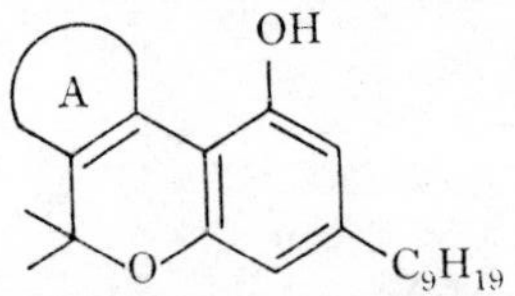

Compound number	Ring A	DOPA 5 mg kg^{-1}	Audiogenic seizure 10 mg kg^{-1}	Mouse fighting 10 mg kg^{-1}	Analgesia ED$_{50}$ (mg kg^{-1})	Sedative–hypnotic mg kg^{-1}	TST	Dog ataxia mg kg^{-1}
120 (XIV)	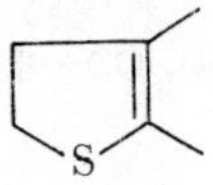	+++	++	++	W(71·8) HP(12·1)	1 2	+30 +31	0·1(+) 10(++)
129	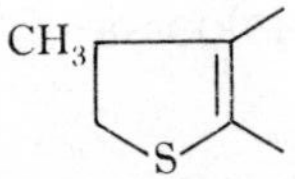	++	++	++	W(4·7) HP(1·4)	0·1 0·25	+21 +50	0·1(++) 1(++)
130	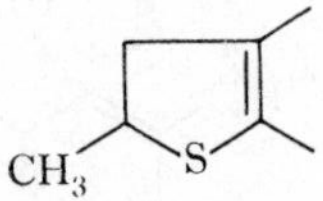	+	+	++	W(34)			10(++)
131	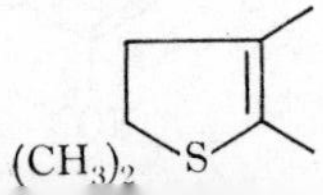	+	+	+	W(>40)			10(++)

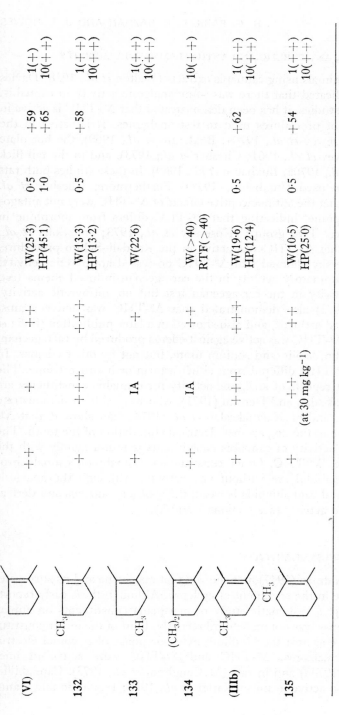

Compound									
(VI)	++	++	+	+	+++	W(25.3) HP(45.1)	0.5 1.0	+59 +65	1(+) 10(++)
132	++	+	+	+++	+++	W(13.3) HP(13.2)	0.5	+58	1(++) 10(++)
133	+	IA	+	IA	+++	W(22.6)	0.5		10(++)
134	++	IA	++	+++	++	W(>40) RTF(>40)	0.5	+62	10(++)
(IIIb)	+	+++	+	+++	+	W(19.6) HP(12.4)	0.5	+62	1(++) 10(++)
135	+	++ (at 30 mg kg⁻¹)	+	++ +++	++	W(10.5) HP(25.0)	0.5	+54	1(++) 10(++)

---

[a] All doses are in mg kg⁻¹ (po); in the DOPA potentiation test, results have been graded as + (slight), ++ (moderate), +++ (marked) increases; in the audiogenic seizure test, + corresponds to 1–33 per cent, ++ (33–66 per cent) and +++ (66–100 per cent) protection after 1 h; in the mouse fighting test, + corresponds to 1–33 per cent, ++ (33–66 per cent), +++ (66–100 per cent) reduction; in the dog ataxia, test, + corresponds to decreased activity only and ++ to decreased activity and ataxia; W, writhing; RTF, rat tail flick; HP, hot plate; TST change in total sleep time; IA, inactive.

[b] Razdan et al. (1976a).

[c] C_9H_{19}, $CH(CH_3)CH(CH_3)(CH_2)_4CH_3$.

4.1   ANALGESIC, ANTIPYRETIC AND ANTIINFLAMMATORY ACTIVITY

Early work in animals using cannabis extracts (Walton *et al.*, 1938; Davies *et al.*, 1946) indicated that there was some analgesic activity in cannabis. Since the early studies, it has been demonstrated that Δ^9-THC is active in a wide variety of procedures used to test analgesics. It is active in the writhing test (Dewey *et al.*, 1970a; Buxbaum *et al.*, 1969), the hot plate procedure (Dewey *et al.*, 1961; Chesher *et al.*, 1973), and in the tail flick test (Dewey *et al.*, 1970a; Buxbaum *et al.*, 1969). In these studies both rats and mice were used (Buxbaum, 1972). Furthermore, Chesher *et al.* (1973) showed that the antinociceptive effects of Δ^9-THC were not antagonized by nalorphine, indicating that Δ^9-THC differs from morphine in these procedures. Two groups (Kosersky *et al.*, 1973; and Sofia *et al.*, 1973) showed that Δ^9-THC was active in the Randall–Sellito procedure, but while Kosersky claimed that Δ^9-THC possessed antipyretic activity, but no antiinflammatory activity in the carrageenan-induced edema test, Sofia found activity in the carrageenan test but no antipyretic activity. Sofia *et al.* (1973) also demonstrated that Δ^9-THC was active against adjuvant-induced arthritis, and also showed in a later publication (Sofia *et al.*, 1974) that Δ^9-THC was active against edema produced by carrageenan, dextran, formalin, kaolin and sodium urate, but not by other edemas. In this respect, Δ^9-THC differed from either aspirin or hydrocortisone. The only nonrodent reports of analgesic activity for cannabis constituents are those of Kaymakcalan and Deneau (1971), who were able to demonstrate activity in cats, and of Kaymakcalan *et al.* (1974) who showed that Δ^9-THC was active in the dog against electrical stimulation of the tooth. The weak analgesic activity of cannabis constituents is found mainly with the active principle, Δ^9-THC. Other constituents, cannabinol, cannabichromene and cannabidol are without any activity. Although the analgesic activity of natural cannabinoids is weak, the synthetic analogs and derivatives show good activity (see sections 7 and 8).

4.2   ANTICONVULSANT ACTIVITY

Loewe and Goodman (1947) first showed that marijuana and its surrogates had some value in the treatment of epilepsy. Although these early reports were promising, a systematic study of marijuana constituents on animal models of epilepsy was not made until recently. Four of the major constituents were active against the hindlimb extensor phase of maximal electroshock-induced seizures. Δ^8-THC and Δ^9-THC were active in mice (Karler *et al.*, 1974a) and in rats (McCaughran *et al.*, 1973). Cannabidiol (CBD) was also active in mice (Karler *et al.*, 1973; Izquierdo and Tann hauser, 1973; Turkanis *et al.*, 1974) and cannabinol is active (Karler *et al.*, 1973). Karler *et al.* (1973), showed that tolerance rapidly developed to the effects of Δ^9-THC, CBD in mice, but since this phenomenon was also observed with diphenylhydantoin (DPH), its relevance to human application is doubtful. Turkanis *et al.* (1974) stated that cannabidiol showed a similar spectrum of activity in mice to diphenylhydantoin. Cannabidiol is devoid of marijuana-like CNS effects in man (Mechoulam, 1970; Hollister, 1973) and is therefore potentially useful therapeutically as an agent for the treatment of Grand Mal. The anticonvulsant effect of diphenyldantoin DPH is potentiated by Δ^9-THC in the electroshock procedure (Radnicki, 1974). Like diphenylhydantoin, Δ^9-THC and Δ^8-THC and CBD were not effective in protecting mice against pentylenetetrazole (PTZ)-induced seizures, and Δ^9-THC actually lowered the threshold for such seizures (Sofia *et al.*, 1971a; Turkanis *et al.*, 1974). Carlini *et al.* (1973) claimed that cannabis extracts and cannabidiol protected mice against PTZ-induced seizures in rats but only at high toxic doses, and Consroe *et al.* (1973) showed that Δ^9-THC afforded no protection against PTZ in rats. Using the hind limb extensor effect of a larger dose of PTZ (110 mg kg^{-1}), Turkanis *et al.* (1974) showed that CBD, like DPH, was effective in blocking this action, whereas Δ^9-THC was only partially active. Δ^8-THC and Δ^9-THC protect against audiogenic seizures in rats (Consroe *et al.*, 1973) and mice (Plotnikoff, 1976). Cannabinoids thus appear to possess a real potential for anticonvulsant activity in humans, with cannabidiol being of particular interest due to its lack of other CNS effects.

4.3 SEDATIVE-HYPNOTIC AND ANESTHETIC ADJUVANT ACTIVITY

Δ^9-THC causes ataxia, catatonia and depression of spontaneous activity in rodents, as well as causing a potentiation of the depressant effects of sedative-hypnotics and anesthetics. Pretreatment of dogs with a Δ^9-THC lowers the minimum alveolar concentration for cyclopropane (Vitez *et al.*, 1973). These effects were produced by low doses of Δ^9-THC and it would appear that this would be a useful application of Δ^9-THC in medicine. Pentobarbital hypnosis was also potentiated by cannabis extracts (Bose *et al.*, 1971) as well as by Δ^9-THC (Kubena and Barry, 1972; Sofia and Barry, 1974), Δ^8-THC (Chesher *et al.*, 1974), and cannabidiol (Paton and Pertwee, 1972). In 1974, Chesher showed that either anesthesia was not significantly prolonged by a cannabis extract. Sofia *et al.* (1974) showed that Δ^9-THC (20 mg kg^{-1}, ip) in mice caused decrease in the anesthetic dose of ketamine, sodium thiopental and the steroidal anesthetic CT 1341. The LD_{50} of these agents was unaffected. Siemens *et al.* (1974) explained the effects on pentobarbital sleeping time as due to an effect on hepatic microsomal oxidase systems, although Caldwell *et al.* (1974), who followed ^{14}C-pentobarbital levels in the blood of the rat following treatment with Δ^9-THC, found that Δ^9-THC did not affect pentobarbital metabolism *in vivo.* Friedman and Gershon (1974) showed the potentiation of ethanol-induced sleeping time in rats by Δ^8-THC. Chronic pretreatment with Δ^8-THC reduced this potentiation, but no effect on ethanol metabolism was observed. Using EEG to study sleep stages in the rat, Morton and Davis (1973) showed that REM sleep is depressed in this species. In REM deprived rats, this REM depression was less. The real significance of the depressant effects of Δ^9-THC is best understood when studies in humans are reviewed (see section 5.3), but animal data suggest that a sedative-hypnotic action is present with cannabinoids, albeit nonbarbiturate-like.

4.4 TRANQUILLIZER ACTIVITY

Δ^9-THC produces a state of tranquillization in animals, with underlying CNS stimulation. Whether Δ^9-THC may be of value in the treatment of psychosis or anxiety states is not known. The results of experiments in aggressive animals are equivocal. Δ^9-THC has been shown to reduce shock-induced aggression in rats (Dubinsky *et al.*, 1973) and mice (Plotnikoff, unpublished data) but other authors have demonstrated an increased fighting (Carder and Olsen, 1972), or no effect (Manning and Elsmore, 1972) in rats. The differences may be dose-related as Dubinsky *et al.* used higher doses than either of the other two groups. Other workers, Garrattini (1965) and Carlini and Masur (1969), have shown a reduced fighting in mice and rats following Δ^9-THC treatment. Dubinsky *et al.* (1973) used several other models of aggression in rats and found that Δ^9-THC increased aggression in starvation-stressed rats or septally lesioned rats. Δ^9-THC does not appear to resemble either the neuroleptics or the benzodiazepines.

4.5 ANTIGLAUCOMA EFFECTS

Marijuana ingestion and the administration of Δ^9-THC have been reported to reduce intraocular pressure in man (Hepler and Frank, 1971; Frank *et al.*, 1972). The infusion intravenously of prostaglandins into rabbits (Chiang and Thomas, 1972) and dogs (Nakano *et al.*, 1972) caused an increased intraocular pressure and recently Green and Podos (1974) have shown that an increase in intraocular pressure was produced in rabbits by infusion of arachidonic acid, a precursor of prostaglandin E_2. In all these cases, Δ^9-THC antagonized the increase in intraocular pressure. This was interpreted as an inhibition of the synthesis of PGE_2 in the eye. Several authors have demonstrated that Δ^9-THC is capable of inhibiting prostaglandin synthesis (Burstein and Raz, 1972; Burstein *et al.*, 1973; Howes and Osgood, 1974a) and it has been proposed that Δ^9-THC produces its antiglaucoma actions by this mechanism. These studies indicate a possible mode of action of Δ^9-THC through the prostaglandins.

4.6 CARDIOVASCULAR ACTIVITY

The cardiovascular actions of Δ^9-THC are dependent on the species of animal, the resting blood pressure and the state of consciousness of the animal. Δ^9-THC has now been shown to produce a short-acting, dose-related tachycardia with no hypotension in the conscious rat (Osgood and Howes, 1975). The SHR rat has been widely used to evaluate antihypertensive effects and Δ^9-THC lowers blood pressure in these animals (Lewis *et al.*, 1974). Further, these authors showed that tolerance did not develop to the hypotensive effects of Δ^9-THC. Other studies have also demonstrated hypotensive effects for Δ^9-THC. Birmingham (1973) showed a hypotensive effect in rats showing adrenal regeneration hypertension and Williams *et al.* (1973) showed that Δ^9-THC blocked the appearance of hypertension in immobilized rats.

The effects of cannabinoids in the anesthetized animal are generally a dose-related decrease in heart rate and a fall in blood pressure in the rat (Milzoff *et al.*, 1971), the cat (Dagirmarjian and Boyd 1962), and the dog (Cavero *et al.*, 1972a; Dewey *et al.*, 1971). In the monkey with no anesthesia but a high mid-brain section, intravenous Δ^9-THC causes a fall in blood pressure (Boyd *et al.*, 1971). The direct effect of Δ^9-THC upon the heart would seem to be one of moderate depression; thus in the presence of this agent left ventricular contractile force in the isolated supported dog heart is decreased but to a lesser degree than in the intact dog (Lahiri *et al.*, 1972). In these experiments, block of peripheral muscarinic receptors (atropine methylnitrate) or β-adrenergic receptors (propranolol) partially prevented the decrease in contractile force. Again, in the isolated guinea pig heart left ventricular pressure, the maximum rate of pressure ride (dp/dt), and oxygen consumption were all depressed (Benmouyal *et al.*, 1971).

Efforts to elucidate the mechanism by which Δ^9-THC lowers heart rate and blood pressure have led to somewhat conflicting results. However, it would appear that a combined block of sympathetic and parasympathetic pathways eliminates or attenuates the bradycardia and hypotension following cannabinoid compounds. Thus ganglionic block plus atropine prevented (Cavero *et al.*, 1971) or diminished (Dagirmanjian and Boyd, 1962) the lowering of heart rate and blood pressure; spinal section accompanying vagotomy also eliminated these effects. On the other hand, pretreatment with atropine and propranolol prevented bradycardia but not hypotension (Cavero et al., 1972b) while the combination of atropine and an alpha-adrenergic blocking agent (phenoxybenzamine) partially eliminated hypotension but not bradycardia (Cavero et al., 1972b). In the urethane anesthetized rat, atropine alone abolished the fall in heart rate seen with Δ^9-THC (Forney and Kiplinger, 1971). These results are difficult to interpret but would seem to indicate both a cholinergic and adrenergic component in the cardiovascular actions of marijuana derivatives.

A number of findings suggest that the bradycardia and hypotension following Δ^9-THC are central in origin: spinal transection markedly reduced the fall in blood pressure observed with Δ^9-THC (Lahiri and Hardman, 1972); no change in heart rate was seen with this agent in the isolated guinea pig heart (Benmouyal et al., 1971) and further, Δ^9-THC, when injected into the vascularly isolated neurally intact head of the dog or cerebral ventricles of the cat, depressed heart rate and blood pressure (Cavero et al., 1972b). Since section at the mid-brain level leads to a fall in blood pressure in the monkey after Δ^9- (or Δ^8-) THC (Boyd et al., 1971) and does not alter the depressor effects in the anesthetized cat (Dagirmanjian and Boyd, 1962), the area of the brain relevant to the actions of cannabinoids in the anesthetized animal may lie below the cortex. Furthermore, Vollimer (1972) showed that perfusion of Δ^9-THC into the lateral ventricle of the cat caused a significant reduction in heart rate but not blood pressure. Studies by this group with ^{3}H, ^{14}C-labelled Δ^9-THC showed that very little drug passed into the peripheral circulation. In man, Δ^9-THC and the more potent benzopyrans possess hypotensive activity (sections 5.2 and 7.1). Thus the results from animal experiments may give misleading data in this instance.

4.7 GASTROINTESTINAL EFFECTS

Detailed gastroentrological data has not been published on the cannabinoids. The charcoal-meal test has been used to demonstrate that Δ^8-THC, Δ^9-THC (Chesher et al., 1973) and cannabidiol (Anderson et al., 1974) cause parallel dose-dependent inhibition of intestinal mobility in mice. The effects of Δ^9-THC and cannabidiol were synergistic. These agents were less potent than morphine in this procedure and were not antagonized by nalorphine. Good activity was evident, however, in doses which produced marked CNS symptomatology. Δ^9-THC does not have any antisecretory activity (Hwang, unpublished data). Neither does it increase gastric secretions.

4.8 ANTICANCER AND IMMUNOSUPPRESSANT ACTIVITY

Recent evidence indicates that Δ^9-THC may have antitumour activity (Harris *et al.*, 1974). Mice given Lewis lung carcinomas were treated daily for 10 days. Doses of 100 mg kg^{-1} of Δ^9-THC were effective in increasing survival times by 36 per cent. However, mice treated with this dose over 20 days showed a shorter survival time, which is thought to be due to the suppression of the immune response by Δ^9-THC (Levy *et al.*, 1974; Petersen *et al.*, 1974). Johnson and Wiersema (1974a) showed that Δ^9-THC inhibited bone marrow leukopoiesis and 11-hydroxy-Δ^9-THC was found to inhibit myelopoiesis (Johnson and Wiersema, 1974b). These reports are preliminary and further work is necessary to determine if Δ^9-THC has a role in cancer chemotherapy, or any potential as an immunosuppressant.

4.9 ANTIFERTILITY ACTIVITY

Δ^9-THC (2·0 mg per rat) suppressed the secretion of luteinizing hormone and suppressed ovulation (Nir *et al.*, 1973, and 1974), but Kiplinger *et al.* (1973) showed that Δ^9-THC did not alter mating or fertility in the rat. Grilly *et al.* (1974) showed that chronic marijuana exposure did not effect reproductive activity in chimpanzees. In the male rat, Δ^9-THC caused a decrease in sexual performance (Merari *et al.*, 1973) and Dixit *et al.* (1974) showed that chronic administration of cannabis extracts (2 mg per day for 45 days) caused a complete arrest of spermatogenisis in mice. The potential use of Δ^9-THC as an antifertility agent is low but it is possible that some of the newer derivatives, analogs, or homologs may possess activity in this area.

4.10 ANOREXIA

Sofia *et al.* (1974) have demonstrated a dose-related anorexia in rats following Δ^9-THC. The potency was approximately half that of dextro-amphetamine.

5 Pharmacology of Δ^9-tetrahydrocannabinol: human studies

5.1 INTRODUCTION

The subjective effect of Δ^9-THC has been described by Isbell *et al.* (1967) and Hollister *et al.* (1968) as a "sleepy, happy high", i.e. initial euphoria followed by a period of sleepiness. Numerous other cannabis constituents and their metabolites have also been studied in man. They all produce a qualitatively similar syndrome with the exception of cannabidiol which appears to have no "marijuana-like" activity (Hollister, 1973). Cannabidiol dimethyl ether and cannabichromene were also reported as inactive (Isbell et al., 1967). Cannabinol is active but only in high doses (Hollister, 1973) of 400 mg orally although in another study (Perez-Reyes et al., 1973a), infusion of cannabinol to a dose of 13·3 mg per 70 kg produced effects on heart rate and the perception of euphoria. Differences in route of administration could account for discrepancies in the dosage. The 11-hydroxy metabolites of Δ^8-THC and Δ^9-THC are active in man (Hollister, 1974). The onset of symptoms was rapid, duration was short but intensity was about 20 per cent greater than THC. The 8-hydroxy metabolites of Δ^9-THC (Wall, 1971) were also active in humans, with the 8α isomer being more potent than the 8β isomer.

5.2   CARDIOVASCULAR EFFECTS

Cannabinoids consistently produce tachycardia in man regardless of their route of administration (Weil et al., 1968; Manno et al., 1970; Hollister, 1973). The peak effect occurs at about 20 minutes after ingestion. The effect is acute and on chronic treatment it disappears. Since tachycardia after marijuana smoking is eliminated by pretreatment of subjects with the β-adrenergic blocking agent, propanolol (Bright et al., 1971), it is possible that this effect may stem from activation of the sympathetic nervous system. Further support for such a mechanism has been presented by Welch et al. (1971) who found a 25–36 per cent depletion of epinephrine from the adrenal gland in the unanesthetized mouse within 10 minutes after administration of Δ^9-THC. In addition, Weiss et al. (1972) reported an increase in urinary excretion of free epinephrine (but not norepinephrine) in human subjects after Δ^9-THC. Moreover, certain of the somatic symptoms described by subjects after Δ^9-THC, such as palpitations, weakness and tremor resemble some of the effects of increased levels of epinephrine in the peripheral circulation.

The effects of cannabinoids on blood pressure in man are more variable and seem to depend on the position of the subject; thus in recumbency there tends to be a slight increase in blood pressure while in the upright subject the blood pressure generally falls after Δ^9-THC (Weiss et al., 1972). However, high doses of Δ^9-THC have been found to increase blood presure in human volunteers (position unspecified) (Johnson and Domino, 1971).

The evidence available from both animal data and human studies, indicate that the cardiovascular effects of Δ^9-THC are probably centrally mediated. Clark et al. (1974) attributed the tachycardia to inhibition of vagal tone. Differences between man and experimental animals do exist. The tachycardia observed in humans has only recently been demonstrated in animals (Osgood and Howes, 1975) and hypotension in normotensive man can only be reproduced in anesthetized, normotensive, experimental animals.

5.3 SLEEP STUDIES

The sleepy period following the initial euphoric effects of Δ^9-THC is best observed at low doses. High doses have been shown to make sleep difficult (Taft and Crawford, 1970). A reduction of REM sleep is observed (Pivik et al., 1972) following Δ^9-THC although Kales et al. (1972) showed that subjects became tolerant to REM depletion. In the normative and REM-deprived subjects there was an increment in stage 4 sleep and a decrement in REM sleep (Pivik et al., 1972). The chronic administration of marijuana has been reported to decrease slow-wave sleep in humans (Williams et al., 1973). In a study by Barratt et al. (1974), using volunteers smoking 0·2 mg kg⁻¹ THC per day, slow-wave sleep was found to increase initially but by the 8th day was significantly depressed and remained depressed for at least three days post drug. These workers found no alterations in REM. In a similar study Freemon (1974) used a dose of 20 mg per subject and found a decrease in REM. Abrupt withdrawal of the drug produced insomnia but no REM rebound.

In acute studies Δ^9-THC has been found to decrease the time needed to fall asleep in healthy insomniacs (Cousens and DiMascio, 1973).

5.4 OTHER THERAPEUTIC STUDIES

The weak analgesic effects of cannabinoids in animals has also been reported in man. Noyes and Bagram (1974) reported several uncontrolled studies where marijuana ingestion was effective in the management of menstrual pain and headache. Subsequently, Brunk et al. (1974) reported that 70 mg of Δ^9-THC produced significant pain relief in patients with metastatic cancer.

In other studies Nahas et al. (1974) demonstrated an impairment of cellular-mediated immunity and cell division in man, confirming previous work in animals. Petersen et al. (1974) showed that cannabis smokers had a reduced level of phagocytic activity. However, a recent study by Silverstein and Lersin (1974) showed that cannabis ingestion did not alter the immune response of patients sensitized to a skin test of 2,4-dinitrochlorobenzene, whereas age-matched cancer patients showed a decreased capacity to be sensitized.

Δ^9-THC may possess some antiasthmatic activity as suggested by studies of Vachon et al. (1973a), Tashkin et al. (1973), Shapiro et al. (1973) and Beaconsfield et al. (1972). A recent study by Davies et al. (1975) failed to show any changes in respiratory parameters following 10 mg of Δ^9-THC.

6 Biochemical pharmacology studies of Δ^9-tetrahydrocannabinol

6.1 EFFECTS ON KNOWN NEUROTRANSMITTERS

The effects of Δ^9-THC on all of the important neurohumoral systems of the brain have been studied. The effects of Δ^9-THC on serotonin (5-HT) have been reported by Holtzman et al. (1969) who found a decrease in whole brain serotonin in mice given doses greater than 5·0 mg kg^{-1} ip. This was accompanied by a significant decrease in norepinephrine following doses of 5·0 mg kg^{-1} and 10 mg kg^{-1} ip or by a significant increase at doses of 200 mg kg^{-1} ip and above. These changes correlated with changes in body temperature. Δ^9-THC is hyperthermic at low doses and hypothermic at higher doses (Sofia, 1972). Ho et al. (1972) confirmed the work of Holtzman by showing a biphasic response of both serotonin and norepinephrine to Δ^9-THC treatment; serotonin was increased by high doses and decreased by doses of less than 2·0 mg kg^{-1} ip of Δ^9-THC.

Δ^9-THC differed from LSD in these experiments while, like LSD, it increased 5-HT at certain doses, there was no concurrent decrease in 5-hydroxyindole-acetic acid (5-HIAA) as seen with LSD.

In rats, high doses of Δ^9-THC caused only a slight increase in serotonin (Schildkraut and Efron, 1971) and Pal and Ghosh (1972) found an increase in urinary 5-HIAA only after repeated doses of 10 mg kg^{-1} ip Δ^9-THC or an acute dose of 100 mg kg^{-1}. At low doses Gallagher et al. (1972) found no effects on either 5-HT or 5-HIAA in rat brain. Those changes which are seen probably reflect only the toxic effects of high doses of Δ^9-THC. Perhaps the most convincing evidence for the involvement of a neuro-humoral agent in the actions of Δ^9-THC is that concerning dopamine. Δ^9-THC causes catalepsy and reduced utilization of dopamine is associated with this state. In addition, drugs which are known to affect cerebral dopamine interact with Δ^9-THC. Howes (1973a) showed that while low doses of Δ^9-THC protected mice against the aggregated toxicity of amphetamine, higher doses potentiated this lethality, and later showed that other agents such as pemoline antagonize many of the effects of Δ^9-THC (Howes, 1973b). Further studies indicated that Δ^9-THC and the water-soluble derivative inhibit the uptake of ^{14}C-dopamine into the crude rat-striatal synaptosomes (Howes and Osgood, 1974a).

Several authors have studied the effects of cannabinoids on dopamine levels in the CNS. All seem to agree that steady-state levels are reduced. Chronic treatment of rats with Δ^9-THC (8 days) reduced endogenous levels of dopamine in the brain stem but not in the fore-brain (Friedman and Gershon, 1972), whereas acute treatment of rats with 10 mg kg^{-1} po Δ^9-THC lowered whole brain dopamine (Graham et al., 1974). These latter authors showed that this treatment did not alter whole brain norepinephrine. Changes in the major metabolites of dopamine have been noted by several authors. Treatment with Δ^9-THC alone did not alter striatal homovanillic acid or dihydroxyphenylacetic acid levels in the rat. However, the decrease in these metabolites caused by amphetamine was altered during Δ^9-THC treatment and the increased dihydroxyphenylacetic acid and homovanillic acid levels following an acute dose of L-dopa (200 mg kg^{-1} ip) were potentiated (Osgood and Howes, 1974b). In contrast to these studies, Friedman and Gershon (1972) were able to demonstrate an elevation in brain homovanillic acid following an acute dose of Δ^9-THC. Δ^8-THC, however, caused an increase in striatal dihydroxyphenylacetic acid with no effects on homovanillic acid (Maitre et al., 1973). All of these data indicate an effect on the dopaminergic system of the brain. Further studies are required to clear up some of the inconsistencies reported.

Following an intravenous dose of ^{3}H-tyrosine in rats treated with either Δ^9-THC or Δ^8-THC, there was an increased accumulation of ^{3}H-norepinephrine (NE) and ^{3}H-dopamine (DA). The accumulation of ^{3}H-NE was most marked in the hypothalamus and of ^{3}H-DA in the corpus striatum. Both cannabinoids caused an accelerated release of newly synthesized DA and NE. The disappearance of NE was the most marked (Maitre et al., 1973).

Repeated administration of Δ^9-THC to rats leads to an increase in the activity of tyrosine hydroxylase with no effects on either tryptophan hydroxylase or DOPA decarboxylase (Ho et al., 1973).

One may conclude that Δ^9-THC affects the catecholamines significantly, possibly altering the distribution of these neurohumorals in the synaptic region. The changes in the metabolites of DA clearly indicate some alteration in the disposition of DA in the striatum.

A recent candidate for the mediation of THCs central effect is phenethylamine (PEA) (Sabelli and Mosnaim, 1974). These authors (Sabelli et al., 1974a) presented evidence to support the hypothesis that phenethylamine and its metabolites modulate affective behavior. They demonstrated (Sabelli et al., 1974b) that in rabbits Δ^9-THC increased the recovery of labelled β-phenethylamine from the brain following intraventricular administration. Δ^9-THC also enhanced the excitatory effect of iontophoretically administered phenethylamine and increased by five- to sixfold the whole brain levels of phenethylamine in rabbits given doses of Δ^9-THC of 30 mg kg^{-1}. Furthermore, the stimulant effects of phenethylamine were enhanced by Δ^9-THC. If one accepts PEA as a neurotransmitter the evidence would appear to be convincing for its role in the mediation of Δ^9-THCs stimulant effects.

Domino (1971) reviewed the effects of Δ^9-THC on acetylcholine (ACh). Increases in whole-brain acetycholine were observed and Δ^9-THC antagonized the hemicholinium-induced reduction of ACh. Brown (1973) showed a small but significant increase in rat brain ACh following a 10·0 mg kg^{-1} ip dose of Δ^9-THC and Karbowski et al. (1975) showed that high doses of Δ^9-THC caused large increases in mouse brain ACh. The meaning of these results is not clear since many CNS depressants are known to increase brain acetylcholine, by nonspecific effects. Δ^9-THC has even been reported to alter levels of brain GABA (Leonard, 1971). The results on all of these neurohumoral agents indicate that there is no clear involvement of any single neurohumoral agent in the actions of Δ^9-THC.

6.2   EFFECTS ON PROSTAGLANDINS AND CYCLIC AMP

There is a growing body of evidence that Δ^9-THC produces many of its actions by an effect on prostaglandin synthesis. There is much circumstantial evidence which would fit this hypothesis. Δ^9-THC, like aspirin and indomethacin, is active in procedures designed to identify anti-inflammatory agents (see section 4.1). Furthermore the potentiation of norepinephrine and the cardiovascular system of the dog (Zitko et al., 1972) may be explained by an effect on prostaglandins. It is well established that the prostaglandins exert a modulating effect on norepinephrine in the cardiovascular system (McGiff, 1975). Inhibition of prostaglandin synthesis by either indomethacin or eicosatetraynoic acid (ETA) caused a potentiation of norepinephrine and of adrenergic nerve stimulation in the dog-paw perfusion experiment (Zimmerman et al., 1973). By analogy with this experiment the potentiation·of epinephrine and norepinephrine by Δ^9-THC could be due to inhibition of prostaglandin synthesis. These observations have been followed up by investigations showing that Δ^9-THC potentiates the hypotensive activity of arachidonic acid, an effect it shares with indomethacin (Howes and Osgood, 1975). Other evidence consistent with the prostaglandin hypothesis is its activity as a bronchodilator, its effects on luteinizing hormone secretion (see section 4.9) and its effects on pentylenetetrazole-induced seizures (see section 4.2).

More direct evidence for the hypothesis is the findings described in section 4.5 which indicate that Δ^9-THC prevents glaucoma due to arachidonic acid, the precursor of PGE$_2$. Direct evidence that Δ^9-THC inhibits prostaglandin synthesis in the sheep, bull seminal vesicle preparations (Burstein and Raz, 1972; Burstein et al., 1973) or the rat corpus striatum (Howes and Osgood, 1974a) has been presented. Crowshaw and Hardman (1974) showed that both Δ^9-THC and 11-hydroxy-THC inhibited PGE_2 synthesis in the rabbit adrenal medulla acetone powder preparation. The levels required to achieve significant inhibition were high (100 mg ml^{-1}). Thus, while much more data must be gathered, the hypothesis that Δ^9-THC may act by inhibiting prostaglandin appears to be valid.

Centrally, Δ^9-THC, by blocking prostaglandin synthesis, would remove its modulating effect on dopamine, explaining many of the previously described observations. The catecholamines and prostaglandin are known to modify cyclic AMP in the brain. Dolby and Kleinsmith (1974) measured the levels of cyclic AMP in the brains of mice and discovered that Δ^9-THC caused a biphasic effect. Low doses (0·1–1·0 mg kg^{-1} ip) caused an elevation of cyclic AMP, whereas doses of 2·0 mg kg^{-1} ip and above caused decreases in cerebral cyclic AMP. These changes occurred in the cortex, cerebellum medulla and the hypothalamus. Askew and Ho (1974) showed that Δ^8-THC but not Δ^9-THC caused a significant increase in cyclic AMP in the rat brain together with a decrease in both adenylcyclase and phosphodiesterase.

Thus Δ^9-THC may exert some of its effects through mechanisms which are very basic to the neuron or other cell. This would account for the wide range of activities observed with this compound. A great deal more data needs to be gathered, however, before one can state that the mechanisms described above account for the action of Δ^9-THC.

7 Pharmacology of carbocyclic (C, H, O) analogs and derivatives

As described in section 1, a series of compounds with the basic structure **III** were synthesized by Adams et al. (1949).

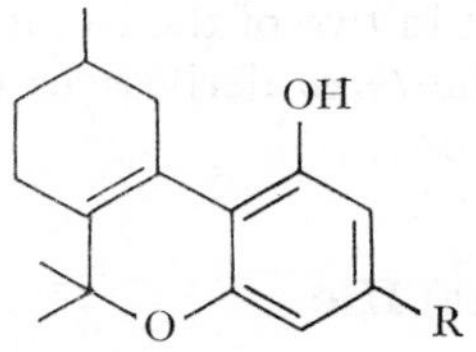

(III)

The group R was altered and a structure–activity relationship was developed using the dog ataxia test as a means of estimating activity. From this study, the most potent member of the series was discovered when

$R=CH(CH_3)CH(CH_3)(CH_2)_4CH_3$. The compound which is referred to as dimethylheptylpyran (DMHP, **IIIb**) has been studied in animals and in man.

7.1 DIMETHYLHEPTYLPYRAN (DMHP)

This agent is qualitatively similar to Δ^9-THC but is generally more potent. It produces the characteristic symptoms of marijuana intoxication in dogs (Hardman *et al.*, 1970; Hardman *et al.*, 1971) as well as CNS depression, hypothermia, hypotension and analgesia in dogs and monkeys. Its analgesic activity was varied and it lacked significant activity in the rat tail-flick test (Howes, unpublished data). DMHP produced marked hypotension in dogs, cats, monkeys, and in man (Hardman *et al.*, 1971). Since DMHP is a diastereoisomeric mixture, *erythro* and *threo* derivatives have been prepared and studied separately. An investigation of these diastereoisomers showed that the $(\pm)$-*threo* derivative was significantly more active than the $(\pm)$-*erythro* diastereoisomer:

	Hot plate ED_{50} (mg kg^{-1}, ip) (Howes)	MES-ED_{50} (Karler, 1973)
$(\pm)$-*erythro*-DMHP	12·0 (1·4–103·2)	24·0 (18·0–32·0)
$(\pm)$-*threo*-DMHP	1·5 (0·9–2·5)	6·8 (5·4–8·5)

Lemberger *et al.* (1974) administered DMHP to healthy male volunteers. The dose used in this study was low (200 μg per 70 kg iv) and no euphoric or dysphoric effects were observed. Some drowsiness did occur but the prominent effects observed were tachycardia and hypotension. Conjuntival injection was not reported in this study. The eight isomers of the acetate of DMHP have also been synthesized (by Aaron and Ferguson, 1968) and studied in man (Sidell *et al.*, 1973). The principal effect seen was hypotension, which was prominent in two of the isomers ($-$)-*threo* and ($+$)-*threo*. The marked activity of the *threo* derivatives over the *erythro* derivatives was also evident in this study.

7.2 SYNHEXYL (PYRAHEXYL) **IIIc**

Synhexyl, synthesized in 1940 by Adams (Adams, 1942), represents the first synthetic cannabinoid administered to man and studied as a potential therapeutic agent. Its pharmacological profile resembles that of Δ^9-THC, and Loewe (1946) found that it had a remarkably high LD_{50} dose. Its euphoric effects indicated that it might be useful in the treatment of mental depression. In a series of studies (Stockings, 1947; Ponce, 1948; Parker and

Wrigley, 1950; Thompson and Proctor, 1953) results were mixed as to its efficacy in this disorder. Thompson and Proctor (1953) felt that it might be useful in treating the alcoholic abstinence syndrome. Loewe and Goodman (1947) showed that synhexyl was active as an anticonvulsant and some studies were undertaken in mentally retarded epileptic children, the results of which were equivocal (Davis and Ramsey, 1949). Himmelsbach (1944) showed some activity in the treatment of opiate withdrawal.

Interest in this compound declined perhaps because of its general lack of specific therapeutic activity, to its resinous and intractable physical characteristics and perhaps because of clinically unacceptable subjective effects.

In 1968, Hollister *et al.* compared synhexyl with Δ^9-THC in man by oral administration. Synhexyl was found to be qualitatively similar to Δ^9-THC but about one-third as active. The onset of symptoms following synhexyl was delayed and its duration was longer, in relation to Δ^9-THC. Euphoria was followed by drowsiness and Hollister described the symptoms of "sleepy, happy high" which along with its physiological effects were clearly similar to Δ^9-THC. Conjuctival injection was observed and tachycardia accompanied by hypotension was characteristically present.

In 1972, Pivik *et al.* demonstrated a similarity between the effects of synhexyl and Δ^9-THC. Synhexyl appears to be less potent but qualitatively similar to Δ^9-THC.

7.3 OTHER CARBOCYCLIC DERIVATIVES OF THC

Numerous other carbocyclic cannabinoids have been synthesized but none have been studied as extensively as DMHP or synhexyl. Adams *et al.* (1949) described a number of side-chain homologs, most of which were only examined in the dog ataxia test. The most interesting activity with carbocyclic derivatives appears to be their anticonvulsant effects. Thus, Garriott *et al.* (1968) described the properties of a series of THC and cannabinoid related compounds. The following phloroglucinol analog showed good anticonvulsant activity in the maximal electroshock procedure:

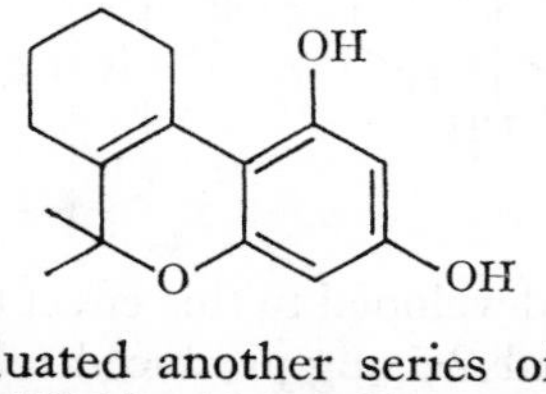

Loewe *et al.* (1946) evaluated another series of synthetic cannabinoids related to DMHP, but DMHP itself turned out to be the most potent of the series:

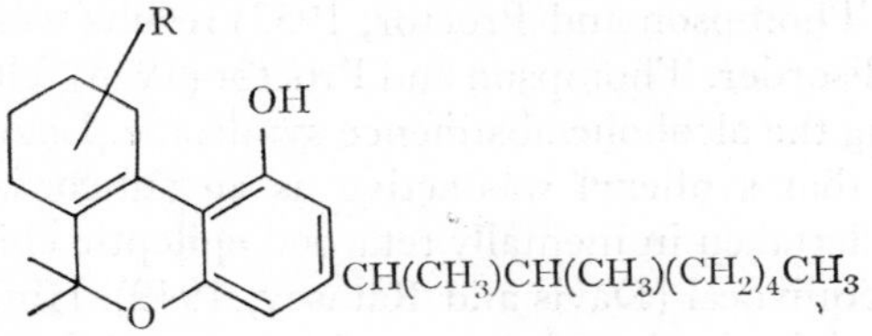

Changing either the length of the aliphatic chain R or its position in the ring or changing the position of the double bond or removing it caused a decreased activity in the rat. These authors also indicated that DMHP may have antiinflammatory, gastric antisecretory and diuretic properties.

Consroe *et al.* (1973), Karler *et al.* (1973, 1974) and Plotnikoff *et al.* (1974, 1975) have carried out detailed studies showing the effects of various carbocyclic (C, H, O) cannabinoids and their water-soluble derivatives in a number of animal procedures designed to show anticonvulsant action. Their data are summarized in Tables 10 to 14. Muscle relaxation was determined using the rotorod procedure (see Table 14). Thus data from both audiogenic and rotorod procedures were compared showing a favorable ratio of activity to toxicity, i.e. a separation of anticonvulsant effects from muscular incoordination. DMHP and several of its water-soluble derivatives (e.g. **1**, Table I) were very active in these procedures, as were some of the newer *p*-fluorophenyl side-chain derivatives (Winn *et al.*, 1976) of DMHP (see **136–138**, Table 13).

Recently a new synthetic carbocyclic benzopyran has been described. Nabilone® (Lilly 109514) inhibits muricide in rats, decreases reactivity in septally lesioned rats at doses of about 1·25 mg kg^{-1} orally (Stark and Archer, 1975). The compound produced hypothermia but after chronic

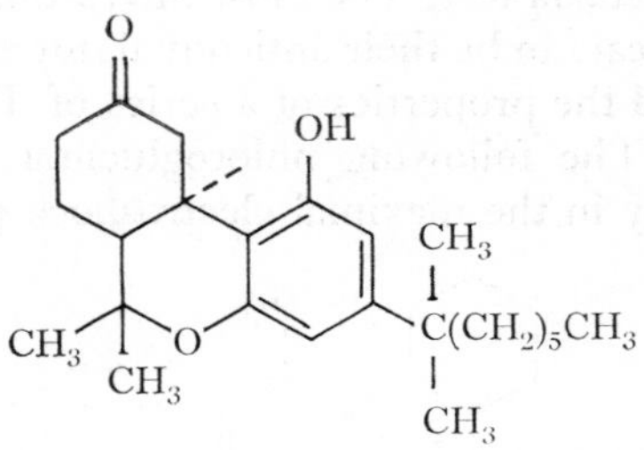

administration tolerance developed to this effect (Page and West, 1975). In human volunteers 1·0 and 2·5 mg produced relaxant and sedative effects in all subjects. At 5 mg kg^{-1}, marked postural hypotension was observed. Euphoria was observed at this dose and administration of 1 or 2 mg twice a

TABLE 10

Summary of literature references to the anticonvulsant effects (mg kg^{-1}) of various cannabis constituents

Compound	Audiogenic[a] seizure test, mouse, oral	Audiogenic[b] seizure test, rat, iv	Supramaximal[a] electroshock test, mouse, oral	Maximal[c] electroshock test, mouse, ip	Supramaximal[a] electroshock test, rat, oral	Maximal[b] electroshock test, rat, iv
Δ^9-THC	5·0 (2·4–7·7)	3·3 (2·0–5·4)	31·9 (29·1–34·5)	80·0 (64–100)	56·4 (36·6–105·8)	4·1 (2·2–7·8)
Δ^8-THC		4·7 (3·1–7·1)				2·6 (1·57–4·29)
Cannabidiol	ED$_{50}$=95·7 (59·7–167·9)			ED$_{50}$=105 (79–104)		
Cannabinol				ED$_{50}$=230 (215–246)		

[a] Plotnikoff et al. (1974, 1976).
[b] Consroe et al. (1973).
[c] Karler et al. (1973, 1974).

TABLE 11

Audiogenic seizure duration studies in mice of selected carbocyclic analogs and derivatives[a]

Structure (compound numbers)	ED_{50} 1 h[b] mg kg^{-1} (95 % CL)	ED_{50} 4 h[b] mg kg^{-1} (95 % CL)	ED_{50} 24 h[b] mg kg^{-1} (95 % CL)
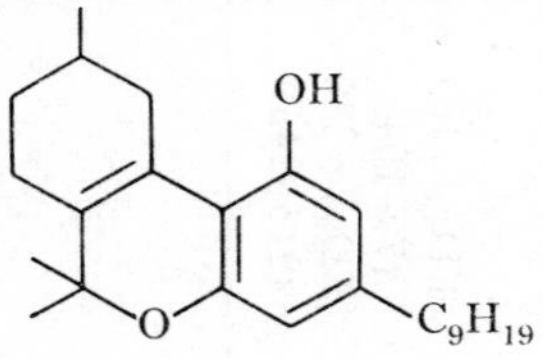 (DMHP (**IIIb**))	6·7 (2·1–11·0)	2·9 (1·8–4·9)	15·1 (8·2–26·3)
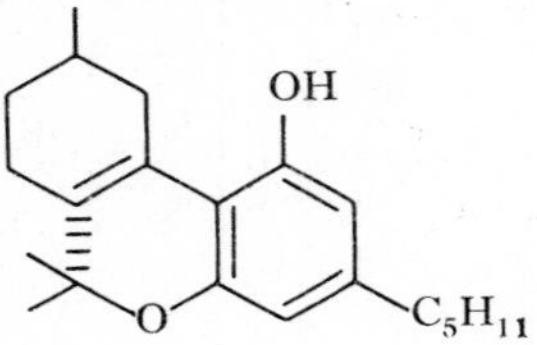 (Δ⁹-THC)	5·0 (2·4–7·7)	38·8 (29·1–49·3)	ED_{50}= > 100
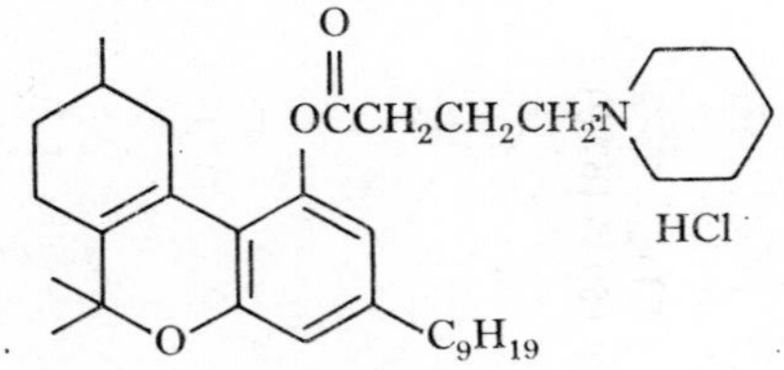 (**1**)	8·5 (5·1–13·8)	2·8 (1·4–6·8)	32·3 (20·0–48·8)
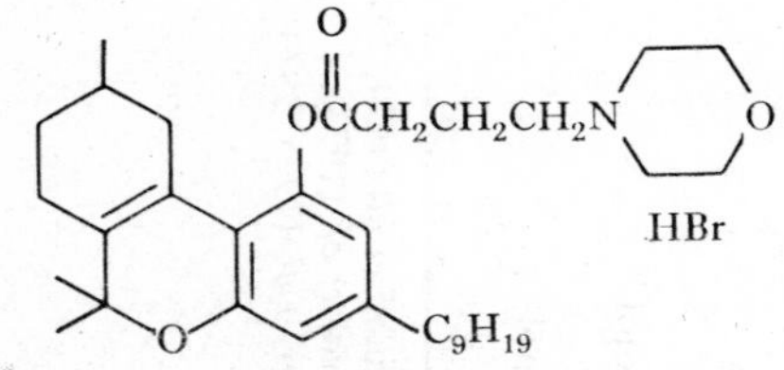 (**2**)	4·2 (2·1–8·0)	2·4 (1·2–5·5)	19·1 (12·5–27·3)

TABLE 11 —*continued*

Audiogenic seizure duration studies in mice of selected carbocyclic analogs and derivatives[a]

Structure (compound numbers)	ED_{50} 1 h[b] mg kg^{-1} (95 % CL)	ED_{50} 4 h[b] mg kg^{-1} (95 % CL)	ED_{50} 24 h[b] mg kg^{-1} (95 % CL)
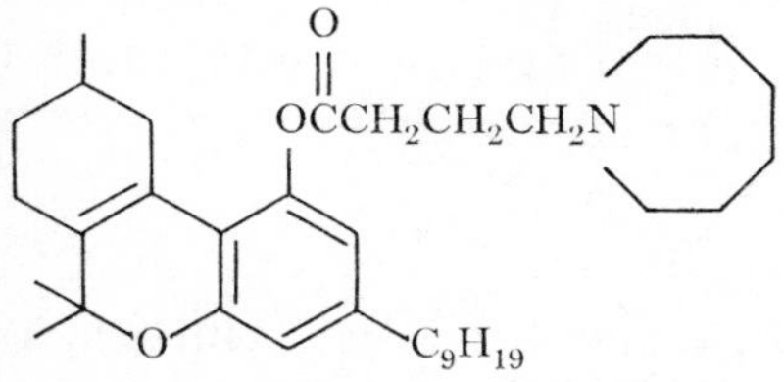 (3)	6·8 (4·1–11·3)	1·1 (0·5–2·4)	$ED_{50} = > 60·0$

[a] Plotnikoff *et al.* (1974).
[b] Oral dose at which 50 per cent of the animals are protected from hindlimb tonic extension.

day for 7 days caused euphoria and dry mouth. Unlike related compounds no tachycardia was observed with this compound (Lemberger and Rowe, 1975a, 1975b). The compound is at present being studied for its anti-anxiety effects.

7.4 WATER-SOLUBLE DERIVATIVES

Δ^9-THC is a sticky, resinous material, which is difficult to handle pharmacologically. An ideal derivative would be one which was water soluble and either retained the profile of Δ^9-THC or was rapidly converted to it. In 1970, two such derivatives (**Vb** and **Va**) were synthesized and tested (Howes, 1970).

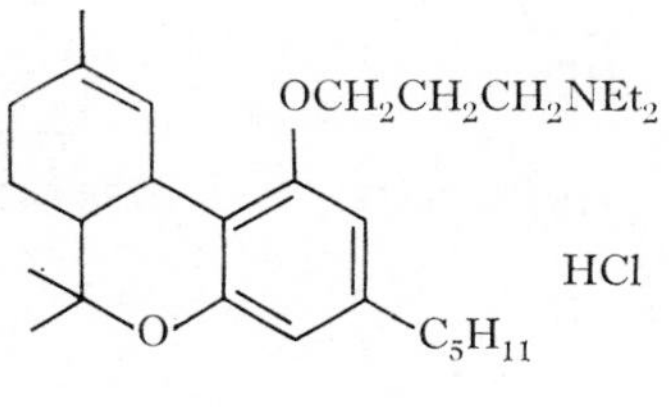

(**Vb**) 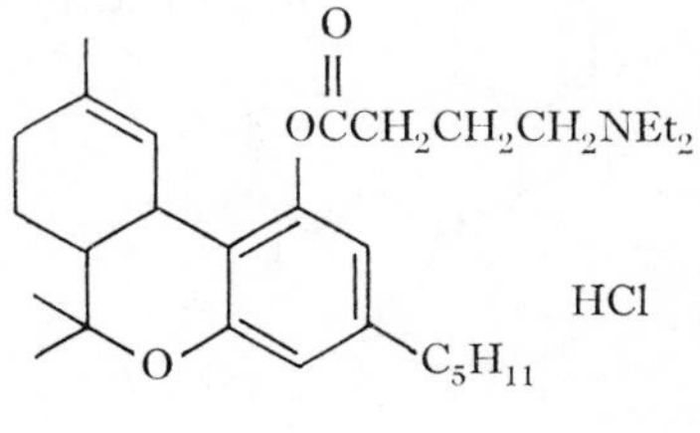   (**Va**)

TABLE 12

Supramaximal electroshock studies in mice of selected carbocyclic analogs and derivatives[a]

Structure (compound number)	ED_{50}, 1 h[b] mg kg^{-1} (95 % CL)	ED_{50}, 4 h[b] mg kg^{-1} (95 % CL)
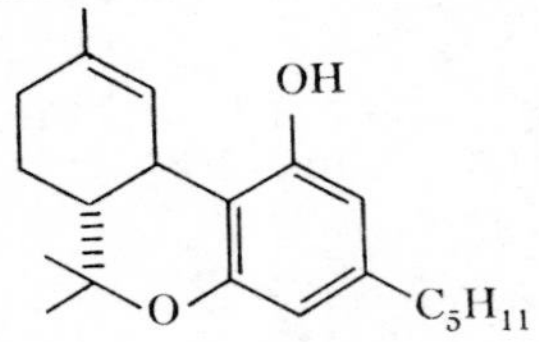 Δ^9-THC	31·9 (29·1–34·5)	101·5 (96·4–106·6)
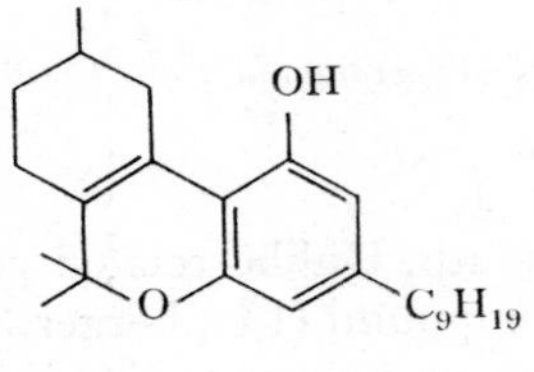 DMHP (IIIb)	300 (estimated)	57·2 (35·1–80·1)
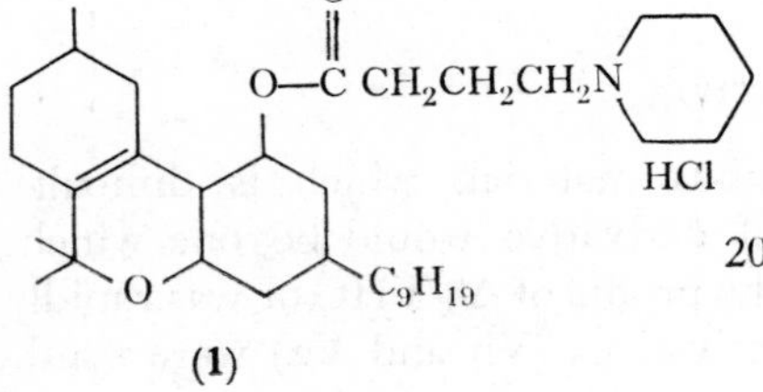 (1)	200	70 (estimated)
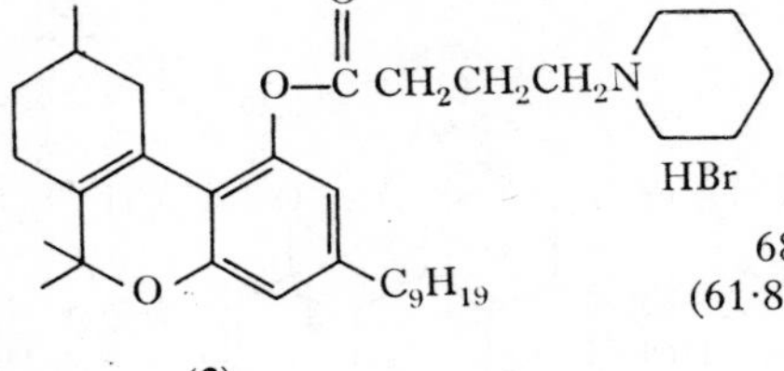 (2)	68·3 (61·8–78·7)	75·9 (58·6–102)

TABLE 12—*continued*

Supramaximal electroshock studies in mice of selected carbocyclic analogs and derivatives[a]

Structure (compound number)	ED_{50}, 1 h[b] mg kg^{-1} (95 % CL)	ED_{50}, 4 h[b] mg kg^{-1} (95 % CL)
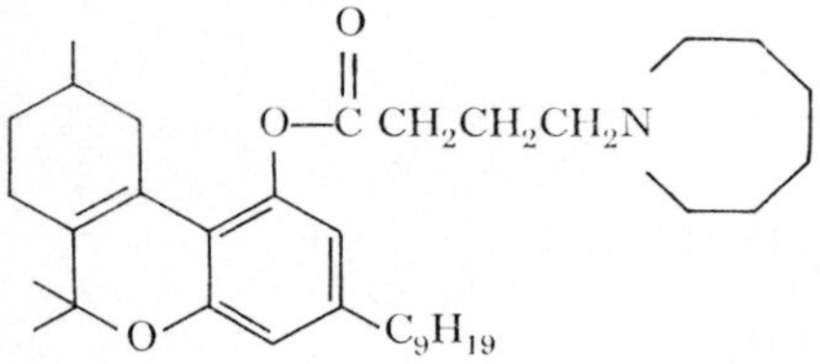 (3)	200	60 (estimated)

[a] Plotnikoff *et al.* (1974, 1976).
[b] Oral dose at which 50 per cent of the animals are protected from hindlimb tonic extension.

The basic ether (**Vb**) was found to be extremely toxic with very little pharmacological similarity with Δ^9-THC. The basic ester (**Va**) was studied and gross symptomatology was found to be similar to Δ^9-THC in dogs and rodents. Subsequently, the compound **IV** was synthesized and studied in a variety of procedures (Zitko *et al.*, 1972). It was similar to Δ^9-THC in the

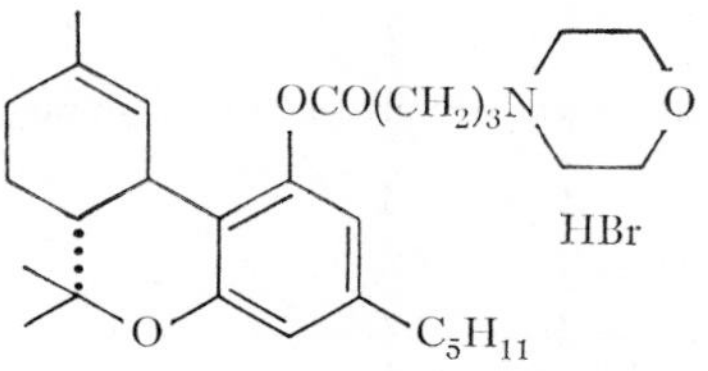

(**IV**)

unanesthetized dog, the rodent, and in the cardiovascular system of the anesthetized dog. The compound has activity in the hot plate test. While definite proof is lacking, it would appear that **IV** is hydrolyzed to Δ^9-THC *in vivo*, although the actions of this derivative *per se* cannot be discounted.

The technique (described in section 2.1) for making water-soluble

TABLE 13

Audiogenic seizure activity in mice of fluorophenyl side-chain derivatives of DMHP[a],

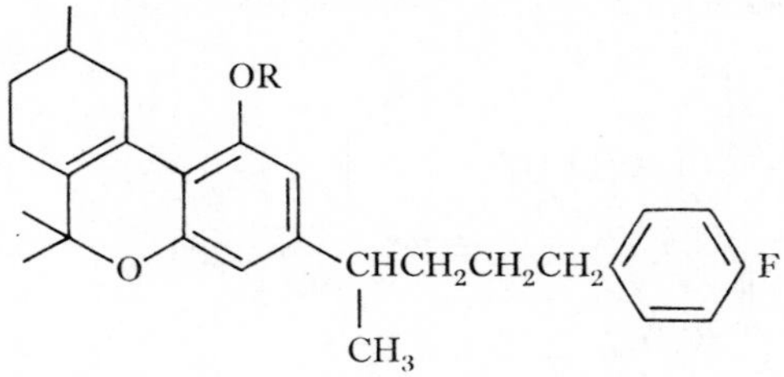

Compound numbers	R	1 h[b] Audiogenic ED_{50} mg kg^{-1}
136	H	2·3 (1·3–4·0)
137	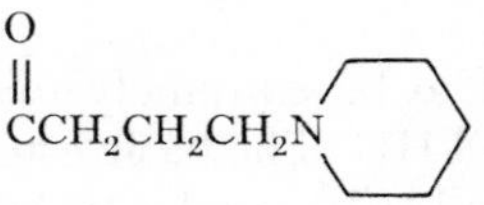 $\overset{O}{\underset{\parallel}{C}}CH_2CH_2CH_2N\!\!\bigcirc$ HCl	7·1 (3·5–16·4)
138	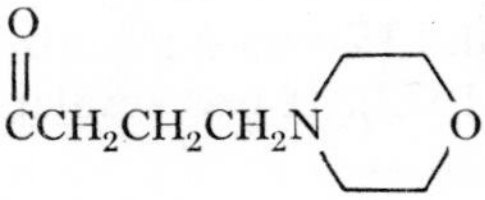 $\overset{O}{\underset{\parallel}{C}}CH_2CH_2CH_2N\!\!\bigcirc\!\!O$ HCl	8·0 (4·7–13·6)

[a] Plotnikoff et al. (1974).
[b] Oral dose (mg kg^{-1}) at which 50 per cent of the animals are protected from tonic extension; 1 h after.

Compound number	R	Mouse hot plate ED_{50}, mg kg,$^{-1}$, po
VI	H	45·1 (28–131)
10		16·0 (9·3–20·6)

derivatives has been applied to other members of the series, with great success. DMHP (**IIIb**) is a resinous material similar to Δ^9-THC. It gave a series of water-soluble salts, which included compound **2** of Table 1. The

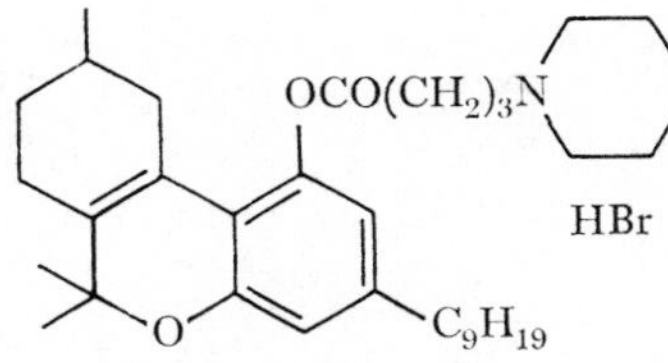

2

general profile of compound **2** was similar to its parent phenol DMHP with the exception that its analgesic activity is enhanced. For example it has an ED_{50} of 4·2 mg kg^{-1} po (2·0–7·0) in the rat tail-flick test (Razdan *et al.*, 1976c). DMHP itself has very little activity in this procedure. This enhancement of activity has also been observed in another carbocyclic series (see Table 2):

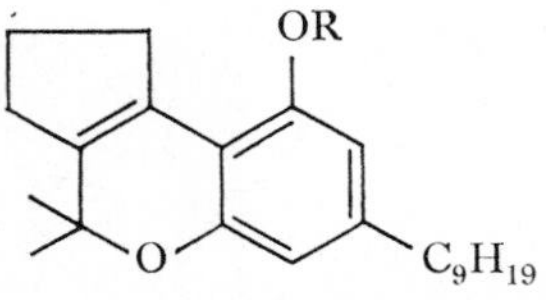

Compound number	R	Mouse hot plate ED_{50}, mg kg^{-1}, po
VI	H	45·1 (28–131)
10	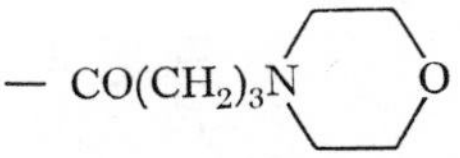 $- CO(CH_2)_3N\diagup O$ HCl	16·0 (9·3–20·6)

For a list of other water-soluble (ester) derivatives and their activities see Tables 7 and 8.

8 Pharmacology of nitrogen and sulfur analogs

The previous sections (4 to 7) were a summary and review of the pharmacology of Δ^9-THC, synthetic carbocyclic (C, H, O) analogs, and their

TABLE 14

Comparison of audiogenic seizure and rotarod duration studies of selected carbocyclic analogs[a]

Structure (compound number)	Audiogenic ED$_{50}$ 1 h mg kg^{-1}	Audiogenic ED$_{50}$ 4 h mg kg^{-1}	Rotarod ED$_{50}$ 1 h mg kg^{-1}	Rotarod ED$_{50}$ 4 h mg kg^{-1}
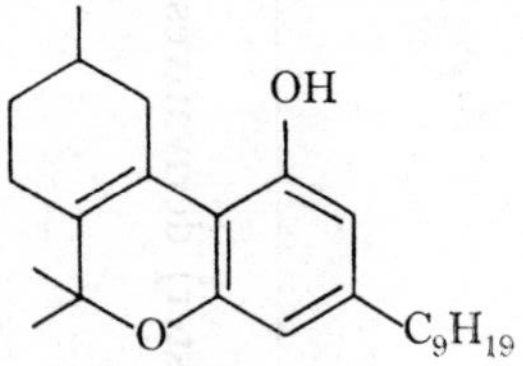 (DMHP (IIIb))	6·7 (2·1–11·0)	2·9 (1·8–4·9)	56·9	23·8
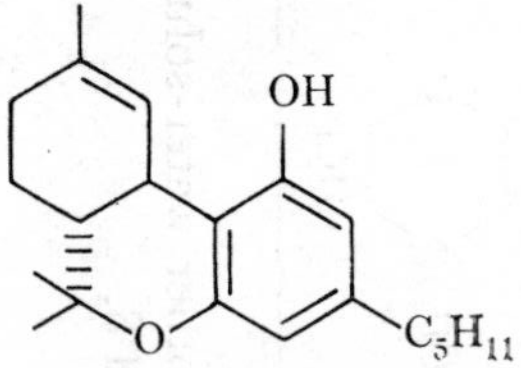 (Δ⁹-THC)	5·0 (2·1–11·0)	38·8 (29·1–49·3)	39·2	80

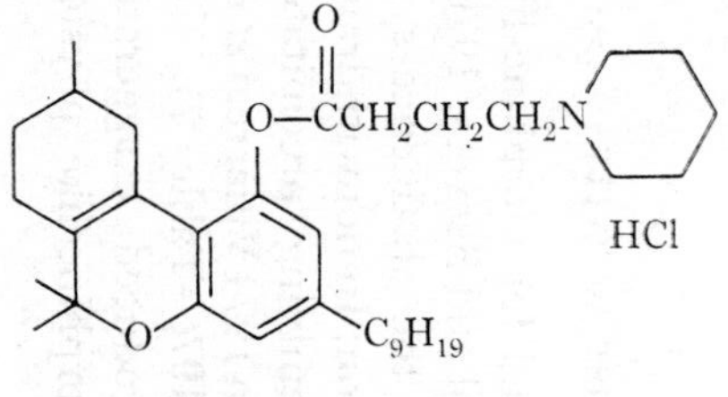

14.1

95.8

2.8
(1.4–6.8)

8.5
(5.1–13.8)

16.1

34.2

2.4
(1.2–5.5)

4.2
(2.1–8.0)

53.7

106.9

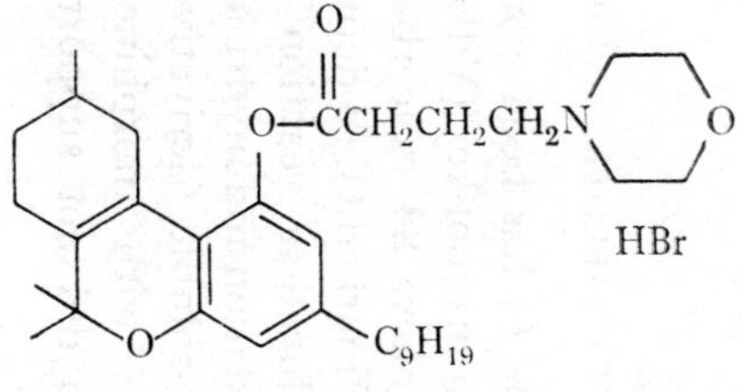

1.1
(0.5–2.4)

6.8
(4.1–11.3)

O=C–CH$_2$CH$_2$CH$_2$N (piperidine) · HCl

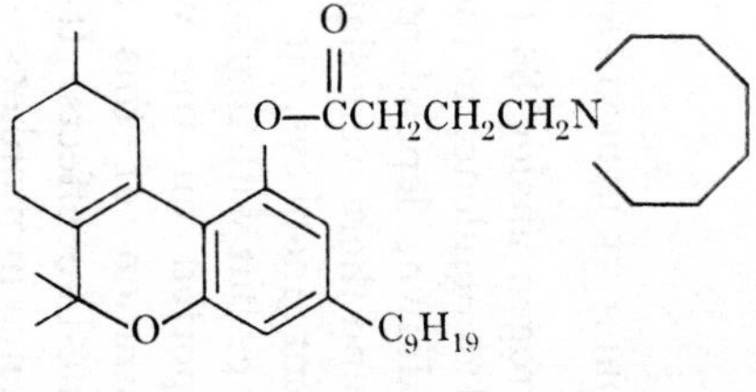

C$_9$H$_{19}$

(1)

O=C–CH$_2$CH$_2$CH$_2$N (morpholine) · HBr

C$_9$H$_{19}$

(2)

O=C–CH$_2$CH$_2$CH$_2$N (azocane)

C$_9$H$_{19}$

(3)

a Plotnikoff et al. (1974, 1976).

water-soluble derivatives. The results presented here summarize recently published work (Dren *et al.*, 1974; Harris and Dewey, 1974; Keats and Romagnoli, 1974; Plotnikoff *et al.*, 1974; Villarreal *et al.*, 1974; Pars *et al.*, 1976; Razdan *et al.*, 1976; and Winn *et al.*, 1976), with the heterocyclic (CHNO, CHOS) analogs.

8.1 ANALGESIC EFFECTS

Where the active principles of cannabis, including Δ^9-THC, show weak and sometimes nondose-related activity, a number of the nitrogen and sulfur analogs have excellent antinociceptive properties in animals. Table 15 lists the ED_{50}s of a variety of such compounds in three analgesic procedures.

The consistently good activity of the *N*-propargyl compounds is noteworthy since these compounds have the phenethylamine configuration found in many CNS-active agents. Conversion to water-soluble derivatives did not significantly alter antinociceptive activity. This is in sharp contrast to what is observed with the DMHP derivative (see section 2.2).

The sulfur heterocyclics are of great interest since they represent some of the most potent analgesic agents known which do not contain a nitrogen. An exception is the five-membered sulfur analog (compound **120**, Table 8) which is only weakly analgesic.

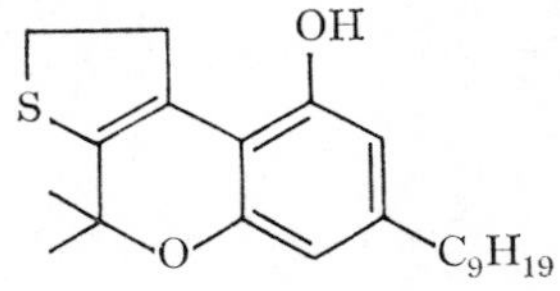

(120)

8.2 MORPHINE DEPENDENCE AND NARCOTIC ANTAGONIST ACTIVITY

The nitrogen analog **84** (Table 6) has been evaluated for morphine-like physical dependence in the Rhesus monkey (Villarreal and Seevers, 1970). In withdrawn, dependent monkeys **84** exacerbated the abstinence syndrome, and there were signs of marked CNS depression. In nonwithdrawn dependent monkeys, it produced a reaction resembling precipitated abstinence but with marked sedation and mydriasis. In 1974 Villarreal *et al.* also reported on the water-soluble derivative (**107**, Table 7). Co-administration of this agent with morphine produced exaggerated morphine-like effects. It also did not support morphine-like physical dependence in monkeys.

TABLE 15

Analgesic activity of selected nitrogen and sulfur analogs[a,b,c]

| Structure (compound number) | ED_{50} mg kg^{-1}, po | | |
	Hot plate[d] (mouse)	Anti-writhing[e] (mouse)	Tail flick[f] (rat)
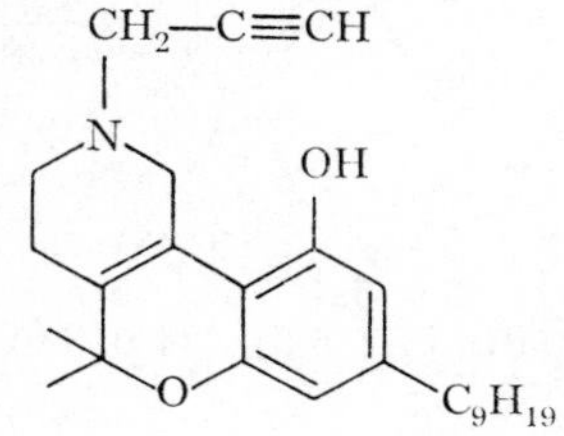 (84)	7·7 (4·1–12·7)	4·3 (3·2–5·9)	13·8 (4·5–23·9)
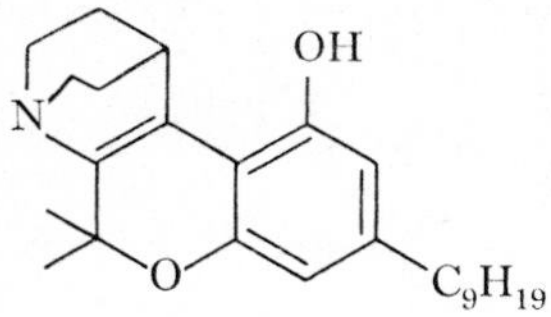 (96)	4·3 (2·8–5·9)	10·3 (7·4–15·8)	27·7 (19·1–43·2)
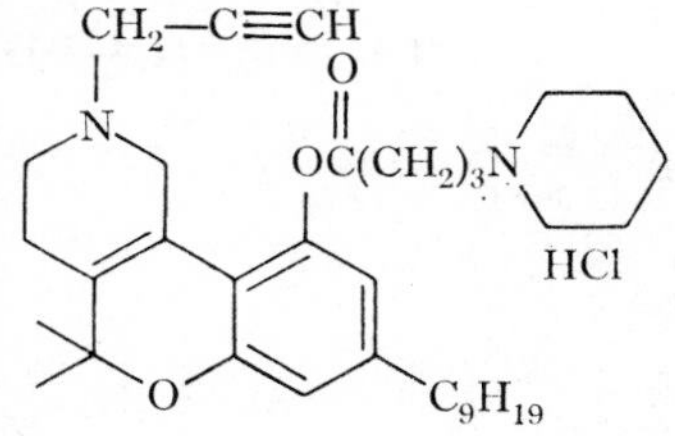 (107)	4·2 (2·0–6·8)	12·0 (9·3–16·9)	12·5 (9·4–15·7)
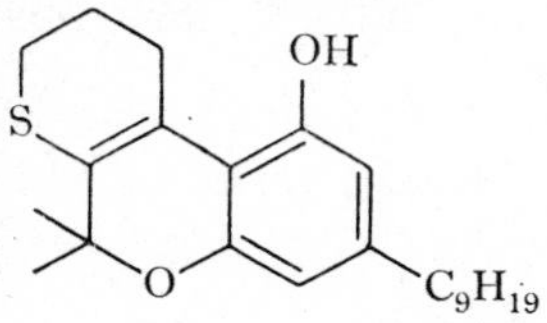 (124)	8·7	10·8 (9·2–12·7)	2·7 (0·9–4·8)

TABLE 15—*continued*

Analgesic activity of selected nitrogen and sulfur analogs [a,b,c]

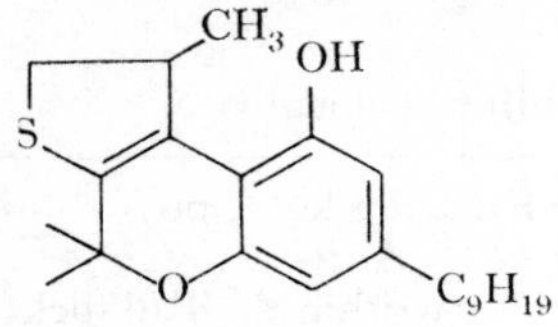

(129)

1·4	4·7	1·4
(0·1–3·5)	(3·0–7·0)	(0·5–2·0)

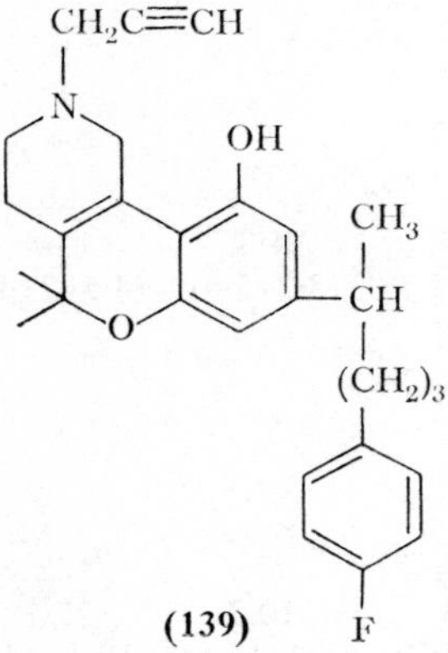

(139)

5·7	5·3	3·7
(2·0–10·0)	(4·2–6·8)	(1·0–8·0)

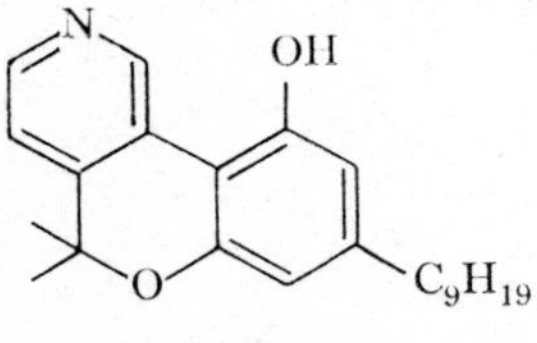

(140)

—	3·3	3·1
	(1·1–39·6)	(1·4–5·1)

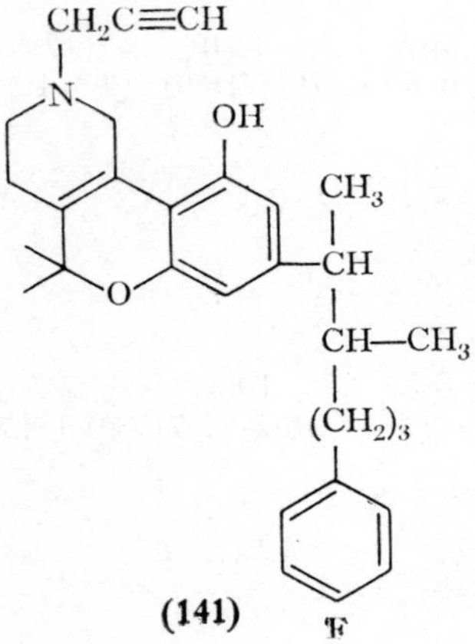

(141)

—	4·4	8·3
	(0·7–9·5)	(3·8–14·9)

TABLE 15—*continued*

Analgesic activity of selected nitrogen and sulfur analogs[a,b,c]

Structure (compound number)	Hot plate[d] (mouse)	Anti-writing[e] (mouse)	Tail flick[f] (rat)
		ED_{50} mg kg^{-1}, po	

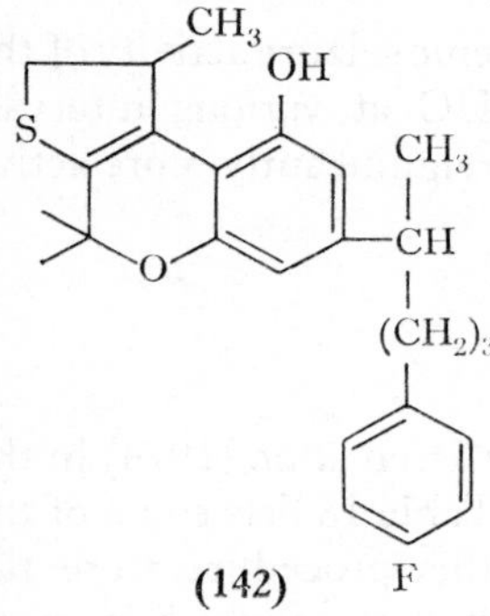

(142)

For compound (142): — , 8·4 (3·1–14·0), —

(143)

For compound (143): — , 7·2 (2·3–12·2), —

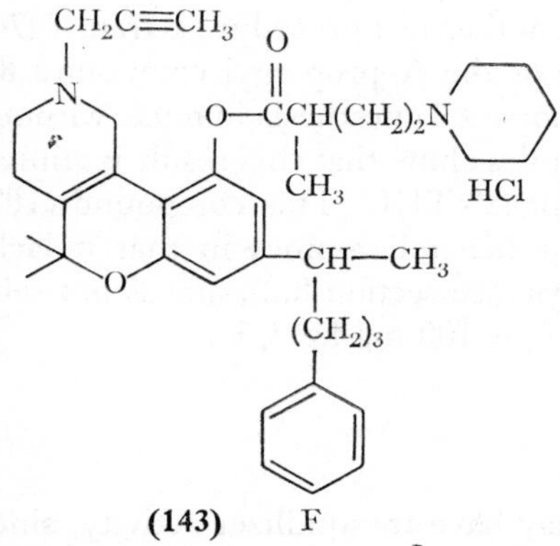

[a] Pars *et al.* (1976).
[b] Razdan *et al.* (1976a, 1976b).
[c] Winn *et al.* (1976).
[d] Harris and Pierson (1962).
[e] Sigmund *et al.* (1957).
[f] D'Amour and Smith (1941).

These reports suggested the possibility of narcotic antagonist activity for the heterocyclic compounds. Thus, in 1974, Harris and Dewey studied a series of nitrogen and sulfur analogs for their ability to antagonize morphine analgesia in the mouse tail-flick procedure. A number of these compounds, including the N-propargyl analog, **84**, showed a prolonged duration of action, with narcotic antagonist-like activity lasting as long as 7 days following a single administration. Results are shown in Table 16.

8.3   ANTICONVULSANT ACTIVITY

Plotnikoff et al. (1974, 1976) compared the audiogenic seizure activity of the N-propargyl compound **84**, DMHP and Δ^9-THC at various intervals following administration. Both DMHP and **84** are significantly more active than Δ^9-THC in this procedure (Table 17).

8.4   SEDATIVE-HYPNOTIC ACTIVITY

A number of heterocyclic analogs were studied by Dren et al. (1974) in the cat and found to increase total sleep time (TST). Table 18 lists some of the active compounds. Most active compounds in this procedure were the bicyclic nitrogen analog **96** and a sulfur analog **129**, both of which increase TST without affecting REM sleep. In another test procedure (Dren, 1974, Table 19) the water-soluble derivative of the N-propargyl compound **84** was shown to potentiate significantly thiopental anesthesia in mice, without affecting thiopental toxicity. Dren's studies show that this result is similar to the findings of Sofia et al. (1974) for Δ^9-THC. This compound (**107**, Table 19) differs from barbiturates or benzodiazepines in that it lacks narcotic-like abuse potential in monkeys (see section 8.2), and is not self-administered by monkeys at doses of 10 or 100 mg kg^{-1}, iv.

8.5   TRANQUILLIZER ACTIVITY

Table 20 lists several analogs which may have tranquillizer activity, since they are active in antagonizing methamphetamine-induced motor activity in the rat (Razdan, 1974).

Clark et al. (1974) found that the pyridyl compound **105** (Table 6) produced a marked depression of locomotor activity, hypothermia and catalepsy, and potentiated barbiturate hypnosis. This analog also reduced conditioned avoidance in rats and reduced aggression in isolated mice.

In a baboon colony with a social hierarchy, compound **105** reduced aggressiveness caused by the intrusion of a human (Clark et al., 1974). In

TABLE 16

Narcotic antagonist properties of selected nitrogen and sulfur analogs[a]

Compound number	R	R_1	R_2	Route	% Antagonism[b] 2-Day	7-Day
84	$CH_2C\equiv CH$	H	C_9H_{19}	po	43	NT[c]
85	$CH_2C\equiv CH$	$COCH_3$	C_9H_{19}	po	33	22
144	$CH_2C_6H_5$	H	$CH(CH_3)_2$	po	65	76
145	$CONH_2$	H	C_9H_{19}	po	46	72

120 (XIV)				po	43	39
				sc	38	NT

	X	Y		Route	2-Day	7-Day
127 (XVIII)	X	Y			31	30
124 (XVII)	S	CH_2		po	35	42
				sc		
	CH_2	S		po	41	20

[a] Harris et al. (1974).
[b] 1 mg kg^{-1} given 2 or 7 days prior to morphine (10 mg kg^{-1}, sc).
[c] Not tested.

TABLE 17

Comparison of the audiogenic seizure activity of compound **84**, DMHP and Δ^9-THC[a]

Structure (compound numbers)	ED_{50} 1 h[b] mg kg^{-1} (95% CL)	ED_{50} 4 h[b] mg kg^{-1} (95% CL)	ED_{50} 24 h[b] mg kg^{-1} (95% CL)
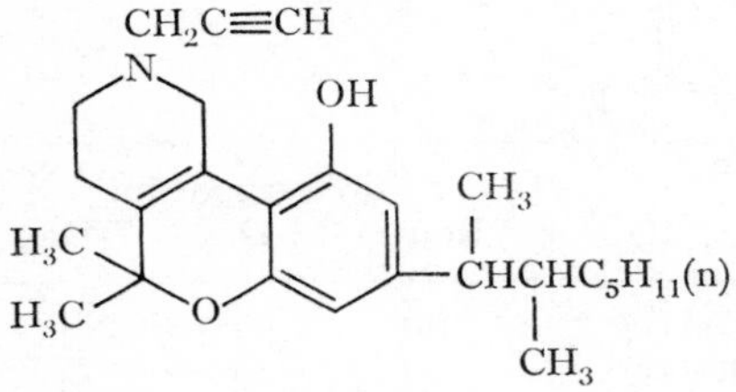 **(84)**	17·1 (9·0–35·0)	11·0 (6·4–19·6)	$ED_{50}=100$
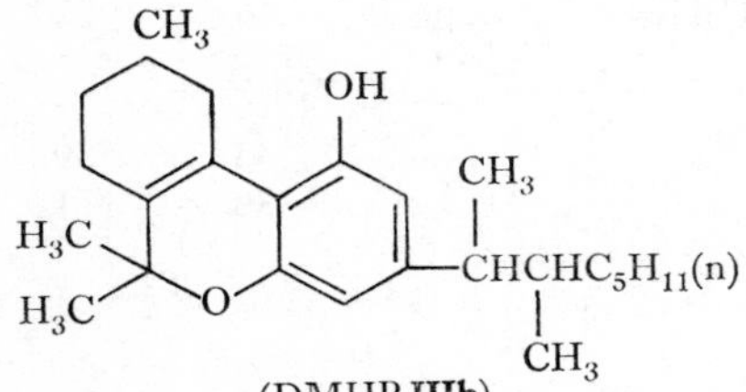 (DMHP **IIIb**)	6·7 (2·1–11·0)	2·9 (1·8–4·9)	15·1 (8·2–26·3)
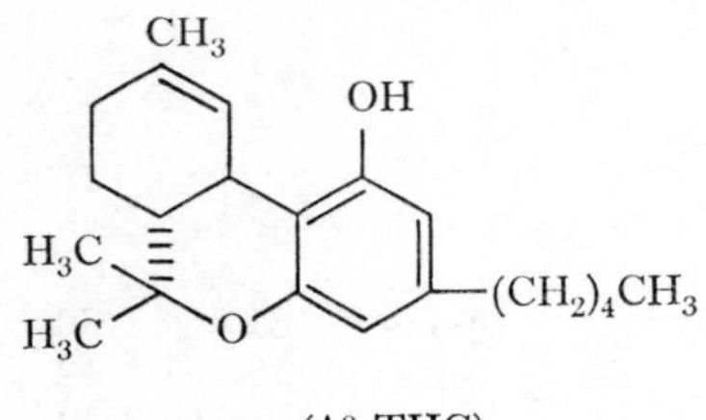 (Δ^9-THC)	5·0 (2·4–7·7)	38·8 (29·1–49·3)	$ED_{50}=100$

[a] Plotnikoff *et al.* (1974, 1976).
[b] Oral dose at which 50 per cent of the animals are protected from hindlimb tonic extension.

TABLE 18

Sedative hypnotic actions of selected nitrogen and sulfur analogs[a]

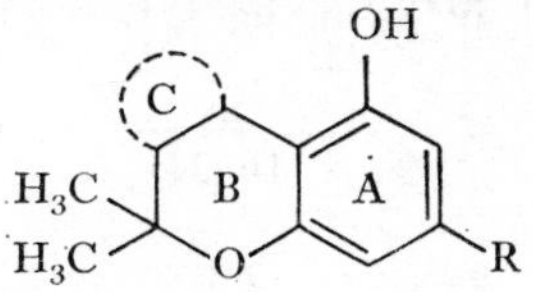

Compound number	C-Ring	R[c]	Dose (mg kg^{-1}, po)	% Increase in TST[b]
84	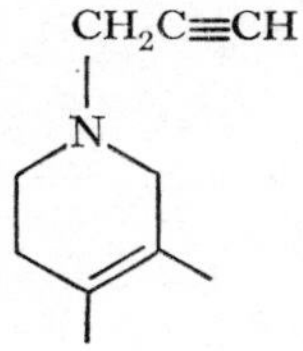 CH$_2$C≡CH N	C$_9$H$_{19}$	0·5	+44
96	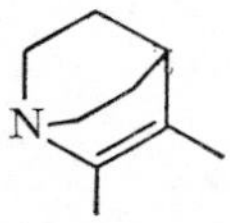 N	C$_9$H$_{19}$	0·5	+71
120	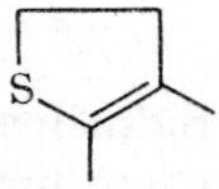 S	C$_9$H$_{19}$	1·0	+30
129	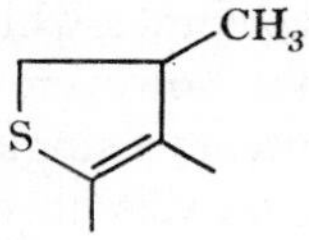 CH$_3$ S	C$_9$H$_{19}$	0·5	+108
124	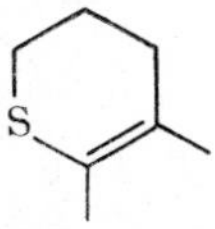 S	C$_9$H$_{19}$	0·5	−3

[a] Dren et al. (1974).
[b] Total sleep time, EEG in cats.
[c] C$_9$H$_{19}$, CH(CH$_3$)CH(CH$_3$)(CH$_2$)$_4$CH$_3$.

TABLE 19

Potentiation of thiopental anesthesia in mice[a]

Compound number	Pre-treatment dose mg kg^{-1}, iv	Thiopental ED$_{50}$ mg kg^{-1}, iv	Thiopental LD$_{50}$ mg kg^{-1}, iv	Therapeutic index
None	—	20 (16–24)	76 (72–80)	3·8
107[b]	1[c]	5·6 (4·8–6·6)	74 (68–81)	13·2
107[b]	5[c]	4·5 (3·6–5·7)	73 (68–79)	16·2

[a] Dren et al. (1974).

[b]

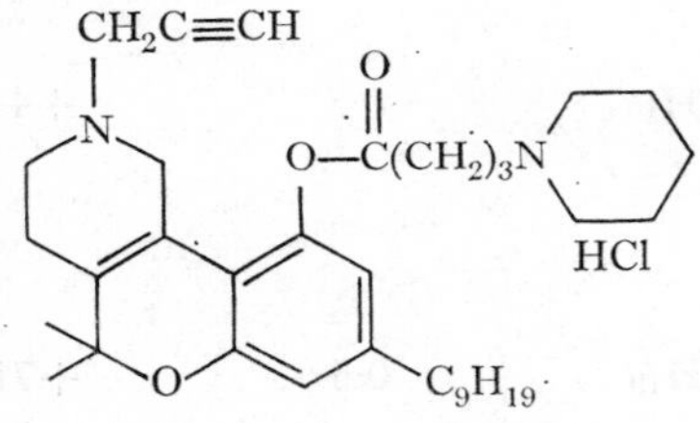

[c] 15 minutes pretreatment time.

isolated mice territorial aggression was reduced. Using a Sidman avoidance procedure in rats **105** reduced all responses at doses where the animals were not sedated. This is in contrast to the benzodiazepines which cause this only at sedative doses. Like the benzodiazepines however, **105** was found to block polysynaptic reflexes. In human volunteers a single dose of 10 mg of compound **105** caused ataxia. No hypotension was observed. In

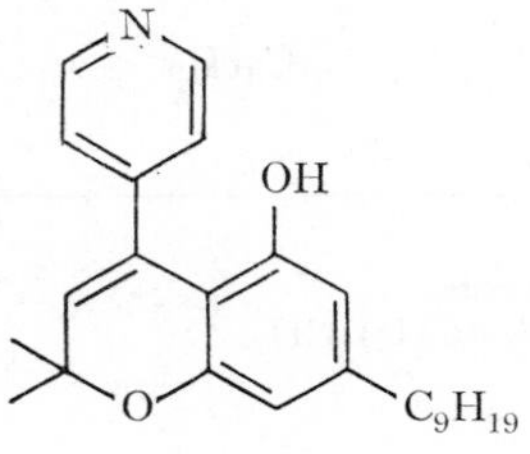

(105)

TABLE 20

Tranquillizer activity of selected nitrogen and sulfur analogs[a]

Structure compound number	Dose mg kg^{-1}, po	% Reversal of meth- amphetamine (rats)	% Reversal of fighting mice
(DMHP (**IIIb**))	5·0 10·0	−62 —	— −92
(Δ⁹-THC)	10·0	—	−68
(84)	10·0	−50	−62
(129)	10·0	−91	−62

TABLE 20 —*continued*

Tranquillizer activity of selected nitrogen and sulfur analogs[a]

Structure compound number	Dose mg kg^{-1}, po	% Reversal of meth- amphetamine (rats)	% Reversal of fighting mice
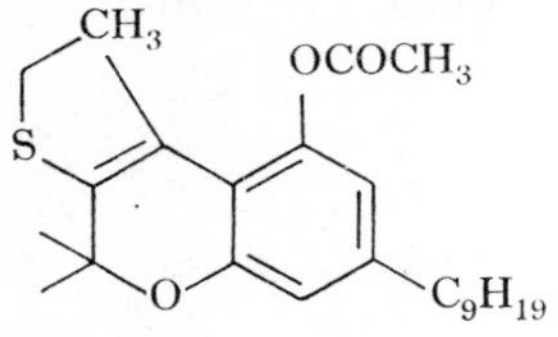 **(146)**	10·0	−70	−89
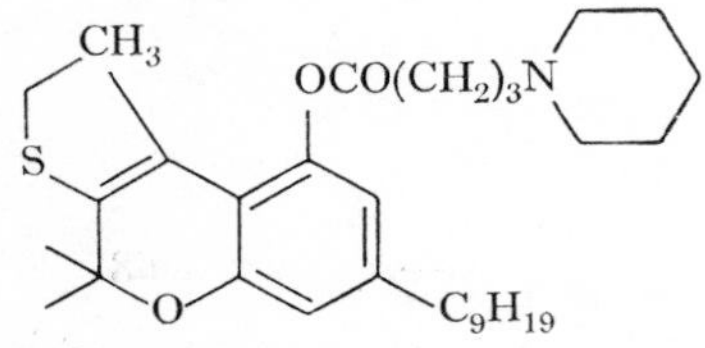 **(147)**	10·0	−88	−100

[a] Razdan *et al.* (1974).

another study in which 5 mg per person per day was given this analog suppressed REM sleep, and caused impaired consciousness. Its activity was described as lying somewhere between the major and the minor tranquillizers.

8.6   CARDIOVASCULAR ACTIVITY

Many of the heterocyclic benzopyrans have demonstrated significant antihypertensive activity in genetically hypertensive rats. Studies to date indicate that this type of activity is accompanied by CNS behavioral effects. However, separation of these two actions has been observed in humans (see Lemberger *et al.*, 1974) with DMHP.

In 1976 Pars *et al.* described some cardiovascular effects of compound **84** and compared it with DMHP (**IIIb**), viz:

Cardiovascular, iv MED   **84**   DMHP
Anesthetized cat, blood pressure and respiration   0·025   0·025
Unanesthetized dog, blood pressure only   0·1   0·4

The piperidino analog **136** was described in detail by Fake *et al.* (1974).

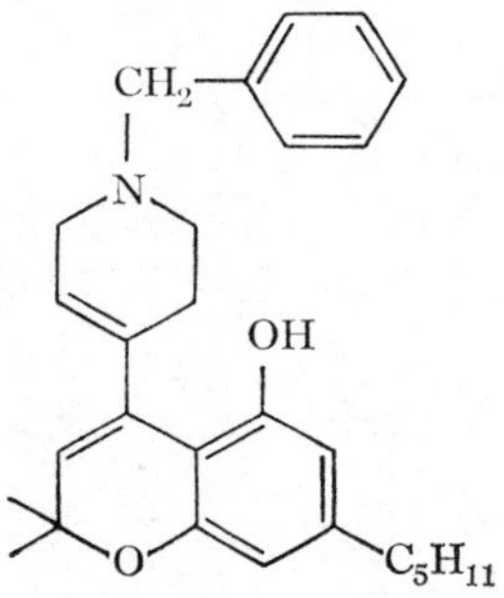

(136)

Using the nephrectomized DOCA-treated hypertensive rat as a model, this agent was active at 100 mg kg^{-1} po, whereas symptoms of CNS behavioral effects were not evident until 800 mg kg^{-1} po had been administered. A structure-activity study of this series revealed **136** as one of the most effective compounds studied (Table 21).

8.7 GASTROINTESTINAL ACTIVITY

The inhibition of gastric motility is also characteristic of some of the nitrogen analogs (Pars *et al.*, 1976). Table 22 shows the activity of some of the most active members of the series. The propargyl compound (**84**) shows the most significant activity in this procedure. The others show effects at such high doses that marked CNS effects occur.

9 Conclusions

9.1 OVERALL STRUCTURE-ACTIVITY RELATIONSHIPS

The synthesis and demonstration of central nervous system (CNS) activity for a wide variety of carbocyclic, and nitrogen- and sulfur-containing benzopyrans has resulted in an expansion of the structure-activity (SAR) conclusions originally put forth by Roger Adams and his co-workers (1949).

TABLE 21

Hypotensive activity of various pyridyl analogs[a]

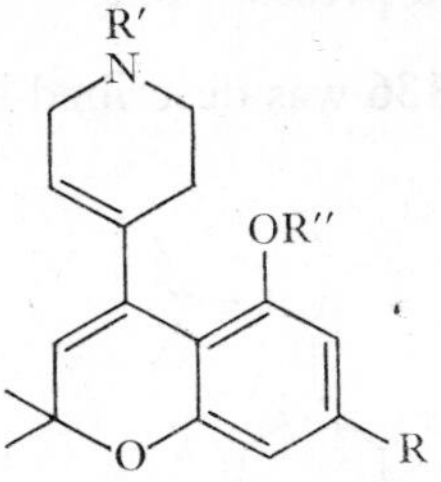

R'	R	R''	% Fall in blood pressure at 100 mg kg^{-1}, po	
			4 h	24 h
$CH_2C_6H_5$	C_4H_9	H	16	6
$CH_2C_6H_5$ (136)	C_5H_{11}	H	23	17
$CH_2C_6H_5$	C_6H_{13}	H	15	26
$CH_2C_6H_5$	C_7H_{15}	H	10	9
$CH_2C_6H_5$	$CH(CH_3)C_5H_{11}$	H	17	17
$CH_2C_6H_5$	$CH(CH_3)CH(CH_3)C_5H_{11}$	H	8	0
CH_3	C_5H_{11}	H	5	11
C_2H_5	C_5H_{11}	H	9	0
C_3H_7	C_5H_{11}	H	8	12
$CH_2CH=CH_2$	C_5H_{11}	H	20	25
$CH_2CH_2C_6H_5$	C_5H_{11}	H	24	27
$CH_2C_6H_5$	C_5H_{11}	CH_3	11	4
$CH_2C_6H_5$	C_5H_{11}	CH_3CO	12	11
$CH_2C_6H_5$	C_5H_{11}	$Et_2N(CH_2)_3CO$	16	11

[a] Clarke et al. (1974).

By using dog ataxia as the principal model of activity, Adams found that characteristic effects are observed when R^2 is a highly branched alkyl with the 1,2-dimethylheptyl showing optimum activity. He further showed that when R^1 is gem-dimethyl, activity is greater than when these (R^1) substituents are higher alkyl, that reduction of the double bond in the C-ring retained activity, and that ring C could be contracted, expanded, or even

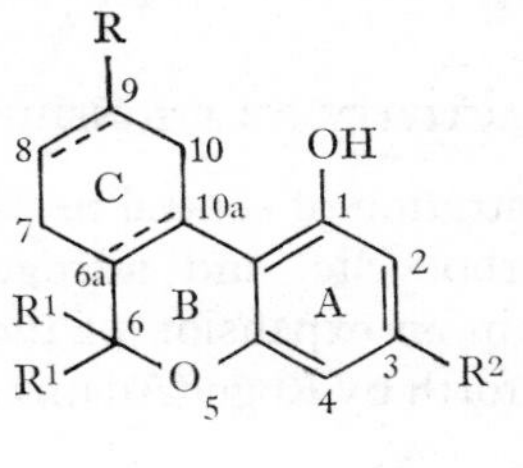

TABLE 22

Antidiarrheal activity of selected nitrogen analogs[a,b]

Structure (compound numbers)	Dose (mg kg^{-1}, po)	% Inhibition (charcoal meal)
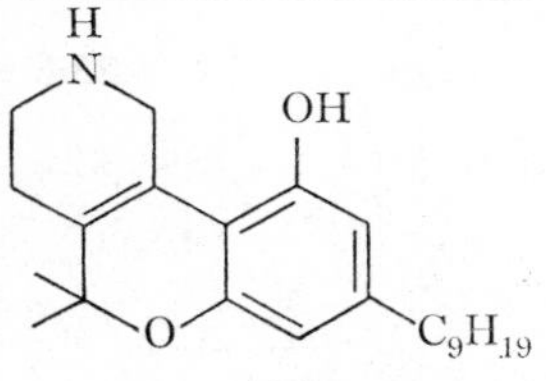 (67)	200 100	23·4 25·4
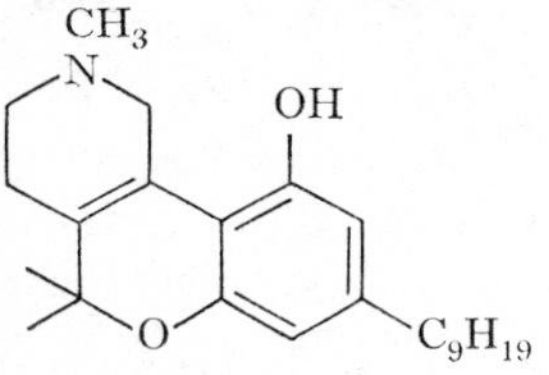 (64)	200 100 10	35·0. 27·4 18·6
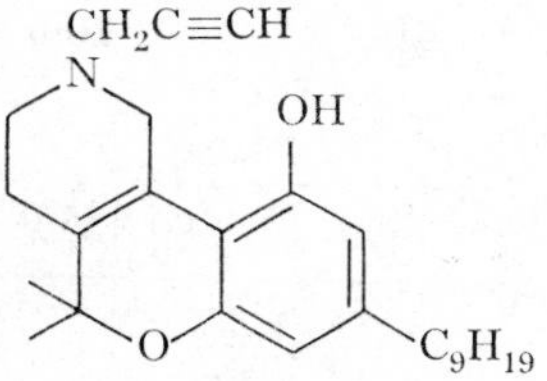 (84)	100 10 2·0 1·0 0·1	66·9 49·6 48·8 39·4 21·0
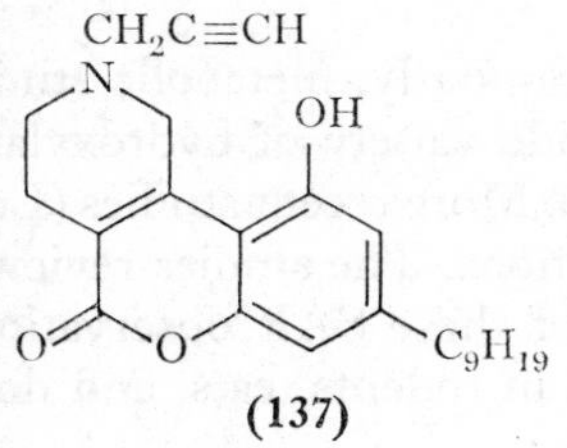 (137)	10	26·1

TABLE 22—*continued*

Antidiarrheal activity of selected nitrogen analogs[a,b]

Structure (compound numbers)	Dose (mg kg^{-1}, po)	% Inhibition (charcoal meal)
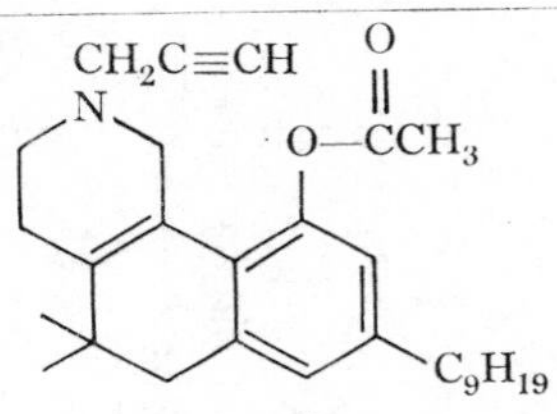 (85)	20	23·5
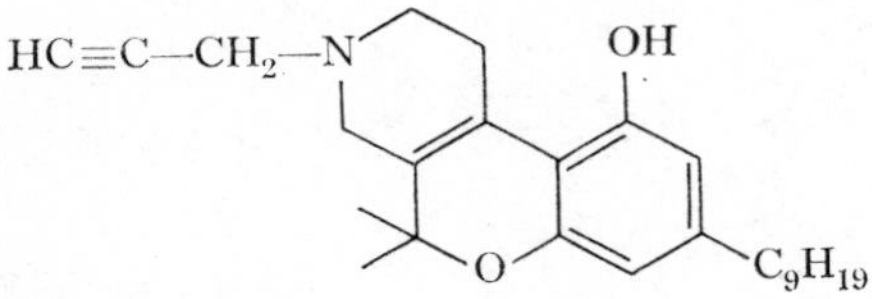 (138)	100	31·6
DMHP	100	36·3
	10	10·0
Diphenoxylate (Lomotil®)	20·0	53·0

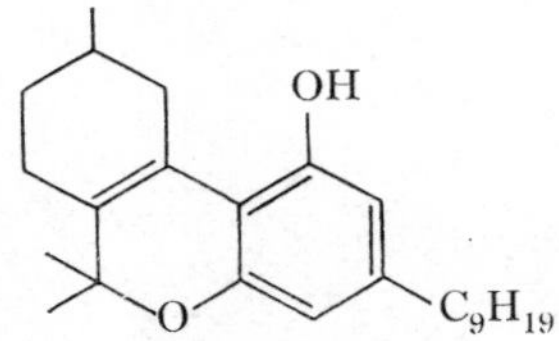

[a] Pars *et al.* (1976).
[b] Pars *et al.*, unpublished work.

opened without entirely eliminating activity. Similarly, metabolic studies have shown that activity is retained with a wide variety of hydroxylated benzopyrans (see, for example, Wall *et al.*, 1971). More recent studies (Loev *et al.*, 1974) have expanded these SAR observations. The studies reviewed in this chapter have also enlarged the scope of these SAR observations. Thus, based on CNS pharmacological profiles in rodents, cats, and dogs, the SAR picture can be summarized as follows:

1. The C-ring in cannabinoids can be substituted by a variety of nitrogen and sulfur-containing rings (tetrahydropyridines, dihydro-

pyrroles, thiopyrans, dihydrothiophenes, etc.) without loss of CNS activity.

2. The 1,2-dimethylheptyl side chain (R^2) produces potent CNS effects as the case with Adams' compounds. Similarly, p-fluorophenyl-alkyl (R^2) aromatic side chains also give good activity.

3. Substituents in close proximity to the phenolic OH in the aromatic A-ring have significant effect on activity, viz.

    a. The OH at position C-1 is in itself necessary for CNS activity.

    b. Methyl substituents in the C-ring significantly alter the activity of both carbocyclic and (C-ring) heterocyclic benzopyrans, particularly in the case of five-membered C-rings.

    c. Esterification of the phenol retains activity and in some carbocyclic as well as heterocyclic structures can lead to greater selectivity of action. Etherification of the phenol eliminates activity.

4. Replacement of one of the R^1 substituents in the B-ring with and hydroxymethyl group retains activity.

5. Oxidation of the C-ring, e.g. the oxo derivative at position C-7, retains CNS activity.

6. In both carbocyclic and heterocyclic analogs, opening the pyran ring (at positions C-5 and C-6) generally decreases activity. An exception is compound **68** (Table 6), where activity is approximately equiactive with DMHP (**IIIb**).

7. With the nitrogen and sulfur analogs, the most active CNS agents, including analgesics, are obtained when the hetero-atom is in a phenethyl orientation, e.g. inserted in place of C-7 or C-9.

8. Planarity of the C-ring is not a necessary criterion for activity. See, for example, the quinuclidine analog **106** (Table 7) and the benzoxocine compounds **65–67** (Table 6).

9.2 MECHANISM OF ACTION

On the basis of biochemical and pharmacology studies carried out to date with both Δ^9-THC and some of the heterocyclic (C-ring) analogs, it is already clear that these cannabinoid-like structures have unique profiles of action, unlike any other class of drugs known.

Biochemical and drug–drug interaction studies have shown the following: cannabinoids inhibit prostaglandin synthesis, potentiate the pressor effects of endogenous amines like norepinephrine, and act synergistically with the stimulant effects of amphetamine. Furthermore, they potentiate the hypotensive effects of arachidonic acid; they potentiate dopaminergic agents such as apomorphine, ephedrine and amantadine, and are themselves antagonized in some animal procedures, by neuroleptics.

Although there is some evidence to suggest that Δ^9-THC produces many of its actions by interacting with prostaglandins, cannabinoids are not aspirin-like. They do exhibit analgesic effects in animals, some interact with and/or block the analgesic action of morphine, and share some other properties of narcotics (e.g. antidiarrheal activity). However, they are not narcotic-like in the rat tail-flick test, do not support morphine dependence in monkeys and are not themselves antagonized by classical narcotic antagonists. Clearly, more work needs to be carried out to establish the mechanism of action for Δ^9-THC and the heterocyclic analogs.

9.3 THERAPEUTIC INDICATIONS

Animal studies to date, particularly among the nitrogen-containing analogs and carbocyclic derivatives, clearly point to therapeutic potential in the area of analgesics and anticonvulsants. Preliminary studies in man have already given some indication of the analgesic potential in this field, both with Δ^9-THC (Brunk *et al.*, 1974) and with a water-soluble nitrogen analog known as SP-106 (compound **107**, Table 7) (Houde and Wallenstein, 1976). The extensive animal studies of Karler *et al.* (1974), Consroe *et al.* (1973), and Plotnikoff (1976) on cannabidiol show a good separation of anticonvulsant properties from other effects. The cardiovascular properties of many of the newer analogs are of potential interest. The findings of Lemberger *et al.* (1974) and Sidell *et al.* (1973) showing hypotensive effects for DMHP, at doses where no CNS effects occur, is noteworthy and will undoubtedly be pursued. Similarly the findings of Lemberger and Rowe (1975) on the potential use of a compound known as Nabilone as a tranquilizing agent is also noteworthy. Other clinical indications suggest possible use as a sedative-hypnotic, as an antiglaucoma agent, and for anti-asthmatic activity. Animal pharmacology studies have also given some indication of therapeutic utility as an antidiarrheal agent. Preliminary reports have also shown certain cannabinoids to have anticancer and immunosuppressant activity.

References

Aaron, H. S. and Ferguson, C. P. (1968). *Journal of Organic Chemistry*, **33**, 684.

Adams, R., Loewe, S., Smith, C. M. and McPhee, W. D. (1942). *Journal of the American Chemical Society*, **64**, 694.

Adams, R., Harfenist, M. and Loewe, S. (1949). *Journal of the American Chemical Society*, **71**, 1624, and earlier papers cited therein.

POTENTIAL CANNABINOID-DERIVED AGENTS

Anderson, P. F., Jackson, D. M. and Chesher, G. B. (1974). *Journal of Pharmacy and Pharmacology*, **26**, 136.
Anker, R. M. and Cook, A. H. (1946). *Journal of the Chemical Society*, **58**.
Archer, R. A. (1974). *In* "Annual Reports in Medicinal Chemistry", (Ed. R. V. Heinzelman), vol. 9, p. 253. Academic Press, New York and London.
Askew, W. E. and Ho, B. T. (1974). *Experientia*, **30**, 879.
Barratt, E. S. and Adams, P. M. (1973). *Journal of Biology and Psychiatry*, **6**, 207.
Barratt, E. S., Beaver, W. and White, R. (1974). *Journal of Biology and Psychiatry*, **8**, 47.
Beaconsfield, P., Ginsburg, J. and Rainsbury, R. (1972). *New England Journal of Medicine*, **287**, 209.
Benmouyal, E., Côte, G. and Morin, Y. (1971). *Clinical Research*, **14**, 758.
Bergel, F. (1965). *In* "Hashish: Its Chemistry and Pharmacology", Ciba Foundation Study Group No. 21 (Ed. G. E. W. Wolstenholme), p. 81. Churchill, London.
Bicher, H. I. and Mechoulam, R. (1968). *Archives Internationales de Pharmacodynamie et de Thérapie*, **172**, 1.
Birmingham (1973). *British Journal of Pharmacology*, **48**, 169.
Boggan, W. O., Steele, R. A. and Freedman, D. X. (1973). *Psychopharmacologia*, **29**, 101–106.
Bose, G. C., Saifi, and Bhagwat, A. W. (1971). *Archives Internationales de Pharmacodynamie et de Thérapie*, **147**, 291.
Boyd, E. S., Boyd, E. H., Muchmore, J. S. and Brown, L. E. (1971). *Journal of Pharmacology and Experimental Therapeutics*, **176**, 480.
Bright, T. P., Kiplinger, C. F., Brown, D., Phillips, U. and Forny, R. B. (1971). National Academy of Science, National Research Council Committee on Problems of Drug Dependence, Annual Report, p. 1737.
Brimblecombe, R. W. (1973). Psychotomimetic Drugs: Biochemistry and Pharmacology. *In* "Advances in Drug Research" (Ed. A. B. Simmonds), vol. 7, p. 165. Academic Press, London and New York.
Brown, D. M. (1973). *Pharmacologist*, **15**, 200.
Brunk, S. F., Noyes, R., Avery, D. H. and Canter, A. (1974). *Journal of Clinical Pharmacology*, **15**, 664.
Burstein, S. and Raz, A. (1972). *Prostaglandins*, **2**, 369.
Burstein, S., Levin, E. and Varanelli, C. (1973). *Biochemical Pharmacology*, **22**, 2905.
Buxbaum, D. M. (1972). *Psychopharmacologia*, **25**, 275.
Buxbaum, D., Sanders-Bush, E. and Efron, D. M. (1969). *Federation Proceedings*, **28**, 735.
Cahn, R. S. (1933). *Journal of the Chemical Society*. p. 1400, and earlier papers cited therein.
Caldwell, B. B., Bailey, K., Anderson, G. and Paul, C. (1974). *Toxicology and Applied Pharmacology*, **29**, 77.
Carder, B. and Olsen, J. (1972) *Physiology and Behaviour*, **8**, 599.
Cardillo, B., Merlini, L. and Servi (1973). *Gazzetta Chimica Italiana*, **103**, 127.
Carlini, E. A. and Masur, J. (1969). *Life Sciences*, **8**, 607.
Carlini, E. A., Leite, J., Tannhauser, M. and Berarci, A. C. (1973). *Journal of Pharmacy and Pharmacology*, **25**, 664.
Cavero, I., Solomon, J., Buckley, J. P. and Jandhyala, B. S. (1972a). 5th International Congress of Pharmacology, No. 228 (Abstract).

Cavero, I., Buckley, J. P. and Jandhyala, B. S. (1972b). *European Journal of Pharmacology*, **19**, 301.
Chesher, G B., Dahl, C. J., Everingham, M., Jackson, D. M., Marchant, W. H. and Starmer, G. A. (1973). *British Journal of Pharmacology*, **49**, 588.
Chesher, G. B., Jackson, D. M. and Starmer, G. A. (1974). *British Journal of Pharmacology*, **50**, 593
Chiang, T. S. and Thomas, R. P. (1972). 5th International Congress on Pharmacology, No. 243 (Abstract).
Clark, S. C., Greene, C., Karr, G. W. and MacCannell, K. L. and Milstein, S. L. (1974). *Canadian Journal of Physiology and Pharmacology*, **52**, 706.
Clark, J., Clark, M. and Cook, A. (1974). Symposium on "Approaches to Centrally Acting Drugs Derived from the Cannabinol Nucleus", presented at the 68th American Chemical Society Meeting, Atlantic City, New Jersey (Abstract).
Cohen, S. and Stillman, R. (eds) (1976). "Therapeutic Aspects of Marihuana". Plenum Press, New York.
Consroe, P. F., Man, D. P., Chin, L. and Picchioni, A. L. (1973). *Life Sciences*, **13**, 429.
Consroe, P. F., Man, D. P., Chin, L. and Picchioni, A. L. (1973). *Journal of Pharmacy and Pharmacology*, **25**, 764.
Cousens, K. and DiMascio, A. (1973). *Psychopharmacologia*, **33**, 355.
Crowshaw, K. and Hardman, H. F. (1974). *Federation Proceedings*, **33**, 1847 (Abstract).
Cushman, M. and Castagnoli, Jr., N. (1973). *Journal of Organic Chemistry*, **38**, 440.
Cushman, M. and Castagnoli, Jr., N. (1974). *Journal of Organic Chemistry*, **39**, 1546.
Dagirmanjian, R. and Boyd, E. S. (1962). *Journal of Pharmacology and Experimental Therapeutics*, **135**, 25.
D'Amour, F. E. and Smith, D. L. (1941). *Journal of Pharmacology and Experimental Therapeutics*, **72**, 74.
Davies, B. H., Radcliffe, S., Seaton, A. and Graham, J. D. P. (1975). *Thorax*, **30**, 80.
Davies, O. L., Raventos, J. and Walpole, A. L. (1946). *British Journal of Pharmacology*, **1**, 255
Davis, J. A. and Ramsey, H. H. (1949) *Federation Proceedings*, **8**, 284 (Abstract).
Deneau, G. A. and Seevers, M. H. (1966). National Academy of Science/National Research Council, Committee on Problems of Drug Dependence, Annual Report, Addendum 2.
Dewey, W. L., Harris, L. S., Howes, J. F., and Kennedy J. S. (1970a). *Pharmacologist*, **11**, 278 (Abstract).
Dewey, W. L., Harris, L. S. Howes, J. F., Kennedy, J. S., Granchelli, F. E., Pars, H. G. and Razdan, R. K. (1970b). *Nature*, **226**, 1265.
Dewey, W. L., Harris, L. S., Ford, R. D., Frankenheim, J. M., McMillan, D. E. and Turk, R. (1971). National Academy of Sciences/National Research Council, Committee on Problems of Drug Dependence, Annual Report, 1092.
Dixit, V., Sharma, V. and Lohiya, N. (1974). *European Journal of Pharmacology*, **26**, 111.
Dolby, T. W. and Kleinsmith, L. J. (1974). *Biochemical Pharmacology*, **23**, 1817.
Domino, E. F. (1971). *Annals of the New York Academy of Sciences*, **191**, 166.
Dren, A. T. (1974). Symposium on "Approaches to Centrally Acting Drugs

Derived From the Cannabinoid Nucleus", presented at the 68th American Chemical Society Meeting, Atlantic City, New Jersey (Abstract).

Dren, A. T., Plotnikoff, N. P., Dodge, P. W. and Terris, B. Z. (1974). *Pharmacologist*, **16**, No. 090 (Abstract).

Dubinsky, B., Robichaud, R. C. and Goldberg, M. E. (1973). *Pharmacology*, **9**, 204.

Fake, C. S., Gardner, T., Mellon, T. and Miller, D. (1974). Symposium on "Approaches to Centrally Acting Drugs Derived from the Cannabinoid Nucleus", presented at the 68th American Chemical Society Meeting, Atlantic City, New Jersey (Abstract).

Forney, R. B. and Kiplinger, G. F. (1971). *Annuals of the New York Academy of Sciences*, **191**, 74.

Frank, I. R., Hepler, R. S., Epps, L., Ungerleider, J. T. and Szara, S. (1972). 5th International Congress on Pharmacology, No. 426 (Abstract).

Freemon, F. R. (1974). *Psychopharmacologia*, **35**, 39.

Friedman, E. and Gershon, S. (1972). 5th International Congress on Pharmacology, No. 439 (Abstract).

Friedman, E. and Gershon, S. (1974). *Psychopharmacologia*, **39**, 193.

Gallagher, D. W., Sanders-Bush, E. and Sulser, F. (1972). *Psychopharmacologia*, **26**, 337.

Garratini, A. (1965). *In* "Hashish: Its Chemistry and Pharmacology", Ciba Foundation Study Group No. 21 (Ed. G. E. W. Wolstenholme), pp. 70–82. Churchill, London.

Garriott, J. C., Forney, R. B., Huges, F. W. and Richards, A. B. (1968). *Archives Internationales de Pharmacodynamie et de Thérapie*, **171**, 425.

Graham, J. D. P., Lewis, M. J. and Williams, J. (1974). *British Journal of Pharmacology*, **52**, 446P.

Greb, W., Bieniek and Korte, F. (1972). *Tetrahedron Letters*, 545.

Green, K. and Podos, S. M. (1974). *Investigative Ophthalmology*, **13**, 422.

Grilly, D., Ferraro, D. P. and Braude, M. C. (1974). *Pharmacology*, **11**, 304.

Hardman, H. F., Domino, E. F., Woods, L. A. and Seevers, M. H. (1970). *University of Michigan Medical Center Journal*, **36**, 238.

Hardman, H. F., Domino, E. F. and Seevers, M. M. (1971). *Pharmacological Reviews*, **23**, 295.

Harris, L. S. and Dewey, W. L. (1974). Symposium on "Approaches to Centrally Acting Drugs Derived from the Cannabinoid Nucleus", presented at the 68th American Chemical Society Meeting, Atlantic City, New Jersey (Abstract).

Harris, L. S. and Pierson, A. K. (1962). National Academy of Sciences/National Research Council Committee on Problems of Drug Dependence, Annual Report, Addendum 1.

Harris, L. S., Razdan, R. K., Dewey, W. L. and Pars, H. G. (1967). *Chimica Therapeutica*, **2**, 167.

Harris, L. S., Munson, A. E., Friedman, M. A. and Dewey, D. L. (1974). *Pharmacologist*, **16**, 390 (Abstract).

Hepler, R. S. and Frank, I. R. (1971). *Journal of the American Medical Association*, **217**, 1392.

Hill, S. Y., Schwin, R., Goodwin, D. W. and Powell, B. J. (1974). *Journal of Pharmacology and Experimental Therapeutics*, **188**, 415.

Himmelsbach, C. K. (1944). *Southern Medical Journal*, **37**, 26.

Hine, B., Friedman, E., Torrelio, M. and Gershon, S. (1975). *Neuropharmacology*, **14**, 607.

Ho, B. T., Taylor, D., Fritchie, D. E., Englert, L. M. and McIssac, W. M. (1972). *Brain Research*, **38**, 163.
Ho, B. T., Taylor, D. and Englert, L. F. (1973). *Research Communications in Chemical Pathology and Pharmacology*, **5**, 851.
Hollister, L. E. (1973). *Experientia*, **29**, 825.
Hollister, L. E. (1974). *Pharmacology*, **11**, 3.
Hollister, L. E. and Gillespie, H. K. (1967). *Clinical Pharmacology and Therapeutics*, **14**, 353.
Hollister, L. E., Richards, R. K. and Gillespie, H. K. (1968). *Clinical Pharmacology and Therapeutics*, **9**, 783.
Holmes and Horton (1967). *In* "Prostaglandin Symposium of The Worcester Foundation For Experimental Biology" (Eds Ramwell and Shaw), p. 21.
Holtzman, D., Lovell, R. A., Jaffe, J. and Freedman, D. X. (1969). *Science*, **163**, 1464.
Hoops, J. W., Bader, H. and Biel, J. H. (1968). *Journal of Organic Chemistry*, **33**, 2995.
Houde, R. W. and Wallenstein, S. (1976). Personal communication.
Houry, S. and Mechoulam, R. (1975). *Journal of Medicinal Chemistry*, **18**, 951.
Houry, S., Mechoulam, R., Fowler, P. J., Macko, E. and Loev, B. (1974). *Journal of Medicinal Chemistry*, **17**, 287.
Howes, J. F. (1970). *Pharmacologist*, No. 324 (Abstract).
Howes, J. F. (1973a). *Research Communications in Chemical Pathology and Pharmacology*, **6**, 895.
Howes, J. F. (1973b). *Research Communications in Chemical Pathology and Pharmacology*, **6**, 901.
Howes, J. F. and Osgood, P. F. (1974a). *Neuropharmacology*, **13**, 1109.
Howes, J. F. and Osgood, P. F. (1974b). *Pharmacologist*, **16**, No. 389.
Howes, J. F. and Osgood, P. F. (1975). Unpublished work.
Indian Hemp Drug Commission Reports. Simla, India (1893–1894).
Irwin, S. (1964). *In* "Animal and Clinical Pharmacologic Technique in Drug Evaluation" (Eds J. A. Nodine and P. E. Siegler), pp. 36–54. Year Book Publishers, Chicago, Illinois.
Isbell, H., Gorodetzky, C. W., Jasinski, D., Claussen, U., Spulack, F. V. and Korte, F. (1967). *Psychopharmacologia*, **11**, 184.
Izquierdo, I. and Tannhauser, M. (1973). *Journal of Pharmacy and Pharmacology*, **25**, 916.
Johnson, R. J. and Wiersema, V. (1974a). *Research Communications in Chemical Pathology and Pharmacology*, **7**, 613.
Johnson, R. J. and Wiersema, V. (1974b). *Research Communications in Chemical Pathology and Pharmacology*, **8**, 393.
Johnson, S. and Domino, E. P. (1971). *Clinical Pharmacology and Therapeutics*, **12**, 762.
Kales, A., Hanley, J., Richler, W., Kanas, N., Baker, M. and Goring, P. (1972). *Psychophysiology*, **9**, 92.
Karbowski, M., Jayoda, A., Dewey, W. L. and Harris, L. S. (1975). *Pharmacologist*, **17**, 254.
Karler, R., Cely, W. and Turkanis, S. A. (1973). *Life Sciences*, **13**, 1527.
Karler, R., Cely, W. and Turkanis, S. A. (1974a). *Research Communications in Chemical Pathology and Pharmacology*, **1**, 353.

Karler, R., Cely, W. and Turkanis, S. A. (1974b). *Research Communications in Chemical Pathology and Pharmacology*, **9**, 23.

Kaymakcalan, S. and Deneau, G. A. (1971). *Pharmacologist*, **13**, 247.

Kaymakcalan, S., Turker, K. and Turker, M. (1974). *Psychopharmacologia*, **35**, 123.

Keats, A. S. and Romagnoli, A. (1974). Symposium on "Approaches to Centrally Acting Drugs Derived from the Cannabinoid Nucleus", presented at the 68th American Chemical Society Meeting, Atlantic City, New Jersey (Abstract).

Kiplinger, M. L., Wright, P. L., Haley, S. L., Plank, J. B., Braude, M. C. and Calandra, J. C. (1973). *Toxicology and Applied Pharmacology*, **25**, 449.

Kolansky, H. and Moore, W. T. (1971). *Journal of the American Medical Association*, **216**, 486.

Kornhaber, A. (1971). *Journal of the American Medical Association*, **215**, 1988.

Kosersky, D. S., Dewey, W. L. and Harris, L. S. (1973). *European Journal of Pharmacology*, **24**, 1.

Kotin, J., Post, R. M. and Goodwin, F. K. (1973). *Archives of General Psychiatry*, **28**, 345.

Kubena, R. K. and Barry, H. (1972). *Nature*, **235**, 397.

La Guardia Report (1939–1944). "The Marihuana Problem in the City of New York. Sociological, Medical and Pharmacological Studies."

Lahiri, P. K. and Hardman, H. F. (1972). 5th International Congress on Pharmacology, No. 796 (Abstract).

Lemberger, L., McMahon, R., Archer, R., Matsumoto, K. and Rowe, H. (1974). *Clinical Pharmacology and Therapeutics*, **15**, 380.

Lemberger, L. and Rowe, H. (1975a). *Pharmacologist*, **17** (Abstract No. 191).

Lemberger, L. and Rowe, H. (1975b). *Clinical Pharmacology and Therapeutics*, **18**, 720.

Leonard, B. E. (1971). *Research Communications in Chemical Pathology and Pharmacology*, **3**, 139.

Levy, J. A., Munson, A. E., Harris, L. S. and Dewey, W. L. (1974). *Pharmacologist*, **16**, No. 393.

Lewis, S. C., Brown, D. J. and Forney, R. B. (1974). *Toxicology and Applied Pharmacology*, **29**, 78.

Loev, B., Bender, P. E., Dowalo, F., Macko, D. E. and Fowler, P. J. (1973). *Journal of Medicinal Chemistry*, **16**, 1200.

Loev, B., Dienel, B., Goodman, M. M. and Van Hoeven, H. (1974). *Journal of Medicinal Chemistry*, **17**, 1234.

Loewe, S. (1946). *Journal of Pharmacology and Experimental Therapeutics*, **88**, 154.

Loewe, S. and Goodman, L. S. (1947). *Federation Proceedings*, **6**, 352.

Maitre, L., Waldmeier, P. and Baumann, P. (1973). *Life Sciences*, **13**, 112.

Manning, F. J. and Elsmore, T. F. (1972). *Psychopharmacologia*, **25**, 218.

Manno, J. E., Keplinger, G. F., Haine, S. E., Bennett, I. F. and Forney, R. B. (1970). *Clinical Pharmacology and Therapeutics*, **11**, 808.

Marihuana and Health (1974). Fourth Report to the US Congress, from the Secretary of Health Education and Welfare, (DHEW) Publication No. (ADM) 75–181.

McCaughran, Corcoran, M. E. and Wada, J. (1973). *Pharmacology, Biochemistry and Behavior*, **2**, 227.

McGiff, J. C. (1975). *Hospital Practice*, April issue, p. 101.

Mechoulam, R. (1970). *Science*, **168**, 1159.

Mechoulam, R. (ed.) (1973). *In* "Marihuana". Academic Press, New York and London.
Mechoulam, R., McCallum, N. K. and Burstein, S. (1976). *Chemical Reviews*, **76**, 75.
Merari, A., Barak, A. and Plaves, M. (1973). *Psychopharmacologia*, **28**, 243.
Merck Index (1950). 7th Edition. Synhexyl, Mild Euphoriant, Anti-Depressant.
Milzoff, J. R., Brown, D. J. and Stone, C. J. (1971). *Federation Proceedings*, **30**, 1381.
Morton, J. E. and Davis, W. M. (1973). *Neuropharmacology*, **12**, 897.
Nahas, G. G., Sucia-Foca, N., Armand, J. P. and Morishima, A. (1974). *Federation Proceedings*, **33**, 1848.
Nakano, J., Chang, A. C. K. and Fisher, R. A. (1972). *Proceedings of the Society for Experimental Biology and Medicine*, **140**, 866.
Neumeyer, J. L. and Shagoury, R. A. (1971). *Journal of Pharmaceutical Sciences*, **60**, 1433.
Nir, I., Agalon, D., Tsafriri, F., Cordova, T. and Linder, H. R. (1973). *Nature*, **244**, 470.
Nir, I., Agalon, D., Tsafriri, F., Cordova, T. and Linder, H. R. (1974). *Israel Journal of Medical Sciences*, **10**, 795.
Noyes, R. and Bagram, D. A. (1974). *Comparative Psychiatry*, **15**, 531.
Noyes, R., Brunk, F. and Bagram, D. A. (1975). *Journal of Clinical Pharmacology*, **15**, 139.
Osgood, P. F. and Howes, J. F. (1974). *Research Communications in Chemical Pathology and Pharmacology*, **9**, 621.
Osgood, P. F. and Howes, J. F. (1975) *Federation Proceedings*, **34**, Abstr. 2970.
Page, J. E. and West, L. E. (1975). *Pharmacologist*, **17** (Abstract No. 192).
Pal, B. and Ghosh, J. J. (1972). *Biochemical Pharmacology*, **21**, 263.
Parker, C. S. and Wrigley, F. (1950). *Journal of Mental Science*, **96**, 276.
Pars, H. G. (1973). *Anesthesiology*, **38**, 519.
Pars, H. G. and Razdan, R. K. (1971). *Annals of the New York Academy of Sciences*, **191**, 15.
Pars, H. G. and Razdan, R. K. (1976). *In* "Therapeutic Aspects of Marihuana" (Eds S. Cohen and R. Stillman). Plenum Press, New York.
Pars, H. G., Granchelli, F. E., Keller, J. K. and Razdan, R. K. (1966). Communication to the Editor, *Journal of the American Chemical Society*, **88**, 3664.
Pars, H. G., Granchelli, F. E., Razdan, R. K., Rosenberg, F., Teiger, D. and Harris, L. S. (1976). *Journal of Medicinal Chemistry*, **19**, 445, and references cited therein.
Paton, W. D. M. and Pertwee, R. G. (1972). *British Journal of Pharmacology*, **44**, 250.
Paton, W. D. M. and Pertwee, R. G. (1973). *In* "Marijuana" (Ed. R. Mechoulam). Academic Press, New York and London.
Perez-Reyes, M., Timmons, M. C., Lipton, M. A., Davis, K. M. and Wall, M. E. (1972). *Science*, **177**, 633.
Perez-Reyes, M., Lipton, M. A., Timmons, M. C., Wall, M. E., Brine, D. R. and Davis, K. H. (1973a). *Clinical Pharmacology and Therapeutics*, **14**, 48.
Perez-Reyes, M., Timmons, M. C., Lipton, M. A., Christensen, M. D., Davis, K. H. and Wall, M. E. (1973b). *Experientia*, **29**, 1609.
Perez-Reyes, M., Timmons, M. C., Davis, K. M. and Wall, M. E. (1973c). *Experientia*, **29**, 1368.

Petersen, B. H., Graham, J., Lemberger, L. and Dalton, B. (1974). *Pharmacologist*, 16, No. 392.

Petrzilka, T. and Lusuandi, W. G. (1973). *Helvetica Chimica Acta*, 56, 510.

Petrzilka, T., Demutta, M. and Lusuandi, W. G. (1973). *Helvetica Chimica Acta*, 56, 519.

Pivik, R. T., Zarcone, V., Dement, W. C. and Hollister, L. E. (1972). *Clinical Pharmacology and Therapeutics*, 13, 426.

Plotnikoff, N. (1976). *In* "Therapeutic Aspects of Marihuana" (Eds S. Cohen and R. Stillman). Plenum Press, New York.

Plotnikoff, N. P., Zaugg, H. E., Petersen, A. C., Arendsen, D. and Anderson, R. F. (1975), *Life Sciences*, 17, 97.

Plotnikoff, N., Zaugg, H., Petersen, H., Anderson, R. and Arendsen, D. (1974). Symposium on "Approaches to Centrally Acting Drugs Derived from the Cannabinoid Nucleus", presented at the 68th American Chemical Society Meeting, Atlantic City, New Jersey.

Ponce, D. A. (1948). *Journal of Neurology, Neurosurgery and Psychiatry*, 11, 271.

Poyser, R. H. and Palfreyman, M. G. (1975). Sixth International Congress on Pharmacology, Helsinki (Abstract No. 1380).

Radnicki, S. W. (1974). *Psychopharmacologia*, 37, 225.

Razdan, R. K. (1973). *In* "Progress in Organic Chemistry" (Eds W. Carruthers and J. K. Sutherland), vol. 8, chapter 3. Butterworths, London.

Razdan, R. K. (1974). Symposium on "Approaches to Centrally Acting Drugs Derived from the Cannabinoid Nucleus", presented at the 68th American Chemical Society Meeting, Atlantic City, New Jersey (Abstract).

Razdan, R. K., Thompson, W. R., Pars, H. G. and Granchelli, F. E. (1967). *Tetrahedron Letters*, 3405.

Razdan, R. K. and Pars, H. G. (1970). *In* "The Botany and Chemistry of Cannabis" (Eds C. R. B. Joyce and S. H. Curry), p. 137. Churchill, London.

Razdan, R. K. *et al.* (1970). National Academy of Sciences/National Research Council, Committee on Problems of Drug Dependence, Annual Report, p. 6860.

Razdan, R. K., Granchelli, F. E. and Pars, H. G. (1972). United States Patent Number 3, 639, 427.

Razdan, R. K., Dalzell, H. C. and Handrick, G. R. (1974a). *Journal of the American Chemical Society*, 96, 5860.

Razdan, R. K., Pars, H. G., Thompson, W. R. and Granchelli, F. E. (1974b). *Tetrahedron Letters*, 4315.

Razdan, R. K., Handrick, G. R., Dalzell, H. C., Howes, J. F., Winn, M., Plotnikoff, N., Dodge, P. W. and Dren, A. T. (1976a). *Journal of Medicinal Chemistry*, 19, 552.

Razdan, R. K., Zitko-Terris, B., Handrick, G. R., Dalzell, H. C., Pars, H. G., Howes, J. F., Plotnikoff, N., Dodge, P., Dren, A. T., Kyncyl, J., Shoer, L. and Thompson, W. R. (1976b). *Journal of Medicinal Chemistry*, 19, 549.

Razdan, R. K., Zitko-Terris, B., Pars, H. G., Plotnikoff, N. P., Dodge, P. W., Dren, A. T., Kyncyl, J. and Somani, P. (1976c). *Journal of Medicinal Chemistry*, 19, 454.

Razdan, R. K., Howes, J. F., Uliss, D. B., Dalzell, H. C., Handrick, G. R. and Dewey, W. L. (1976d). *Experientia*, 32, 416.

Sabelli, M. C. and Mosnaim, D. (1974). *American Journal of Psychiatry*, 131, 695.

Sabelli, M. C., Pedemonte, W. A., Whalley, C., Mosnaim, A. D. and Vasquez, P. J. (1974a). *Life Sciences*, 14, 169.

Sabelli, M. C., Vazquez, A. J., Mosnaim, A. D. and Madrid-Pedemonte, L. (1974b). *Nature*, **248**, 144.

Schildkraut, J. J. and Effron, D. H. (1971). *Psychopharmacologia*, **20**, 191.

Schwin, R. (1973). *Journal of the American Medical Association*, **194**, 223.

Shapiro, B. J., Rashkin, D. P. and Frank, I. M. (1973). *Annals of Internal Medicine*, **78**, 832.

Sidell, F. R., Pless, J. E., Neitlich, H., Sussman, P., Copelan, H. M. and Sim, V. M. (1973). *Proceedings of the Society for Experimental Biology and Medicine*, **142**, 867.

Siegmund, E., Cadmus, R. and Lu, G. (1957). *Proceedings of the Society of Experimental Biology and Medicine*, **95**, 729.

Siemens, A. J., Kalant, H., Khanna, J. M., Marshman, J. and Ho, G. (1974). *Biochemical Pharmacology*, **23**, 477.

Silverstein, J. and Lersin, M. (1974). *Science*, **186**, 740.

Sofia, R. D. (1972). *Research Communications in Chemical Pathology and Pharmacology*, **4**, 281.

Sofia, R. D. and Barry, M. III (1974). *Psychopharmacologia*, **39**, 213.

Sofia, R. D. and Knobloch, L. C. (1974). *Archives Internationales de Pharmacodynamie et de Thérapie*, **207**, 270.

Sofia, R. D., Kubena, R. and Barry, M. III (1971a). *Journal of Pharmacy and Pharmacology*, **23**, 889.

Sofia, R. D., Solomon, T. and Barry, M. III (1971b). *Pharmacologist*, **13**, 246.

Sofia, R. D., Nalepa, S. D., Harakal, J. J. and Vassar, H. B. (1973). *Journal of Pharmacology and Experimental Therapeutics*, **186**, 656.

Sofia, R. D., Nalepa, S. D., Vassar, H. B. and Knobloch, L. C. (1974). *Life Sciences*, **15**, 251.

Stark, P. and Archer, R. A. (1975). *Pharmacologist*, **17** (Abstract No. 190).

Stockings, G. T. (1947). *British Medical Journal*, **1**, 918.

Stoelting, R. K., Martz, R. C., Gardner, M. D., Creasser, E., Brown, D. J. and Forney, R. B. (1973). *Anesthesiology*, **38**, 521.

Taft, C. T. and Crawford, H. J. (1970). *Psychophysiology*, **1**, 348.

Tashkin, D. P., Shapiro, B. J. and Frank, I. M. (1973). *New England Journal of Medicine*, **289**, 336.

Thompson, L. J. and Proctor, R. C. (1953). *North Carolina Medical Journal*, **14**, 520.

Todd, A. R. *et al.* (1943). *Journal of the Chemical Society*, p. 286, and earlier papers cited therein.

Turkanis, S. A. (1974). *Federation Proceedings*, **33**, 541.

Turkanis, S. A., Cely, W., Olsen, D. and Karler, R. (1974). *Research Communications in Chemical Pathology and Pharmacology*, **8**, 231.

Uliss, D. B., Razdan, R. K. and Dalzell, H. C. (1974). *Journal of the American Chemical Society*, **96**, 7372.

Uliss, D. B., Dalzell, H. C., Handrick, G. R., Howes, J. F. and Razdan, R. K. (1975). *Journal of Medicinal Chemistry*, **18**, 213, and references cited therein.

Vachon, L., Fitzgerald, M. Y., Solliday, N. M., Gould, I. A. and Gaensler, E. A. (1973a). *New England Journal of Medicine*, **288**, 985.

Vachon, L., Fitzgerald, M. Y., Gould, I. A., Gaensler, E. A. and Solliday, N. H. (1973b). *American Review of Respiratory Diseases*, **107**, 1099.

Villarreal, J. E. and Seevers, M. H. (1970). National Academy of Sciences/

National Research Council, Committee on Problem of Drug Dependence, Annual Report, Addendum 1.

Villarreal, J. E., Seevers, M. H. and Swain, H. M. (1974). Symposium on "Approaches to Centrally Acting Drugs Derived from the Cannabinoid Nucleus", presented at the 68th American Chemical Society Meeting, Atlantic City, New Jersey (Abstract).

Vitez, T. S., Eger, E. I., Miller, R. D. and Way, W. L. (1973). *Anesthesiology*, **38**, 525.

Vollmer, R. R. (1972). *Journal of Pharmacy and Pharmacology*, **26**, 186.

Wall, M. E. (1971). *Annals of the New York Academy of Sciences*, **191**, 23.

Walton, R., Martin, L. and Keller (1938). *Journal of Pharmacology*, **62**, 239.

Weil, A. T., Nilson, J. and Zinberg, N. E. (1968). *Science*, **162**, 1234.

Weiss, J. L., Cardon, P. V., Lemberger, L., Tamankin, N. R. and Watanabe, A. M. (1972). *Clinical Pharmacology and Therapeutics*, **13**, 671.

Welch, B. L., Berger, M. J., Mersilia, F. S. and Welch, A. S. (1971). *Research Communications in Chemical Pathology and Pharmacology*, **2**, 382.

Williams, R. B., Kopin, I. J., Lamprecht, F., Ng, L. K. Y. and Roth, K. (1973). *Psychopharmacologia*, **28**, 269.

Wilson, R. S. and May, E. L. (1974). *Journal of Medicinal Chemistry*, **17**, 475.

Wilson, R. S. and May, E. L. (1975). *Journal of Medicinal Chemistry*, **18**, 700.

Winn, M., Arendsen, D., Dalzell, H. C., Dodge, P., Dren, A., Dunnigan, D., Hallas, R., Hwang, K., Kyncl, J., Lee, Y. H., Plotnikoff, N., Razdan, R. K., Young, P. and Zaugg, H. (1976). *Journal of Medicinal Chemistry*, **19**, 461.

Zimmerman, B. G., Gomer, S., Kraft, E. and Ryan, M. J. (1973). *Journal of Pharmacology and Experimental Therapeutics*, **18**, 315.

Zitko, B. A., Howes, J. F., Dalzell, B. C., Dalzell, H. C., Dewey, W. L., Harris, L. S., Pars, H. G., Razdan, R. K. and Sheehan, J. C. (1972). *Science*, **177**, 442.

Biologically Active
Benzo[b]thiophene Derivatives. II

TALMAGE R. BOSIN, PhD, and ERNEST E. CAMPAIGNE, PhD

*Department of Pharmacology, School of Medicine and Department of Chemistry,
Indiana University, Bloomington, Indiana, USA*

1 Introduction

The first extensive review on the subject of biologically active benzo-
[b]thiophene derivatives appeared 7 years ago (Campaigne *et al.*, 1970).
Other brief reviews (Campaigne *et al.*, 1969, 1973a) have appeared describing new biological activities within this class of compounds and there have
been numerous reports describing the biochemical, physiological, and
toxicological activities of these compounds.

The purpose of this chapter is to review the recent literature describing biological activities exhibited by compounds possessing the benzo[*b*]-thiophene nucleus **(1)**. To facilitate the presentation and understanding of this material, this chapter has been organized into sections describing

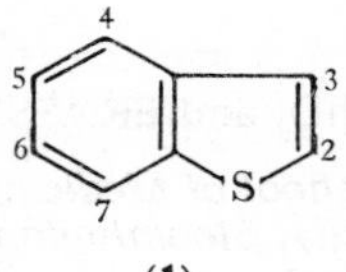

(1)

biochemical, physiological, toxicological, and pharmacological activities. The discussion will be restricted to those benzo[*b*]thiophene derivatives for which biological data is available.

2 Biochemistry

2.1 ENZYME STUDIES

Aromatic L-amino acid decarboxylase (aromatic L-amino acid carboxy-lyase, EC 4.1.1.28) is an enzyme which decarboxylates the L-isomers of 3,4-dihydroxyphenylalanine (DOPA), 5-hydroxytryptophan (5-HTP), phenyl-alanine, tryptophan, and tyrosine thereby producing the corresponding amine. Bosin *et al.* (1974a) studied the substrate specificity of hog kidney aromatic L-amino acid decarboxylase, using the racemic benzo[*b*]thiophene **(2)** and 1-methylindole **(3)** analogs of tryptophan **(4)**. Neither **2** nor **3** produced detectable decarboxylation under conditions which produced significant rates of decarboxylation of **(4)**. In addition, both **2** and **3** were found to inhibit the decarboxylation of **4** and phenylalanine by the enzyme

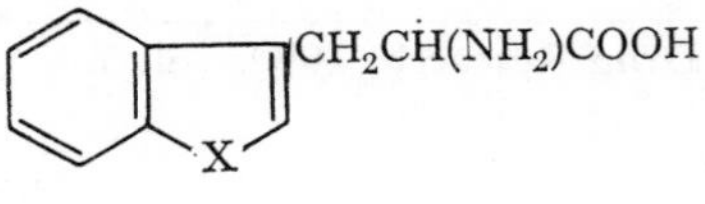

CH₂CH(NH₂)COOH

(2)   X=S
(3)   X=NCH₃
(4)   X=NH

system *in vitro*. Subsequent studies (Maickel *et al.*, 1975) of the de-carboxylation of DOPA demonstrated that the benzo[*b*]thiophene analogs of α-methyltryptophan **(5)** and 5-hydroxytryptophan (5-HTP) **(6)** could function as inhibitors as shown in Table 1. Shetty (1969) had shown that

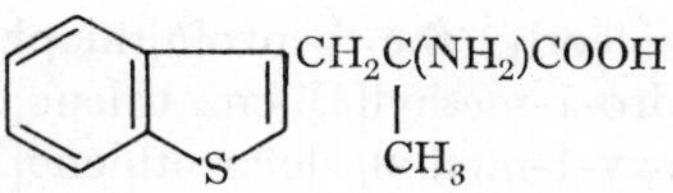

$CH_2C(NH_2)COOH$ with CH_3 substituent

HO ... $CH_2CH(NH_2)COOH$

(5) 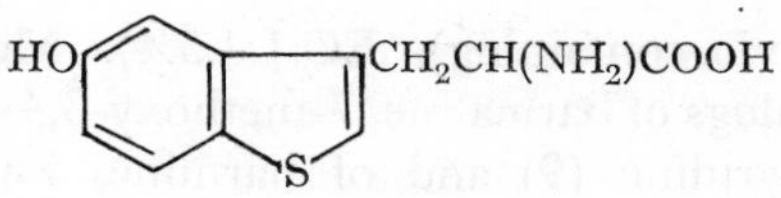   (6)

6 failed to produce any sympathomimetic effects in rats pretreated with iproniazid, in contrast to 5-HTP which produced a profuse sympathomimetic response. Compound **6** was found not to mimic 5-HTP, i.e. was not a substrate for aromatic L-amino acid decarboxylase, and failed to inhibit the effects of 5-HTP (Shetty, 1969).

TABLE 1

Comparison of the inhibitory effects of indole, 1-methylindole and benzo[b]thiophene analogs on the decarboxylation of tryptophan, phenylalanine, and dihydroxyphenylalanine

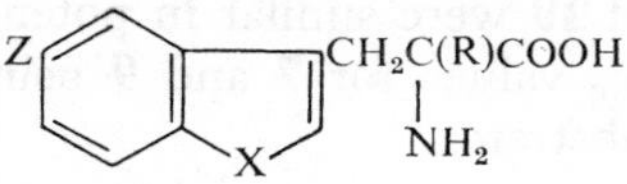

$CH_2C(R)COOH$ with NH_2

X	Inhibitor R	Z	Substrate	K_i (M)
S	H	H	Tryptophan	$0·5 \times 10^{-3}$
NCH$_3$	H	H	Tryptophan	$4·5 \times 10^{-3}$
S	H	H	Phenylalanine	$0·6 \times 10^{-3}$
NCH$_3$	H	H	Phenylalanine	$1·5 \times 10^{-3}$
NH	H	H	Phenylalanine	$1·3 \times 10^{-3}$
S	H	H	DOPA	$1·9 \times 10^{-3}$
NCH$_3$	H	H	DOPA	$8·0 \times 10^{-3}$
S	CH$_3$	H	DOPA	$7·0 \times 10^{-4}$
NH	CH$_3$	H	DOPA	$3·7 \times 10^{-4}$
S	H	OH	DOPA	$5·8 \times 10^{-5}$
NH	H	OH	DOPA	$2·1 \times 10^{-4}$
α-Methyl-DOPA			DOPA	$7·7 \times 10^{-4}$

From Bosin et al. (1974a) and Maickel et al. (1975).

In 1958, Freter *et al.* reported that the harmala alkaloids, harmaline (**7**) and harmine (**8**), were active reversible inhibitors of the enzyme monoamine oxidase (MAO) (amine: oxygen oxidoreductase (deaminating)

(flavin-containing), EC.1.4.3.4). More recently, the benzo[b]thiophene analogs of harmaline, 7-methoxy-3,4-dihydro-1-methyl[1]benzothieno[2,3-c]pyridine (9) and of harmine, 7-methoxy-1-methyl[1]benzothieno[2,3-c]pyridine (10) have been prepared (Bosin et al., 1972a) and evaluated as MAO inhibitors (Bosin et al., 1972b; Clements, 1975; Burkard and Kettler, 1975). When tested in vitro as inhibitors of rat liver MAO, with

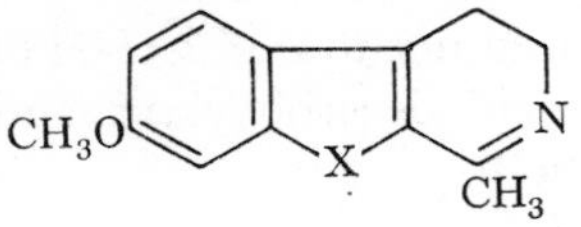

(7) X=NH   (8) X=NH
(9) X=S   (10) X=S

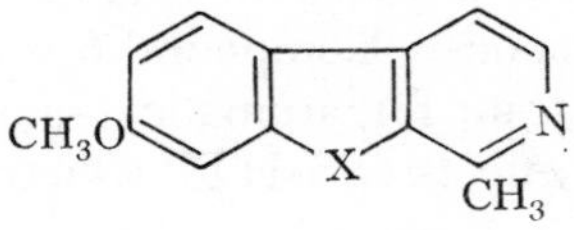

tryptamine as a substrate, compound 9 was 50 times more potent than 7, while compounds 8 and 10 were similar in potency (Table 2). Clements (1975) found similar I_{50} values for 7 and 9 using rat liver MAO with kynurenamine as the substrate.

TABLE 2

Comparison of various MAO inhibitors[a]

Compound (number)	I_{50} (M)
Harmaline (7)	$3 \cdot 9 \times 10^{-5}$
Harmaline-S (9)	$7 \cdot 8 \times 10^{-7}$
Harmine (8)	$7 \cdot 0 \times 10^{-6}$
Harmine-S (10)	$9 \cdot 1 \times 10^{-6}$
Pargyline	$3 \cdot 4 \times 10^{-5}$
Tranylcypromine	$3 \cdot 3 \times 10^{-5}$

[a] Rat liver MAO using tryptamine as the substrate; each value is the mean of 6 determinations and I_{50} values were determined by linear regression analysis.
From Bosin et al. (1972b).

Determination of the partition coefficients of 7 and 9 indicated that replacement of the indolic nitrogen with sulfur significantly increased the lipid solubility of the molecule, as reflected in its physiological disposition. Following administration of a single dose (30 mg kg⁻¹, ip) to mice, the plasma half-life of 7 was 93 minutes, while that of 9 was 40 minutes. The comparable half-lives of 7 were greater in all tissues than those of 9. Tissue to plasma ratios at 2 hours ranged from 6·4 (heart) to 56·0 (lung) for 7 and 2·2 (heart) to 19·8 (lung) for 9.

Administration of a single dose (30 mg kg⁻¹, ip) of 7 or 9 to mice resulted in elevated brain levels of serotonin (5-HT) (11) (Table 3). Compound 9 produced higher levels of 5-HT at all time points except 8 hours. Similar results have been obtained in the rat (Burkard and Kettler, 1975).

TABLE 3

Influence of harmaline and harmaline-S on mouse brain serotonin[a]

| | Harmaline | | Harmaline-S | |
Time (h)	Brain 5-HT ($\mu g\ g^{-1}$)	% of control	Brain 5-HT ($\mu g\ g^{-1}$)	% of control
0	0·47	100	0·47	100
1	0·57	122	0·62	132
2	0·56	121	0·70	151
4	0·75	160	0·88	175
8	0·75	160	0·69	150
24	0·44	94	0·63	135

[a] Groups of 4 mice were given harmaline or harmaline-S (30 mg kg^{-1}, ip) at time = 0. Each value is the mean of 2 assays of 2 brains each.
From Bosin et al. (1972b).

Compounds 7 and 9 have been compared both in vitro and in vivo using 5-HT (the preferred substrate for type A MAO) and tyramine (a substrate of equal activity for types A and B MAO) (Burkard and Kettler, 1975). Both compounds were more powerful inhibitors of 5-HT than tyramine in vitro; and 9 appeared to be a stronger inhibitor of brain MAO than 7. In vivo, 7 showed similar ED$_{50}$ values for brain and liver, while 9 was about 5 times more potent in the brain than in the liver. Thus, of the various known MAO inhibitors only clorgyline and 9 have greater potency in the brain than in the liver.

Phenylethanolamine N-methyltransferase (PNMT) (S-adenosyl-L-methionine: phenylethanolamine N-methyltransferase, EC 2.1.1.28) is an enzyme, highly localized in the adrenal medulla, which catalyzes the terminal step in epinephrine biosynthesis (Axelrod, 1962). 3-Methyl-1,2,3,-4-tetrahydro[1]benzo[b]thieno[3,2-c]pyridine (12) has been shown to be a potent competitive inhibitor of PNMT (Pendleton et al., 1974) in vitro with respect to norepinephrine ($I_{50} = 7 \times 10^{-7}$ M), but uncompetitive with

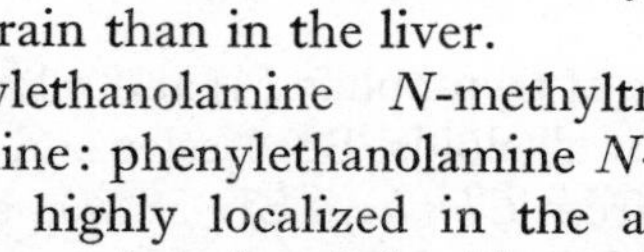

(11) X=NH
(13) X=S

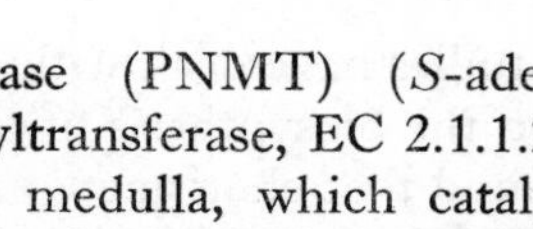

(12)

respect to S-adenosylmethionine. In the rat, **12** selectively reduced the adrenal content of epinephrine upon chronic oral administration; adrenal norepinephrine (NE) levels and heart and brain catecholamine content were not altered.

Ceruloplasmin (monophenol, dihydroxyphenylalanine: oxygen oxidoreductase, EC 1.14.18.1) is a copper-containing enzyme possessing oxidizing properties which was first isolated by Holmberg and Laurell (1948). The substrate specificity of the enzyme has been studied by Barrass et al. (1973) using some 5-HT analogs, including the benzo[b]thiophene analog (**13**). Compound **13** was found to be a very poor substrate for the enzyme and had no effect on the ceruloplasmin-mediated oxidation of 5-HT or norepinephrine (NE). This study demonstrated the importance of the indole nucleus in determining substrate specificity towards ceruloplasmin.

A kinetic study of the enzymatic hydrolysis of adenosine 3',5'-cyclic monophosphate by phosphodiesterase extracted from ox heart revealed 5-chloro-3-(2-dimethylaminoethyl)benzo[b]thiophene (**14**) and N-(4-bromo-2-benzo[b]thienyl) guanidinium toluene-p-sulfonate (**15**) to be marked noncompetitive inhibitors of the enzyme (Ramsden, 1970).

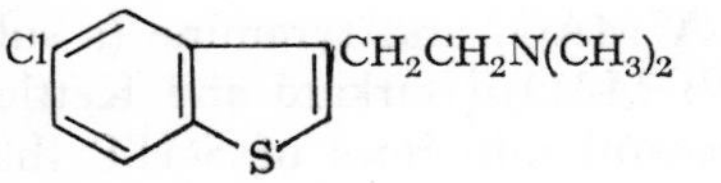

(**14**) 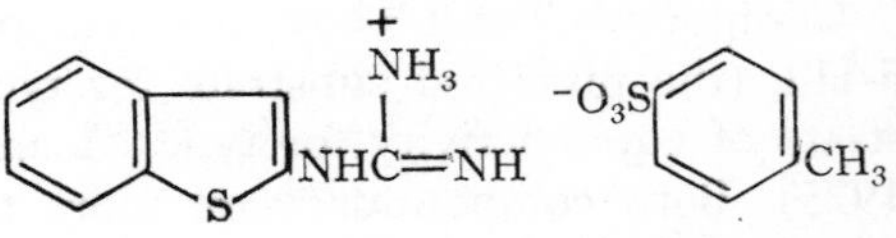   (**15**)

2.2 BIOSYNTHESIS STUDIES

Several studies have dealt with the role of tryptophan (**4**) and related compounds in the biosynthesis of the ergot alkaloids. Sproessler and Lingens (1970) found that chorismate mutase from *Claviceps* SD 58 was activated by **4**, while the benzo[b]thiophene analog of tryptophan (**2**) was inactive. In a related study, Eberspacher et al. (1970) observed that **2** did not inhibit the tryptophan-sensitive isozyme of 3-deoxy-D-arabino-2-heptulosonic acid (DAHP) synthetase in *Claviceps* SD 58 of ergot. More recently, Krupinski et al. (1976) have found that both **2** and **4** enhance ergot alkaloid production in both normal and high phosphate cultures. This effect was shown to more directly relate to increased dimethylallyltryptophan (DMAT) synthetase activity than to the de-regulation of the tryptophan biosynthetic enzymes. Compound **2** was ineffective in the end-product regulation of tryptophan biosynthesis, and was not a substrate for DMAT synthetase, although it did induce *de novo* enzyme synthesis.

2.3 DRUG METABOLISM AND DISPOSITION

Several investigations of the metabolic fate of benzo[b]thiophene derivatives reported since the first review have dealt with the metabolism of the pesticide Mobam, 4-benzo[b]thienyl methylcarbamate (16). In rats, two urinary metabolites, 4-benzo[b]thienyl β-glucoronide (18) and 4-benzo[b]-thienyl sulfate (19), accounted for 83 per cent of the excreted ^{14}C-

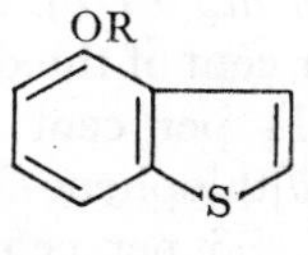

OR

(16) R=CONHCH₃ (18) R= COOH

(17) R=H

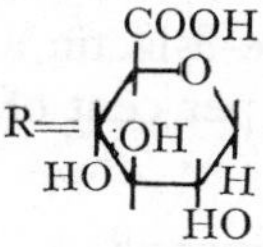

(19) R=SO₃H

compounds from rats dosed at 2·0 mg kg^{-1} and 87 per cent at 13·0 mg kg^{-1} (Robbins *et al.*, 1969). The metabolism of 16 has also been studied in dairy goats and the lactating cow (Robbins *et al.*, 1970). In the latter, two urinary metabolites, 18 and 4-benzo[b]thienyl sulfate 1-oxide (20), accounted for 88–91 per cent of the radioactivity excreted in the urine. In milk, however, 20 accounted for 96–98 per cent of the radioactivity. The degradation of 16 by ruminal bacteria has been shown to produce 4-hydroxybenzo[b]thiophene (17); further degradation of the methylcarbamate moiety of 16 (Williams and Stolzenberg, 1972) leads to carbon dioxide and polar products.

The metabolism of the sulfur analog of N,N-dimethyltryptamine, 3-(2-dimethylaminoethyl)benzo[b]thiopene (21) has been studied *in vitro* and *in vivo* in the rat (Harrison, *et al.*, 1974). Using a rat liver microsomal preparation, the major pathways for the metabolism of 21 were 6-hydroxyl-

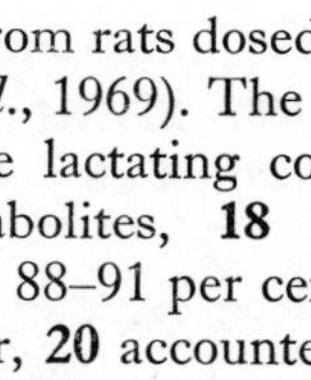

SO₃H

R

Z

(20)

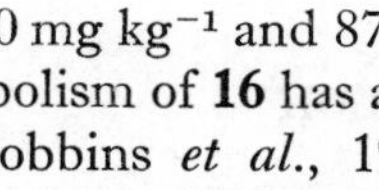

(21) R=CH₂CH₂N(CH₃)₂; Z=H

(22) R=CH₂CH₂N(CH₃)₂; Z=OH

(23) R=CH₂CH₂NHCH₃; Z=H

(24) R=CH₂COOH; Z=H

ation to **22** and *N*-dealkylation to **23**; subsequent oxidation by MAO yielded **24**. Following the ip administration of **21** to rats, a single acidic urinary metabolite consisting of 25 per cent of the dose was isolated and identified as **24**. Metabolites were identified by combination of mass specrometry, nuclear magnetic resonance spectroscopy, thin-layer chromatography, and liquid scintillation counting.

The metabolic fate of the benzo[*b*]thiophene analog of tryptophan (**2**) has been investigated (Bickers *et al.*, 1976). Administration of **2** (100 mg kg^{-1}) ip to rats resulted in 76 per cent of the dose appearing in the 24-hour urine sample; it consisted of 11 per cent tritiated water, 21 per cent unchanged **2**, 14 per cent benzo[*b*]thiophene-3-pyruvic acid (**25**), 5 per cent benzo[*b*]thiophene-3-lactic acid, 1·3 per cent benzo[*b*]thiophene-3-acetic acid (**24**), and 47 per cent of the glycine conjugate of **24** (**27**).

(2)	R=CH$_2$CH(NH$_2$)COOH
(25)	R=CH$_2$COCOOH
(26)	R=CH$_2$CH(OH)COOH
(27)	R=CH$_2$CONHCH$_2$COOH

(28)	X=NH
(29)	X=S

The comparative physiological disposition of melatonin (**28**) and its benzo[*b*]thiophene isostere (**29**) in the rat has been reported (Maickel *et al.*, 1974). When administered iv to rats, both **28** and **29** disappeared from plasma and tissues by first-order decay. The dispositions of **28** and **29** were similar, with the higher lipid solubility of **29** (benzene: pH 7·4 distribution values, **28** = 8·2; **29** = 610) resulting in higher tissue to plasma ratios, especially in adipose tissue, kidney, liver, and longer half-lives in plasma and tissues. These results suggest that both the endogenously occurring indole compound **28** and the foreign benzo[*b*]thiophene analog **29** are handled in a similar manner.

2.4 BIOGENIC AMINE STUDIES

Recently, 5,6-dihydroxytryptamine (**30**) has been reported to have a preferential degenerative effect on central indoleamine-containing neurons. Intraventricular injections of **30** in the rat depleted brain and spinal cord 5-HT (Baumgarten *et al.*, 1972). The sulfur analog of **30**, 3-(2-aminoethyl)-5,6-dihydroxybenzo[*b*]thiophene (**31**) as well as 3-(2-aminoethyl)-5,6-¡sopropylidenedioxybenzo-[*b*]thiophene (**32**) have been synthesized (Campaigne *et al.*, 1973b). Donelson (1976) studied the comparative neuro-chemical and behavioral effects of compounds **30–32**, and related indole derivatives which included 5-hydroxy-6-methoxytryptamine (**33**), 5-methoxy-6-hydroxytryptamine (**34**), and 5,6-dimethoxytryptamine (**35**). These data are summarized in Table 4 and reveal dramatic changes in the neurochemical and behavioral properties of **30** when either the indole nucleus is replaced by benzo[*b*]thiophene or the hydroxyl groups are methylated.

2.5 PROTEIN SYNTHESIS STUDIES

Incorporation of amino acid analogs into cellular proteins constitutes a measure of the structural similarity of the analog to the natural substrate. Hall *et al.* (1974) have examined the ability of some tryptophan analogs, including compounds **2** and **3**, to support protein synthesis in a tryptophan auxotroph of *E. coli.* They found the analogs to be noninhibitory to growth and capable of supporting limited protein synthesis. Compounds **2** and **3** were less effective as measured by ^{3}H-leucine incorporation and β-galactosidase synthesis, than was 5-fluorotryptophan.

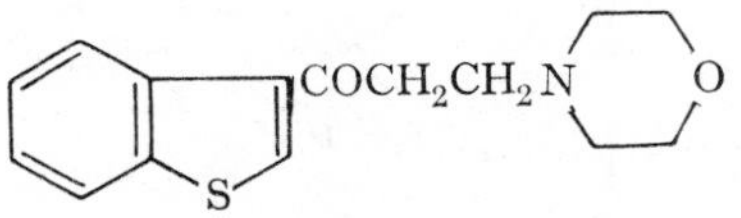

(36)

Kiechle (1974) has investigated the mode of action of 3-(β-morpho-linopropionyl) benzo[*b*]thiophene (**36**) in uninfected and T$_4$-infected *E. coli B*. As a result of the tight interregulation of DNA, RNA, and protein synthesis in uninfected *E. coli B*, the same relative inhibition of each of these three processes was observed at concentrations similar to those used to reduce the rate of cell growth. However, in T$_4$-infected *E. coli B* two distinct direct inhibitory sites of action were demonstrated for **36**; a primary site inhibiting replication and a secondary site inhibiting translation. No direct inhibitory effect against RNA synthesis was noted.

3 Physiology

3.1 ISOLATED SMOOTH MUSCLE STUDIES

Benzo[*b*]thiophene derivatives have been used in several attempts to characterize the tryptamine and serotonin receptors. Pinder *et al.* (1971)

TABLE 4

Summary of neurochemical and behavioral effects of 5,6-dihydroxytryptamine and related derivatives and analogs[a]

Compound	Dose and route	Neurochemical effects	Behavioral effects
(30) HO HO ─ indole ─ CH$_2$CH$_2$NH$_2$ (N–H)	80 µg, intraventricular	Prolonged, moderate (15–40%) ↓ in brain 5-HT; transient (10–25%) ↑ at 2 h followed by (20–30%) ↓ in 5-HIAA; transient (15–30%) ↓ in brain NE. At 2 h (55–60%) ↓ in spleen and heart NE; heart levels returned to control levels by 16 h while spleen persisted up to 16 h. At 2 h (50%) ↓ in spleen 5-HT which persisted to 24 h.	Initial behavioral depression, 30–45 min, then explosive jumping and erratic running behavior, convulsive episodes, vocalization. Peripheral sympathomimetic symptomology, e.g. exopthalmos, piloerection.
(31) HO HO ─ benzothiophene ─ CH$_2$CH$_2$NH$_2$ (S)	100 µg, intraventricular; 30 mg kg^{-1}, ip	No effect on brain 5-HT; ↑ 5-HIAA levels 2–4 days post-injection; transient (25%) ↓ in NE for several hours post-injection. At 2 h (55–60%) ↓ in heart and spleen NE; control levels were attained at 24 h. No effect on spleen 5-HT.	Behavioral depression lasting up to 30 min post-injection; sedation, animal lying prone. Peripheral sympathomimetic symptomology, e.g. exopthalmos, piloerection. No lethality at these doses.

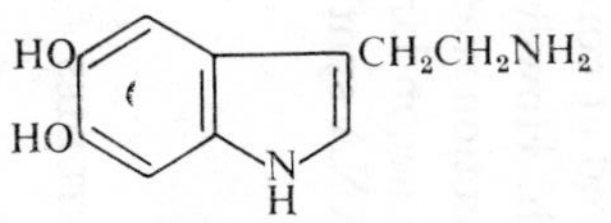

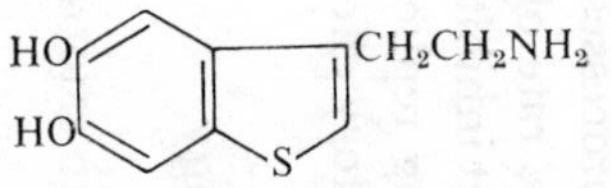

Structure	Dose, route	Neurochemical effects	Behavioral effects
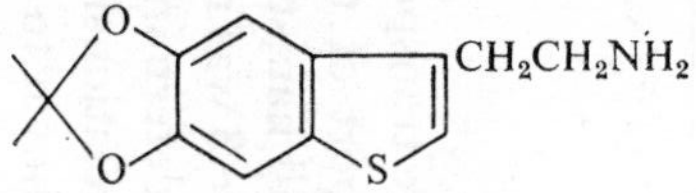 (32)	100 μg, intraventricular	Complex neurochemical effects: At 2 h (33%) ↑ and at 48 h (40%) ↓ in 5-HT levels. At 2 h (35%) ↓ in 5-HIAA and slight ↓ in NE levels.	Increased motor activity; cage circling with periodic pauses, lasting 2 hours following injection. No deaths.
	40 mg kg⁻¹, ip (LD$_{33}$ 4 h; LD$_{100}$ 16 h)	At 2 h (30%) ↓ in brain NE but no effect on brain 5-HT or 5-HIAA. No significant effect on peripheral monoamines.	Behaviorally depressed, stuporous animal soon after injection, increased lethality with time.
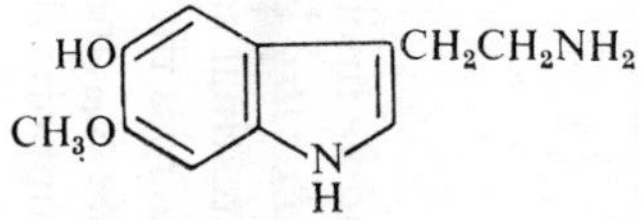 (33)	100 μg, intraventricular	No effect on brain levels of 5-HT or NE at 2 h post-injection; (25%) ↑ in 5-HIAA.	Brief, periodic (3–8 min) convulsive episodes within 15 min injection, associated with erratic running behavior, vocalization; followed by period of increased alertness and responsivity. No deaths.
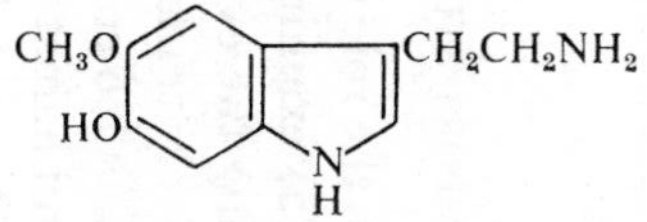 (34)	100 μg, intraventricular	No effect on brain levels of 5-HT or NE at 2 h post-injection; (25%) ↑ in 5-HIAA.	Some increased exploratory activity within 15 min of injection, but otherwise did not differ from control animals. No deaths.
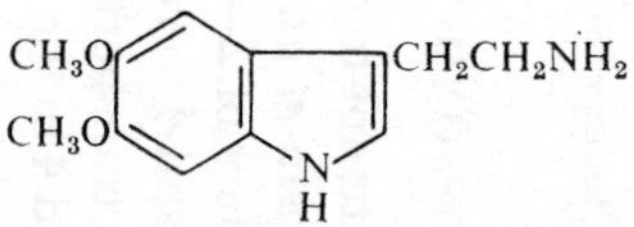 (35)	100 μg, intraventricular	No effect on NE or 5-HIAA in brain at 2 h post-injection. Apparent ↑ in 5-HT, however 35 interfered with the 5-HT assay method.	Disoriented, groping behavior; animal exhibits much rotational behavior and is hyper-reactive to sensory stimulation; decreased rectal temperature; no deaths at this dosage level.

^{a} After Donelson (1975).

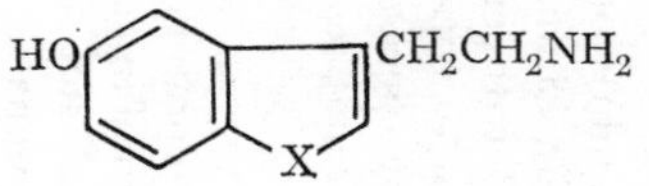

(11) X=NH   (37) X=O
(13) X=S   (38) X=CH$_2$

studied the benzo[*b*]thiophene (13), benzofuran (37) and indene (38) isoteres of 5-HT (11) using a rat stomach fundus preparation. They found the order of potency, as determined by pD$_2$ values, to be 11> 38> 13> 37. Kyburz (1974) obtained similar results for 11 and 13 in the isolated rat stomach fundus. In an attempt to assess the specificity of the 5-HT isosteres for the 5-HT receptor in the rat stomach fundus, the degree of blockade produced by phenoxybenzamine was investigated. In the presence of phenoxybenzamine blockade, the isosteres were shown to be less specific than the parent compound. Table 5 summarizes these data.

TABLE 5

Activity of 5-HT and its isosteres as agonists and degree of blockade by phenoxybenzamine on the rat stomach fundus strip

Compound	Agonist activity			Blockade by phenoxybenzamine, 1.84×10^{-4} M for 20 min	
	Relative intrinsic ($\pm$ SE)	pD$_2$ ($\pm$ SE)	Slope	Bath concentration of agonist, M	% Block of agonist response ($\pm$ SE)
11	1·00	7·59 ($\pm$0·14)	1·00	3.5×10^{-6}	95·67 ($\pm$0·67)
37	0·84 ($\pm$0·04)	4·94 ($\pm$0·11)	0·98	1.8×10^{-3}	67·66 ($\pm$2·4)
13	1·08 ($\pm$0·09)	6·13 ($\pm$0·16)	0·73	7.8×10^{-4}	70·6 ($\pm$4·3)
38	0·96 ($\pm$0·09)	6·60 ($\pm$0·53)	0·62	7.5×10^{-4}	78 ($\pm$5·07)

From Pinder *et al.* (1971).

3.2 INTESTINAL TRANSPORT STUDIES

In an attempt to define the role of the indole nucleus in the active transport of 4, Bosin *et al.* (1975) examined the *in vitro* intestinal transport of the DL-isomers of 2–4, using the everted intestinal sac of the rat and hamster. Both 2 and 4 were actively transported across the intestine, while 3 was not actively transported. Table 6 contains the K_m and V_{max} values determined for 2 and 4 in the rat and hamster, and supports the bioisosteric relationship which exists between 2 and 4. The active transport of 4 was shown to be competitively inhibited by 2, suggesting a similar carrier, while 3 was found not to be an inhibitor of the transport of 4, suggesting little or no interaction with the carrier. The absorption of isomers and analogs of 4 by rat and hamster small intestines have also been examined using an *in situ* perfusion technique (Bosin *et al.*, 1974b). In both rats and hamsters, the relative absorption rankings are in the order: L-4 > DL-2 > DL-4 > DL-3 > D-4. These results indicate that compounds DL-3 and D-4, which are not actively transported by the isolated everted intestinal sac, are significantly absorbed from an intestinal segment containing an intact blood supply on the serosal side.

TABLE 6

K_m and V_{max} for the intestinal transport of tryptophan and its benzo[*b*]thiophene analog in the rat and hamster

Compound number	Species	K_m, mM	V_{max}, μmol g^{-1} per 30 min
4	Rat	1·70	2·91
2	Rat	2·30	4·10
4	Hamster	1·96	3·33
2	Hamster	2·49	4·63

From Bosin *et al.* (1975).

3.3 MELANOPHORE STIMULATING ACTIVITY

Reed (1968) proposed a role for melatonin (28) in the control of circadian pigment changes in the Australian pencil fish, *Nannostomers beckfordi anomalus*. He found that exogenous 28 induced rapid, complete night coloration in the pencil fish, which could be used to assay melanophore stimulating activity. Campaigne and Dinner (1970) synthesized the benzo[*b*]thiophene analog of melatonin (29); the same laboratory also prepared 4-methoxy-3-(2-acetamidoethyl)benzo[*b*]thiophene (39) (Campaigne and Rogers, 1973a and 1973b) and 6-methoxy-3-(2-acetamidoethyl)-benzo[*b*]thiophene (40) (Bosin *et al.*, 1972a). These compounds have been screened by Reed (1974) for melanophore-stimulating activity in the pencil fish; the results appear in Table 7. As can be seen, 29 has approximately one-tenth the activity of 28 in the pencil fish, while the 4- and 6-methoxy analogs (39, 40) are virtually inactive.

3.4 PLATELET AGGREGATION INHIBITION

Several benzo[*b*]thiophene derivatives have been found to be potent inhibitors of platelet aggregation *in vitro*. Kikugawa and Ichino (1973)

TABLE 7

Comparison of the effects of melatonin and benzo[b]thiophene analogs on pencil
fish melanophores

Compound number	MED μg per fish
28	0·0001
29	0·001
39	0·1
40	1·0

From Reed (1974).

described a series of benzo[b]thiophene derivatives (41–44) which possessed
strong inhibitory activity. Compound 43 was the most active compound
and possessed a relative potency of 1·0 when compared to 10^{-4} M adenosine
in the same preparation of platelet-rich citrated plasma.

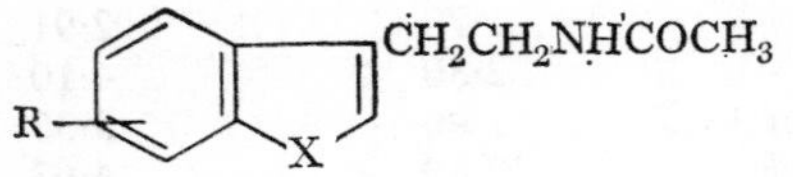

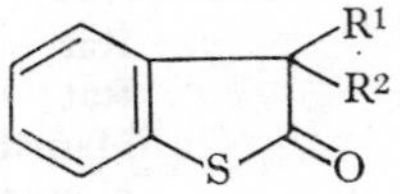

(28) X=NH; R=5-OCH₃	(41) R¹=OH; R²=p-CH₃C₆H₄NH—
(29) X=S; R=5-OCH₃	
(39) X=S; R=4-OCH₃	(42) R¹=OH; R²=—N O
(40) X=S; R=6-OCH₃	
	(43) R¹R²=CHCOC₆H₅
	(44) R¹R²=CHCOCH₃

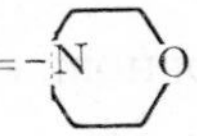

Elslager *et al.* (1972) have evaluated some [1]benzo[b]thieno[3,2-b]-
quinoline derivatives for their inhibitory activity on platelet aggregation.
Compound 45 was the most active inhibitor, producing 62 per cent inhibition of ADP-induced platelet aggregation at a concentration of 10^{-5} M
in vitro. A series of benzothieno[3,2-d]pyrimidines have also been claimed

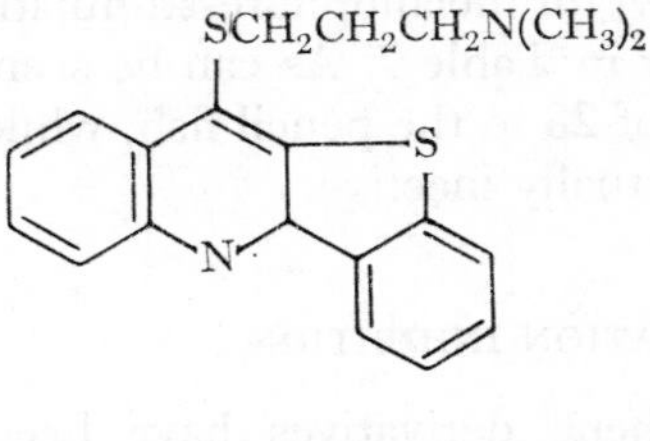

(45)

to possess useful platelet aggregation inhibitory activity (DeAngelis and Hess, 1972).

3.5 BIOGENIC AMINE UPTAKE, INHIBITION AND DISPLACEMENT

It is generally accepted that the process of re-uptake serves as a major mechanism for the inactivation of synaptically released catecholamines (Axelrod, 1971). The central nervous system has a 5-HT accumulation system which has several properties in common with the catecholamine uptake system (Shaskan and Snyder, 1970); however, it is not known whether this system represents a major mechanism for the inactivation of synaptically released 5-HT. Heikkila and Cohen (1974) have investigated the ability of the benzo[b]thiophene isostere of serotonin (13) to inhibit biogenic amine accumulation into rat brain tissue slices. They found 13 to be a potent inhibitor of ^{3}H-5-HT and ^{3}H-dopamine accumulation into rat brain slices with ED_{50} of 4.7×10^{-7} M and 5.0×10^{-6} M, respectively.

Costa et al. (1976) have studied the ability of 5-HT, 13, dopamine, tyramine and related fluoro-derivatives to displace ^{14}C-5-HT from labeled platelet vesicles in vitro. The data shown in Table 8 reveal 13 to possess weaker ability to displace ^{14}C-5-HT from the platelet vesicles than 5-HT.

TABLE 8
Displacement ability of ^{14}C-5-HT from platelet vesicles by select compounds

Pre-treatment	5-HT	13	Dopamine	6-Fluoro-dopamine	Tyramine	3-Fluoro-tyramine
None	1·18	0·562	0·963	0·513	0·578	1·10
Deprenyl	1·20	0·628	2·20	1·88	1·00	0·761

Values are expressed as mol $\times$ 10^{18} of ^{14}C-5-HT displaced from platelet vesicles during a 10-min incubation at 37°C. Concentrations of the compounds were 1×10^{-5}M and that of deprenyl 1×10^{-4} M. Each value represents the mean of four experiments. From Costa et al. (1976).

Buckpitt et al. (1976) examined the ability of 13 to influence the localization of ^{3}H-5-HT in the mouse lung in vivo. In mice pretreated with 13 (80 μg kg^{-1}, iv, 1 h prior to 75 μg kg^{-1} ^{3}H-5-HT) or post-treated with 13 (80 μg kg^{-1}, iv, 11 h after 75 μg kg^{-1} ^{3}H-5-HT), there was no significant change in ^{3}H-5-HT in the lungs when compared to control mice for periods up to 48 h after administration of ^{3}H-5-HT.

4 Toxicology

Since the last review of this subject (Campaigne et al., 1970) several reports have described toxicological studies of benzo[b]thiophene (1) and its biologically active derivatives. Lagno and Sviridor (1972) found that the LD_{50} values for 1 when administered orally to mice and rats were 1·26 and 0·96 g kg^{-1}, respectively. Compound 1 caused excitation of the animals and fatty infiltration of the liver. When administered orally at 0·2 g kg^{-1} per day to rats for 2 months, 1 caused decreased leukocyte and erythrocyte counts and increased weights of the liver, heart, and kidneys.

The comparative acute oral toxicity of 4-benzo[b]thienyl methylcarbamate, Moban® (16), in six species of birds has been reported (Tucker and Halgele, 1971). They found that the sensitivity of any one species to 16 did not differ statistically from that of any other species.

A comparative toxicological study in mice of biologically active indole, benzo[b]thiophene, and 1-methylindole compounds has been reported (Bosin et al., 1976a). LD_{50} values were determined for each compound and overt behavior was measured in animals at doses equal to or less than the LD_{50}. The data, as summarized in Table 9, shows several trends. With the exception of the 1-methylindole analog of tryptophan, the amino acids, acetic acids and their 5-hydroxylated derivatives are the least toxic compounds of all those studied. Melatonin and serotonin, and their benzo[b]thiophene analogs, as well as tryptophol and its benzo[b]thiophene and 1-methylindole analogs are of relatively moderate toxicity. The differences from one compound to another in each of these triads are not very striking, except in the case of the 1-methylindole analog of tryptophan which is a quite toxic compound.

Among the unsubstituted amines, the toxicity of any series followed the sequence: 1-methylindole > benzo[b]thiophene > indole; across these series, the toxicity also followed the order: tertiary amine > secondary amine > primary amine. These relationships are not directly correlated with physicochemical properties such as pK_a or lipid solubility which have been reported by Chiu et al. (1973).

5 Pharmacology

5.1 ANTIFERTILITY AGENTS

A number of triaryl ethylene derivatives have shown potent antifertility activity in rodents as a result of their estrogenic and/or estrogen antagonist activities. Crenshaw et al. (1971) have prepared a series of 2,3-diaryl benzo[b]thiophene derivatives of general structure (46) which may be viewed as cyclized triaryl ethylenes. The most active member of the series was 6-methoxy-3{p-[2-(N-pyrrolidyl)ethoxy]phenyl}-2-phenylbenzo[b]thiophene (47). Estrogenic and antiestrogenic activities were determined for 47 by uterine weight responses in immature 21-day-old mice and rats.

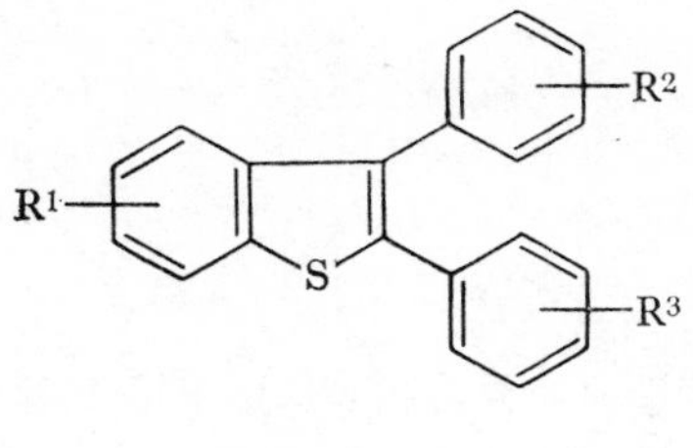

(46)

Compound **47** exhibited potent uterotropic activity in the mouse; at 1 μg per mouse **47** had activity approximating 1 μg of ethinyl estradiol while at 0·1 μg, **47** was less potent than 0·1 μg of ethinyl estradiol. In immature female rats, doubling of uterine weight was seen at 10 μg per rat and no further increase in uterine weight was seen at doses of **47** 200-fold higher.

The antifertility activity of **47** in the mouse closely paralleled its estrogenicity; MED_{100} was 0·1 mg kg^{-1}. The gonadotropin inhibitory activity of **47** was determined by oral administration to 28-day-old male rats for 7 days. At 5 mg kg^{-1} there was an insignificant reduction in testes weight, although the ventral prostate and seminal vesicles were significantly reduced in weight. No dose-response could be established due to toxicity encountered at 20 mg kg^{-1}.

Crenshaw and Luke (1969) have reported the synthesis of B-nor-6-thiaequilenin, ($\pm$)-*trans*-1,2,3,4,5,10-hexahydro-8-hydroxy-3-methyl-3*H*-benzo[*b*]indeno[5,4-*d*]-thiophene-3-one (**48a**) and related compounds (**48b–f**).

In immature mice dosed orally over a 3-day period, compounds **48(a–d)** showed approximately 0·1 per cent the estrogenicity of 17-α-ethinyl-estradiol, while compounds **48e** and **48f** were more active, showing

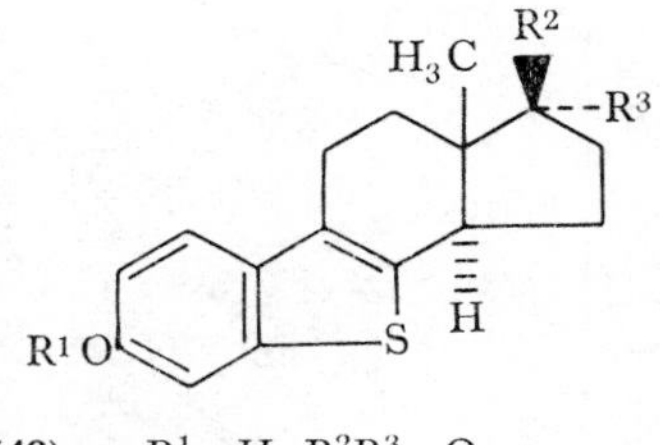

(48) a $R^1=H$; $R^2R^3=O$
     b $R^1=CH_3$; $R^2R^3=O$
     c $R^1=CH_3$; $R^2=OH$; $R^3=H$
     d $R^1=H$; $R^2=OH$; $R^3=H$
     e $R^1=CH_3$; $R^2=OH$; $R^3=C\equiv CH$
     f $R^1=H$; $R^2=OH$; $R^1=C\equiv CH$

TABLE 9

LD$_{50}$ values and overt behavior for indole, benzo[b]thiophene and 1-methylindole derivatives

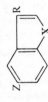

Common name of indolic compound	X	Z	R	LD$_{50}$[a] (mg kg^{-1}, ip)	Overt behavior[b]
Tryptophan	NH	H	CH$_2$CH(NH$_2$)COOH	>500	N
	S	H		>500	N
	NCH$_3$	H		286	N
5-Hydroxytryptophan	NH	HO		486	S-1
	S	HO		429	S-1
Indole-3-acetic acid	NH	H	CH$_2$COOH	>500	S-1
	S	H		>500	S-1
	NCH$_3$	H		>500	S-1
5-Hydroxyindole-3-acetic acid	NH	HO		1125	S-1
	S	HO		668	S-1
5-Methoxyindole-3-acetic acid	NH	CH$_3$O		98	H-1
	S	CH$_3$O		168	S-1
Tryptamine	NH	H	CH$_2$CH$_2$NH$_2$	285	H-2
	S	H		147	H-2
	NCH$_3$	H		109[c]	S-1
5-Hydroxytryptamine	NH	HO		528	S-1
	S	HO		454	S-1
5-Methoxytryptamine	NH	CH$_3$O		176	N
	S	CH$_3$O		192	S-1

NN-Dimethyltryptamine	NH	H	$CH_2CH_2N(CH_3)_2$	117	H-2
	S	H	$CH_2CH_2N(CH_3)_2$	110	H-2
	NCH_3	H	$CH_2CH_2N(CH_3)_2$	61	H-3
Bufotenin	NH	HO	$CH_2CH_2N(CH_3)_2$	196	H-1
	S	HO	$CH_2CH_2N(CH_3)_2$	149	H-1
5-Methoxy-*NN*-dimethyltryptamine	NH	CH_3O	$CH_2CH_2N(CH_3)_2$	126	H-1
	S	CH_3O	$CH_2CH_2N(CH_3)_2$	182	H-2
N-Methyltryptamine	NH	H	$CH_2CH_2NHCH_3$	158	H-1
	S	H	$CH_2CH_2NHCH_3$	147	H-1
	NCH_3	H	$CH_2CH_2NHCH_3$	98[c]	H-1
Melatonin	NH	CH_3O	$CH_2CH_2NHCOCH_3$	478	N
	S	CH_3O	$CH_2CH_2NHCOCH_3$	412	N
Tryptophol	NH	H	CH_2CH_2OH	351	S-2
	S	H	CH_2CH_2OH	> 300[c]	S-3
	NCH_3	H	CH_2CH_2OH	> 500[c]	S-2

[a] Deaths were recorded in the 4-h period after dosage. Each value represents a minimum of 20 mice per dose and 7 doses unless otherwise indicated.

[b] N, normal; S, sedated; H, hyperactive; degrees of sedation or hyperactivity indicated by 1, slight; 2, moderate; 3, pronounced.

[c] 10 mice/dose.

approximately 0·3 per cent the estrogenicity of 17α-ethinylestradiol. Compounds **48a**, **48c**, **48f** afforded complete protection against pregnancy in mice following oral dosing at 50 mg kg^{-1} on days 1 through 4 post coitum; incomplete protection was seen at lower doses. Compounds **48b**, **48c**, and **48d** afforded incomplete protection at 50 mg kg^{-1}. The standard, 17α-ethinylestradiol, was active at 0·1 mg kg^{-1} in this test (Crenshaw, 1976).

In an extension of the thiaequilenin work, Crenshaw *et al.* (1972) have synthesized a series of tetrahydrodibenzothiophenecarboxylic acids and evaluated their antifertility activity. Compounds **49** and **50** were the most active compounds, preventing pregnancy in the rat at doses of 1 mg kg^{-1}. In certain postcoital dosing regimens, **49** and **50** were found to be considerably more active in preventing or terminating pregnancy in the rat than would be predicted on the basis of their estrogenicity in immature rats. The Raney nickel desulfurization of these tetrahydrodibenzothiophenecarboxylic acids produced compounds which are weak estrogens (Crenshaw *et al.*, 1973). In extending this finding of potent estro-

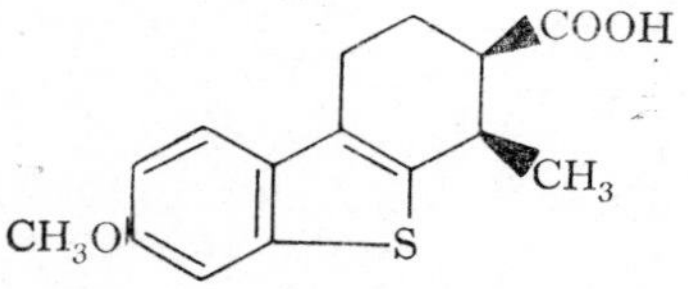

(49) 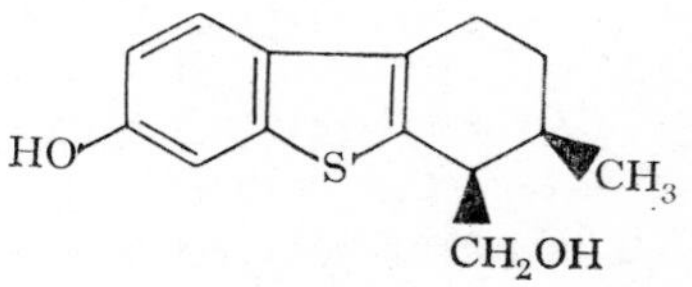   50

genicity associated with compounds such as **51** (Crenshaw *et al.*, 1974), Crenshaw (1976) returned to the benzo[*b*]thiophene series and evaluated the estrogenic activity associated with **52** and **53**.

In immature rats dosed orally over a 3-day period, compound **53** was approximately 10 per cent as estrogenic as 17α-ethinylestradiol while compound **52** was less than 0·1 per cent as estrogenic. Compound **53** afforded complete protection against pregnancy in rats following oral dosing at 1 mg kg^{-1} on days 1 through 5 post coitum; compound **52** afforded no protection at 25 mg kg^{-1}. The MED$_{100}$ for 17α-ethinylestradiol was 0·2 mg kg^{-1} (Crenshaw, 1976).

Gaind and Mathur (1971) have studied the antifertility effects of some 4-aminobenzo[*b*]thiophene and 4-keto-4,5,6,7-tetrahydrobenzo[*b*]thiophene derivatives in rats and found 35–50 per cent reduction in pregnancies when dosed day 1–7 at 20 mg kg^{-1}.

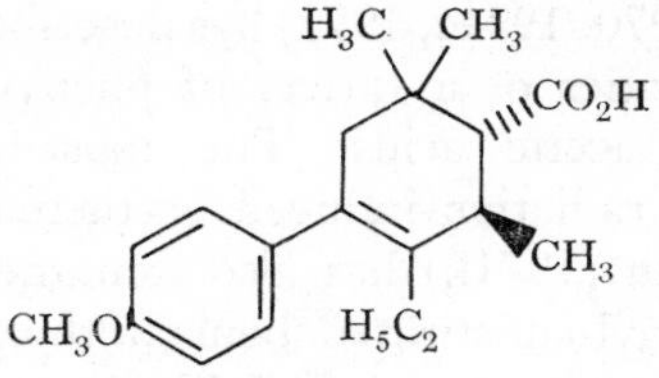

51

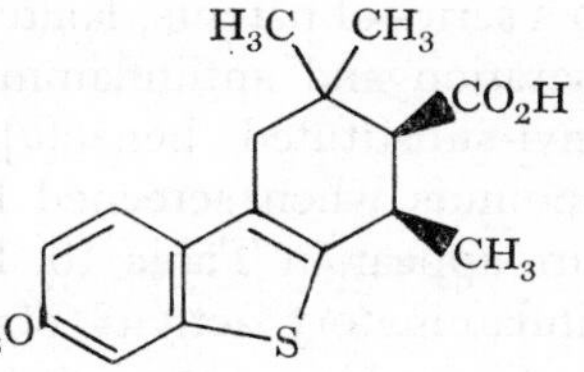

52

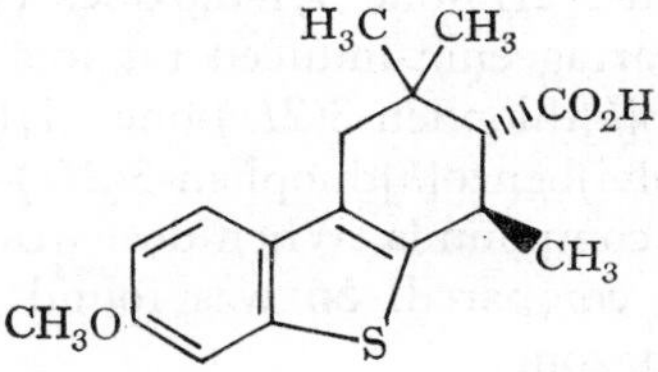

53

5.2 ANTIINFLAMMATORY AGENTS

In recent years there has been considerable interest in the antiinflammatory properties of benzo[b]thiophene derivatives. Descamps et al. (1973) prepared a series of benzo[b]thiophene-2 and 3-acetic acid derivatives, the most active of which were 5-bromo-3-methylbenzo[b]thiophene-2-acetic acid (54) and 5-chloro-3-methylbenzo[b]thiophene-2-acetic acid (55). The latter compound, 55, was the subject of a detailed pharmacological study

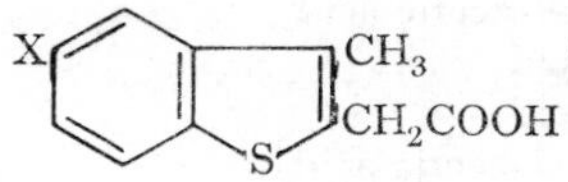

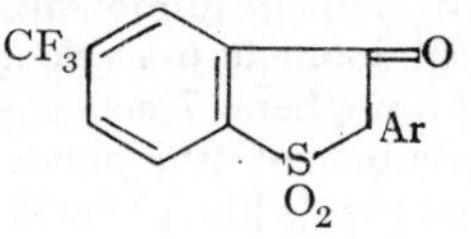

(54) X=Br   (56) Ar=C_6H_5
(55) X=Cl   (57) Ar=p-$CH_3C_6H_4$

(Colot et al., 1974). Compound 55 was shown to possess antiinflammatory and antiarthritic properties in rats when administered orally or used topically and showed activity comparable to phenylbutazone in the carrageenin or uv-induced erythema screens. Compound 55 was found to exhibit moderate gastric ulcerogenic properties and a low acute toxicity, both of which were minimal at the dose-exhibiting antiinflammatory properties.

In a series of patents, Kaltenbronn (1970, 1971a, 1972) has described the preparation and antiinflammatory activities of a variety of phenyl- and thienyl-substituted benzo[b]thiophene acetic acids. The most active compounds when screened by the uv radiation-induced erythema procedure appear in Table 10. Kaltenbronn (1971b) has also examined the antiinflammatory activity of some phenyl-substituted benzo[b]thiophene derivatives. Using the same test procedure 4-phenyl-7β-hydroxyethylbenzo[b]thiophene and 3-phenyl-7-N,N-dimethylaminoethylbenzo[b]-thiophene were each found to have minimum effective doses of 0·2 mg kg⁻¹.

Antiinflammatory activity has also been demonstrated in a series of 2-arylbenzo[b]thiophen-3(2H)-one 1,1-dioxides (Lombardino and Wiseman, 1970). In the carrageenin-induced rat foot edema test 5-trifluoromethyl-2-phenylbenzo[b]thiophen-3(2H)-one 1,1-dioxide (56) and 5-trifluoromethyl-2(p-tolyl)benzo[b]thiophen-3(2H)-one 1,1-dioxide (57) were the most potent compounds. When dose–response curves for 56 and phenylbutazone were compared, 56 was found to be 1·24 times more potent than phenylbutazone.

Several reports have appeared indicating the presence of antiinflamma-

TABLE 10

Antiflammatory activity of benzo[b]thiophene acetic acid derivatives

Compound	Minimum effective dose, mg kg⁻¹
4-Phenylbenzo[b]thiophene-2-acetic acid	6·2
7-Phenylbenzo[b]thiophene-3-acetic acid	0·1
7-Phenylbenzo[b]thiophene-4-acetic acid	0·1
7-(m-Tolyl)benzo[b]thiophene-4-acetic acid	3·1
α-Methyl-7-phenylbenzo[b]thiophene-4-acetic acid	0·4
2-Phenylbenzo[b]thiophene-6-acetic acid	12·5
3-Phenylbenzo[b]thiophene-7-acetic acid	0·4
3-(p-Fluorophenyl)benzo[b]thiophene-7-acetic acid	3·1
α-Butyl-3-phenylbenzo[b]thiophene-7-acetic acid	6·2
4-Phenylbenzo[b]thiophene-7-acetic acid	0·2
2-Methyl-7-phenylbenzo[b]thiophene-4-acetic acid	0·4
7-Cyclohexylbenzo[b]thiophene-3-acetic acid	3·1
3-(5-Bromo-2-thienyl)benzo[b]thiophene-7-acetic acid	3·1
4-(5-Bromo-2-thienyl)benzo[b]thiophene-7-acetic acid	3·1
7-(2-Thienyl(benzo[b]thiophene-4-acetic acid	0·8
α-Methyl-7-(2-thienyl)benzo[b]thiophene-4-acetic acid	0·8
3-(2-Thienyl)benzo[b]thiophene-7-acetic acid	0·4
4-(2-Thienyl)benzo[b]thiophene-7-acetic acid	0·8
4-(5-Chloro-2-thienyl)benzo[b]thiophene-7-acetic acid	3·1

From Kaltenbronn (1970, 1971a, 1972).

tory activity among some benzo[*b*]thieno[2,3-*d*]pyrimidine derivatives (Centre d'Etudes pour l'Industrie Pharmaceutique, 1971; Manhas *et al.*, 1972). In the carrageenin-induced edema test in mice, 2-methyl-3-(*p*-tolyl)-4-oxo-3,4,5,6,7,8-hexahydrobenzo[*b*]thieno[2,3-*d*]pyrimidine (58) was shown to produce 30 per cent inhibition following an oral dose of 80 mg kg^{-1} (Manhas *et al.*, 1972).

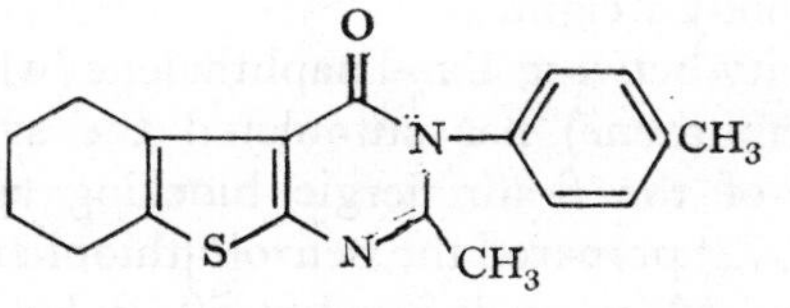

(58)

5.3 CARDIOVASCULAR AND DIURETIC AGENTS

In the past several years a number of reports have appeared describing cardiovascular and diuretic effects associated with benzo[*b*]thiophene derivatives. Several of these reports have dealt with the preparation of a series of 3-(4-dialkylaminoalkoxy-3,5-disubstituted)benzoylbenzo[*b*]-thiophenes (Claeys *et al.*, 1972; Gubin *et al.*, 1975). Two of these derivatives, 2-ethyl-3-(3,5-dibromo-4-γ-di-*n*-propylaminopropoxy)benzoyl-benzo[*b*]thiophene (59) and 2-methyl-3-(3,5-dimethyl-4-γ-dibutyl-aminopropoxy)benzoylbenzo[*b*]thiophene (60) have undergone detailed

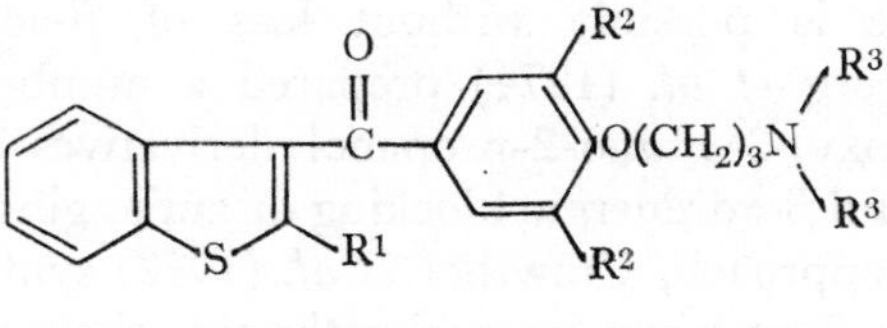

(59) $R^1=C_2H_5$; $R^2=Br$; $R^3=n-C_3H_7$
(60) $R^1=CH_3$; $R^2=CH_3$; $R^3=n-C_3H_9$

pharmacological evaluations which have indicated antiadrenergic and antianginal activities (Charlier *et al.*, 1973, 1975). In the anesthetized dog, both 59 and 60 induced a decrease in myocardial oxygen consumption due mainly to a slowing of the heart rate and a reduction in the total vascular resistance. Both compounds also increased coronary arterial blood flow without decreasing cardiac output. Compounds 59 and 60 possessed antiadrenergic effects not due to β-adrenergic receptor blockade. Vaughan Williams and Polster (1974) have compared the effects of **59** on cardiac muscle to those of the clinically useful antianginal agent, aminodarone. They found that **59**, when administered for a period of 6 weeks to rabbits at a dose of 20 mg kg^{-1} per day, prolonged the plateau of the intracellularly recorded action potential, in a manner similar to aminodarone. In contrast to aminodarone, **59** did not cause a reduction in heart weight when expressed as a percentage of body weight.

The close similarity between **1** and naphthalene (which is the basis of the trivial name thianaphthene) has stimulated the synthesis of benzo[*b*]-thiophene analogs of the β-adrenergic blocking agent propranol (**61**). Chodnekar *et al.* (1972) prepared the benzo[*b*]thiophene analog of propranolol (**62**). Compound **61**, when infused at 50 μg kg^{-1} min^{-1}, produced a 45 per cent inhibition of isoproterenol-induced tachycardia in the cat, while **62** produced a 42 per cent inhibition at the same dose. These results

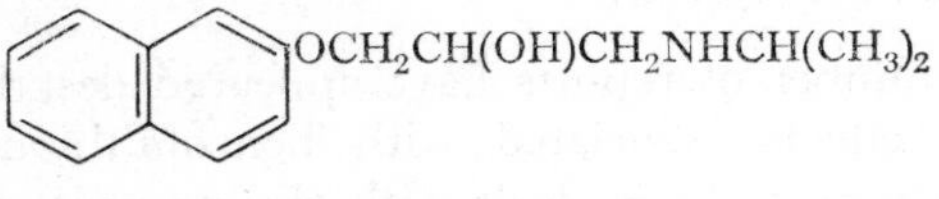

OCH$_2$CH(OH)CH$_2$NHCH(CH$_3$)$_2$

(**61**)

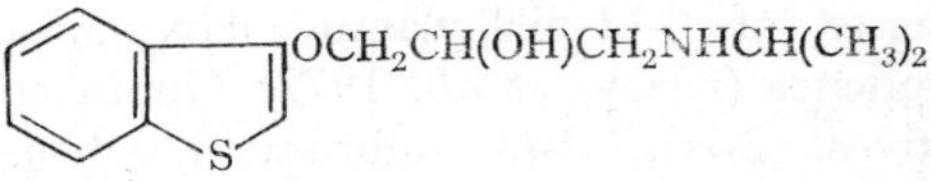

OCH$_2$CH(OH)CH$_2$NHCH(CH$_3$)$_2$

(**62**)

indicate that replacement of the naphthalene ring systems by that of benzo[*b*]thiophene is possible without loss of β-adrenergic blocking activity. Goldenberg *et al.* (1974) prepared a number of 1-(2-alkyl-3-benzo[*b*]thiophenoxy)-3-amino-2-propanol derivatives (**63**) related to **61** and found no useful β-adrenergic blocking or antianginal properties. In an extension of this approach, Crowther *et al.* (1972) synthesized a series of benzo[*b*]thiophene derivatives possessing the side chain of **61**; evaluation of their β-adrenergic blocking activity yielded the data presented in Table 11.

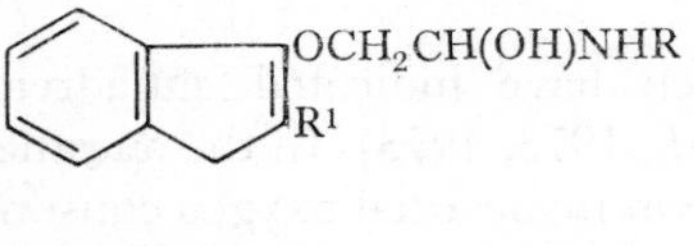

OCH$_2$CH(OH)NHR
R^1

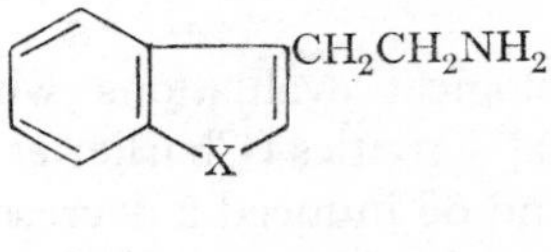

CH$_2$CH$_2$NH$_2$
X

(**63**)   R and R^1 = alkyl and aryl

(**64**)   X = NH
(**65**)   X = NCH$_3$
(**66**)   X = S

TABLE 11

β-Adrenergic blocking activities of some benzo[b]thiophene derivatives related to propranolol

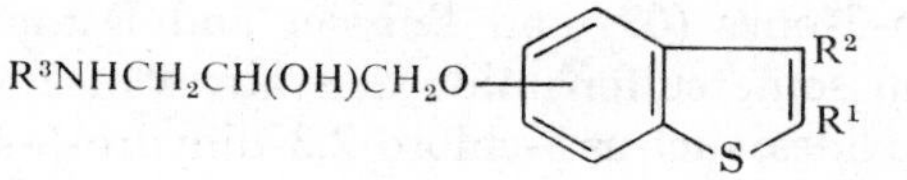

$R^3NHCH_2CH(OH)CH_2O$—

Compound			Position of side chain	Infusion rate, μg per kg^{-1} per min	% Inhibition of tachy-cardia
R^1	R^2	R^3			
H	H	$CHMe_2$	4	2·5	89
H	H	CMe_3	4	1	52
H	H	cyclopentyl	4	20	62
H	H	$CHMe_2$	5	10	52
H	H	CH_2CH_2Me	5	50	29
H	H	$CH_2CH{=}CH_2$	5	5	58
H	Me	$CHMe_2$	7	40	63
H	Me	CMe_3	7	20	83
	Propranolol			50	45

From Crowther *et al.* (1972).

The pressor affects of tryptamine (**64**) and its 1-methylindole (**65**) and benzo[b]thiophene (**66**) analogs have been studied in the intact anesthetized rat (Bosin *et al.*, 1976b). Methylation of **64** at the 1-position to produce **65** resulted in little effect on its potency as a pressor agent, while substitution of a benzo[b]thiophene nucleus (**66**) decreased the pressor activity. The order of activity was shown to be **65** > **64** > **66**. Pretreatment of animals with reserpine reduced the absolute pressor effect of **64** and **66** while increasing the effect of **65**. Pretreatment with phenoxybenzamine reduced the absolute effect of all three compounds.

The antihypertensive properties of some 2-imidazolinylaminobenzo[b]-thiophenes (**67**) and (**68**) have also been reported (Hess and Nelson, 1971). Following oral doses of 100–2000 μg kg^{-1} to dogs, compounds **67** and **68** lowered the blood pressure by 15–55 mm within 2–4 hours.

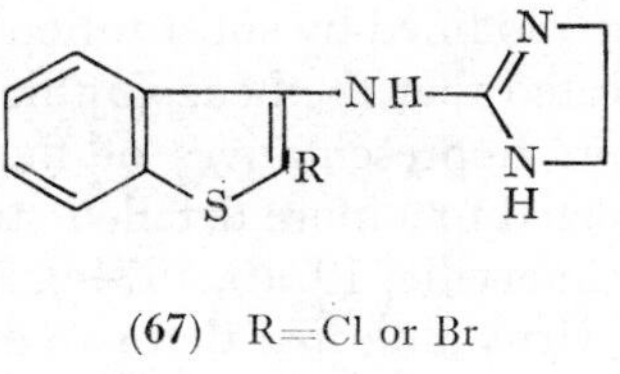

(67) R=Cl or Br

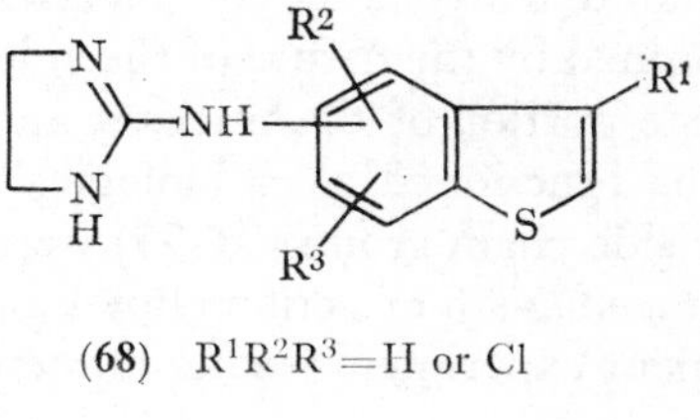

(68) $R^1R^2R^3$=H or Cl

Several benzo[b]thiophene derivatives which exhibit antihypertensive and diuretic properties have appeared in the recent patent literature. Suh (1970b) reported the presence of diuretic activity in some cyclopenta[b]-benzo[b]thiophen-3-ones (69) and Boissier and Ratouis (1970) reported similar activity in some sulfonamide derivatives of 2,3-dihydrobenzo[b]-thiophene 1,1-dioxides, such as 5-chloro-2,3-dihydro-6-sulfamoylbenzo[b]-thiophene 1,1-dioxide (70).

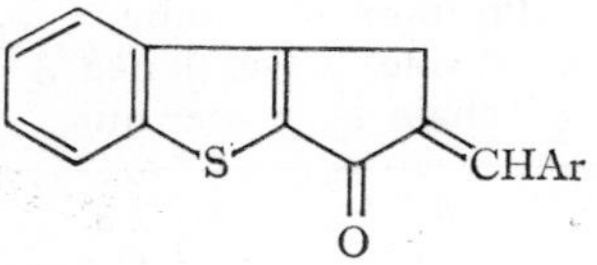

                    (69) 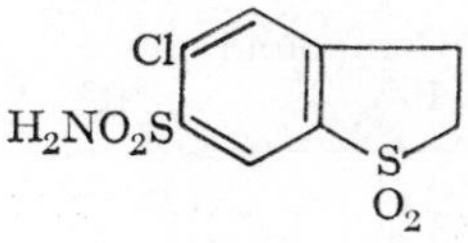   (70)

5.4   CHEMOTHERAPEUTIC AGENTS

The design, synthesis and pharmacological evaluation of potential chemotherapeutic agents has been an active area of research in the past few years; benzo[b]thiophene derivatives exhibit antiviral and antifungal activities.

Stimulated by the antiviral activity present in thiosemicarbazone derivatives such as N-methylisatin β-thiosemicarbazone (methisazone), Dickinson et al. (1973) prepared a series of benzo[b]thiophene-2- and -3-carboxaldehyde thiosemicarbazones. These compounds were screened in vitro against the IHD strain of vaccinia virus and the PR8 strain of influenza A virus. Activity was calculated as the percentage inhibition of virus multiplication produced by the compound when compared with replicate, untreated, but infected control preparations. Table 12 summarizes the results obtained against vaccinia; none of the derivatives demonstrated significant activity against influenza A virus.

Boyd and Sommerville (1974a, 1974b, 1974c) assessed the antiviral properties of 179 benzo[b]thiophene derivatives reported by Chapman et al. (1974). Considerable activity towards influenza A_2 and vaccinia viruses was found (Boyd and Sommerville, 1974a). The antiviral activity was determined by the nature of the side chain, modified by substitution in the benzene portion of the nucleus, and indicated that the benzo[b]thiophene nucleus functioned as a biological carrier. Representatives of the most active side chain group (71–77) were subjected to a more detailed study of their mechanism of action (Boyd and Sommerville, 1974b, 1974c). Timed treatment experiments using influenza A_2 virus indicated that two distinct

TABLE 12

Activity of benzo[*b*]thiophenecarboxaldehyde thiosemicarbazones against vaccinia virus

R^1	R^2	Dose (M)	Inhibition (%)	Dose (M)	Inhibition (%)
H	H	10^{-4}	97·5	10^{-4}	85·8
H	Me	10^{-3}	—	10^{-3}	94·4
		10^{-5}	97·0		
H	Cl	10^{-4}	98·0		
Me	H	10^{-3}	98·8	10^{-4}	96·0
Me	Me	10^{-5}	64·5	10^{-3}	99·3
Me	Cl	10^{-3}	97·4	10^{-3}	96·5
SMe	H	10^{-3}	98·5	10^{-5}	87·0
SMe	Me			10^{-4}	94·0
SMe	Cl			10^{-4}	93·0
Ph	H	10^{-5}	73·4	10^{-5}	60·0
Ph	Me			10^{-4}	33·0
Ph	Cl	10^{-3}	0	10^{-4}	68·0
Ph	Br			10^{-4}	18·0
Cl	H			10^{-4}	59·1
Br	H	10^{-5}	63·2	10^{-3}	66·0
Br	Me	10^{-3}	100		
Br	Me	10^{-4}	96·0		
Br	Me	10^{-5}	91·7		
OCH$_3$	H			10^{-3}	98·0
N-Methylisatin β-thiosemicarbazone (Methisazone)				10^{-5}	97·3

From Dickinson *et al.* (1973).

types of activity were present. One occurred early in the virus growth cycle at a time similar to inhibition by adamantylamine. The second type inhibited a metabolic event after viral uncoating, but before the earliest time at which nuclear antigen inhibition by *p*-fluorophenylalanine could be demonstrated. Compounds **72** and **75** indicated the first type of activity, while **71** and **74** demonstrated the second type of activity (Boyd and Sommerville, 1974b). Similar timed experiments with vaccinia virus indicated that each derivative inhibited vaccinia virus at a different point in the replication cycle. Compounds **75** and **77** were found to act early in the

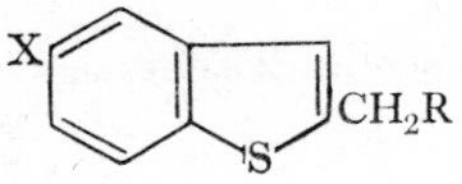

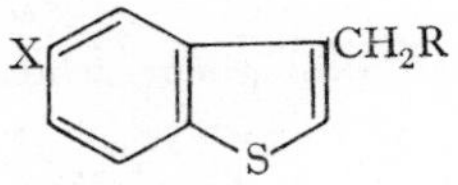

(71) X=Cl; R=N(CH₃)₂

(72) X=Br; R=N

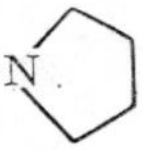

(73) X=Cl; R=N
$$R=N \begin{array}{c} C_2H_5 \\ CH_2CH_2OH \end{array}$$

(74) X=Cl; R=N(C₂H₅)₂

(75) X=Cl; R=N   O

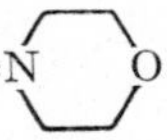

(76) X=I; R=N

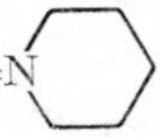

(77) X=Cl; R=NHCN(CH₃)₂
‖
NH

growth cycle while **73** acted 2–3 hours later. The actions of **76** corresponded closely to that of 5-iodo-2'-deoxyuridine.

Antiviral activity has also been claimed in the patent literature (Lwoff *et al.*, 1970a, 1970b) for 2,3-dihydrobenzo[*b*]thiophene-2,3-dione thiosemicarbazone (**78**) and amidinohydrazones of 2,3-dihydrobenzo[*b*]thiophene-2,3-dione (**79**) and 4,5,6,7-tetrahydrobenzo[*b*]thiophene-4-one (**80**). These compounds were active against poliomyelitis viruses type 1, and strain Sabin LSc2ab and G81.

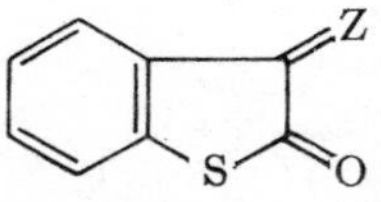

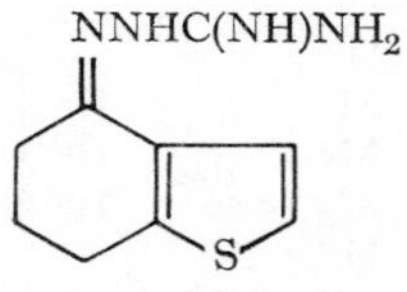

(78) Z=NNHCSNH₂   (80)
(79) Z=NNHC(NH)NH₂

A number of reports have also appeared describing antifungal activity among select benzo[*b*]thiophene derivatives. Chandler and Florestano (1971a, 1971b, 1971c) have found significant antifungal activity for methyl-5-chloro-3-hydroxy-benzo[*b*]thiophene-2-carboxylate (**81**) and related compounds. An ointment containing 0·1 per cent of **81** totally suppressed skin infection due to *Trichophyton mentagrophytes* in the guinea pig. Saraf (1971) has reported antifungal and muscle relaxant activity at low doses of the benzo[*b*]thiophene derivative, 5-bromo-*N*-ethyl-*N*-(2-fluoroethyl)-3-aminomethylbenzo[*b*]thiophene (**82**). Lastly, fungicidal properties have

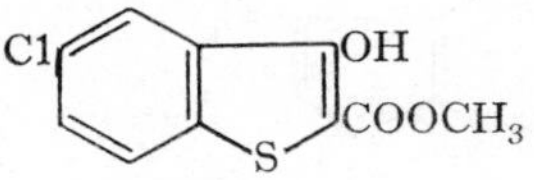

(81) 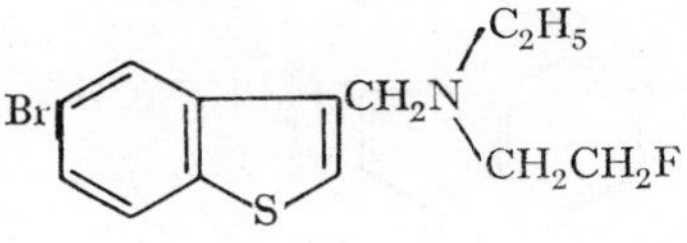   (82)

been claimed for a series of 2- or 3-arylthiobenzo[b]thiophene 1,1-dioxides (Von Schmeling *et al.*, 1970).

Antibacterial activities have also been reported for benzo[b]thiophene derivatives. Webber *et al.* (1971) prepared a series of 3-methoxymethyl-7-acylaminocephalosporins, including the benzo[b]thiophene derivative (83),

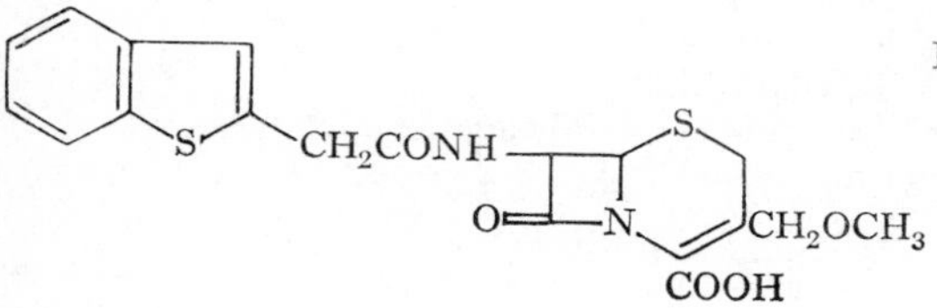

(83) 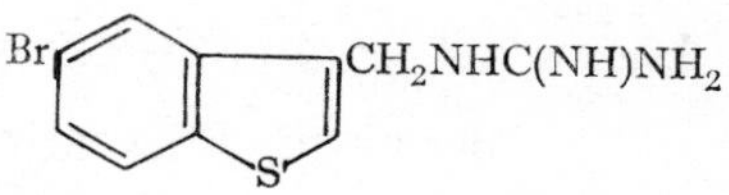   (84)

which was found to be a potent inhibitor of penicillin-resistant *Staphylococcus aureus* but had no effect on Gram-negative bacteria. Chapman *et al.* (1974) have shown that 5-bromo-3-guanidinomethylbenzo[b]thiophene (84) inhibited the growth of *Staphylococcus aureus* at a concentration less than 0·35 μg ml^{-1}.

5.5 CENTRAL NERVOUS SYSTEM AGENTS

Centrally active benzo[b]thiophene derivatives have contributed significantly to the pharmacological activities associated with this heterocycle (Campaigne *et al.*, 1969, 1970, 1973a). In continuing studies of the synthesis and pharmacological properties of benzo[b]thiophene isosteres of biologically active indole derivatives, Campaigne and Rogers (1973a, 1973b) synthesized 3-(2-dimethylaminoethyl)-4-hydroxybenzo[b]thiophene (86), the sulfur analog of psilocin (85), and some related compounds (87–89). Chapman *et al.* (1972) and Neidlein and Gehringer (1974) have also reported the synthesis of 86. Beck (1973) has examined the central effects of 86–89 on pentobarbital-sedated male albino rabbits as determined by amplitude analysis of the cortical electroencephalogram (EEG).

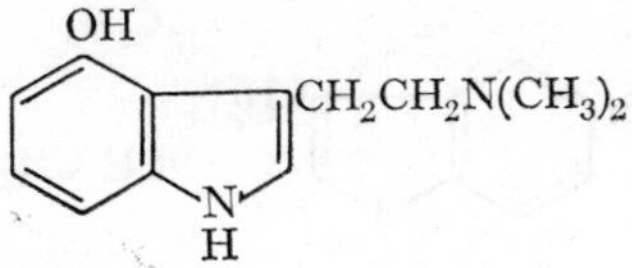

OH
⟨structure⟩ CH$_2$CH$_2$N(CH$_3$)$_2$
N
H

(85)

OR'
⟨structure⟩ CH$_2$CH$_2$NR$_2$
S

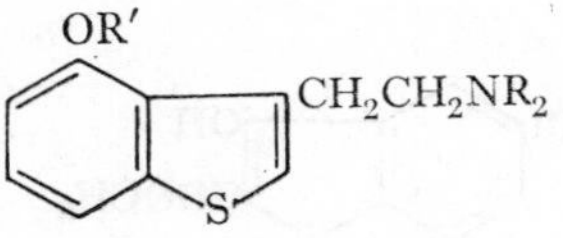

(86) R=CH$_3$; R'=H
(87) R=H; R'=H
(88) R=H; R'=CH$_3$
(89) R=CH$_3$; R'=CH$_3$

These data appear in Table 13 along with related benzo[b]thiophene and indole derivatives. The tertiary amine derivatives of benzo[b]thiophene produced increased sedation while the corresponding indole and primary amine derivatives of either heterocycle caused stimulation.

TABLE 13

Quantitative EEG analysis of some benzo[b]thiophene isosteres

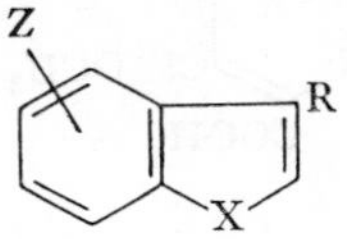

Z
⟨structure⟩ R
X

X	Compound R	Z	Dose mg kg^{-1}	% Reversal of phenobarbital-induced sedation
NH	CH$_2$CH$_2$NH$_2$	H	1·0	54·2
S	CH$_2$CH$_2$NH$_2$	H	1·0	83·2
S	CH$_2$CH$_2$N(CH$_3$)$_2$	H	1·0	−107·2[a]
S	CH$_2$CH$_2$NH$_2$	4-OH	1·0	59·2
NH	CH$_2$CH$_2$N(CH$_3$)$_2$	4-OPO$_3$H	0·27	50·0
S	CH$_2$CH$_2$N(CH$_3$)$_2$	4-OH	1·0	−27·7[a]
S	CH$_2$CH$_2$NH$_2$	4-OCH$_3$	1·0	31·1
S	CH$_2$CH$_2$N(CH$_3$)$_2$	4-OCH$_3$	1·0	−26·0[a]
NH	CH$_2$CH$_2$N(CH$_3$)$_2$	5-OCH$_3$	0·08	50·0

[a] Sedating.
From Beck (1973).

Humber et al. (1975) have described the synthesis and pharmacology of a novel class of antidepressants which are 1-aminoalkyl-1,3,4,9-tetra-hydropyrano[3,4-b] indoles. Extending this finding to benzo[b]thiophenes, they prepared and evaluated a series of 1H[1]benzothieno[2,3-c]pyrans (90) (Dobson et al., 1975). The acute toxicities of compounds 90 were determined in albino mice and the LD$_{50}$ determined from 5-day mortality

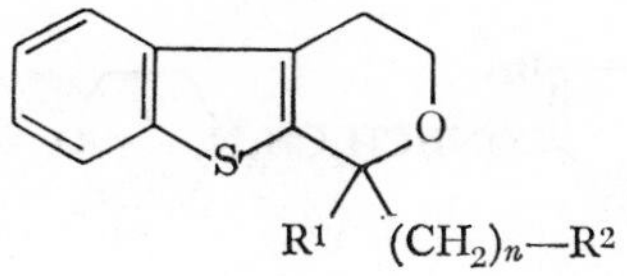

(90) R^1=H, CH_3; n=1,2; R^2=NH_2, $NHCH_3$, $N(CH_3)_2$

data. Antidepressant activity was assessed by measurement of the ability of these compounds to prevent reserpine-induced ptosis following an ip dose. Table 14 summarizes the acute toxicity and antidepressant activity of these 1H[1]benzo[b]thieno[2,3-c]pyran derivatives along with the known antidepressants amitriptyline and imipramine. Wright and Brabander (1970) have claimed in a patent that a series of amides of benzo[b]thiophene-2-

TABLE 14

Toxicity and antidepressant activity of some 1H[1]benzo[b]thieno[2,3-d]pyran derivatives

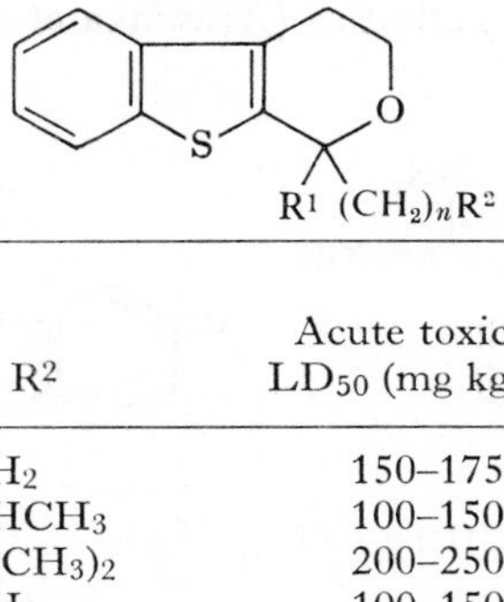

| Compound | | | Acute toxicity | Prevention of reserpine-induced |
R^1	n	R^2	LD_{50} (mg kg^{-1})	ptosis ED_{50} (mg kg^{-1})
H	1	NH_2	150–175	1·0
H	1	$NHCH_3$	100–150	1·75
H	1	$N(CH_3)_2$	200–250	0·85
H	2	NH_2	100–150	> 30·0
H	2	$N(CH_3)_2$	150–200	> 45·0
CH_3	3	$N(CH_3)_2$	100–150	9·6
Amitriptyline			94	4·7
Imipramine			115	6·0

From Dobson et al. (1975).

carboxylic acids, such as 3-bromo-2-(N-morpholinoethyl)benzo[b]thiophene carboxamide (91), possessed antidepressive and anticonvulsive activity.

Several reports have evaluated the antiaggressive activity of select benzo[b]thiophene derivatives. Suh (1972) has prepared and evaluated the

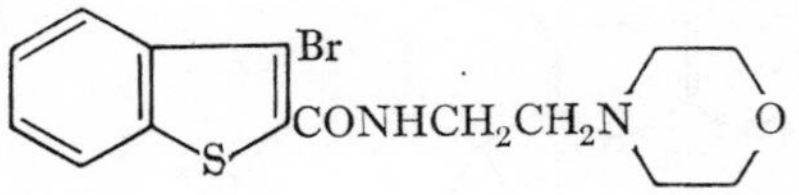

(91)

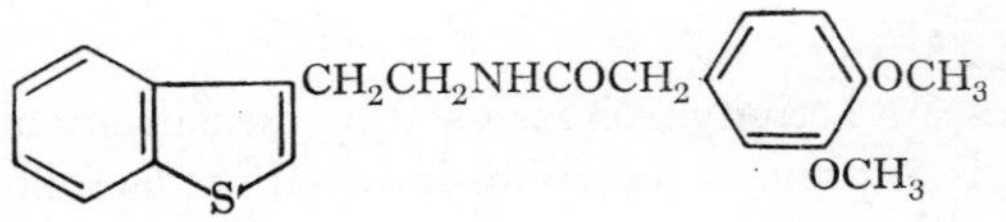

(92)

antiaggressive activity of a series of amides of 2-(3-benzo[b]thienyl)-ethylamines. Compound **92**, at a dose of 5 mg kg^{-1}, was able to reduce the aggressiveness and fighting of mice by 50 per cent. A series of 4-benzo[b]-thienyloxyalkyl amidoximes (**93**) have been prepared and found to possess very weak antiaggressive activities (Areschka *et al.*, 1975).

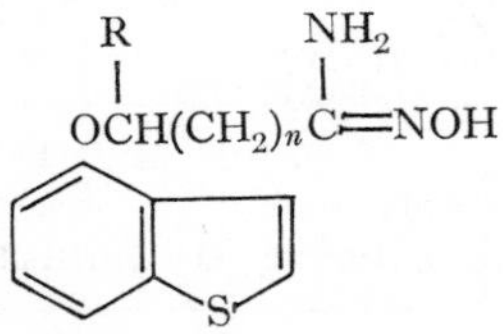

(93)   R=H, CH$_3$; $n=0,1$ 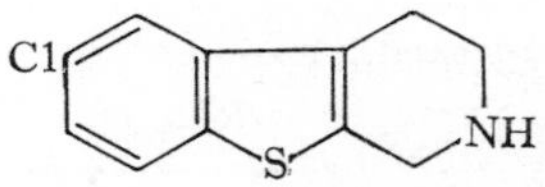   (94)

The behavioral effects of a potential antipsychotic agent, 6-chloro-1,2,3,4-tetrahydrobenzo[b]thieno[2,3-c]pyridine (**94**), have been studied in mice, rats, and squirrel monkeys (Miller *et al.*, 1971). In the mouse, **94** produced mild CNS depression, reducing both reactivity and spontaneous motor activity; spontaneous motor activity was depressed by doses $\geqslant$ 5 mg kg^{-1} ip. In the rat and squirrel monkey, similar depressant activities were found.

Central nervous system depressant activity has also been claimed, in patents, for a series of N-[4-phenyl-1-piperazinyl)alkyl]benzo[b]thiophene-2-carboxamides (**95**) (Wright and Brabander, 1972, 1973) and 3-substi-tuted-2,3-dihydro-1H-cyclopenta[b]benzo[b]thiophenes (**96**) (Suh, 1970a).

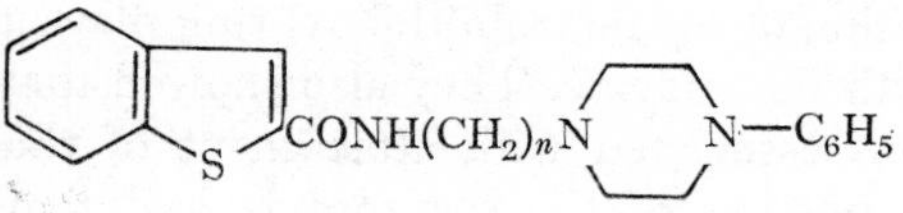

(95) $n=2,3$ 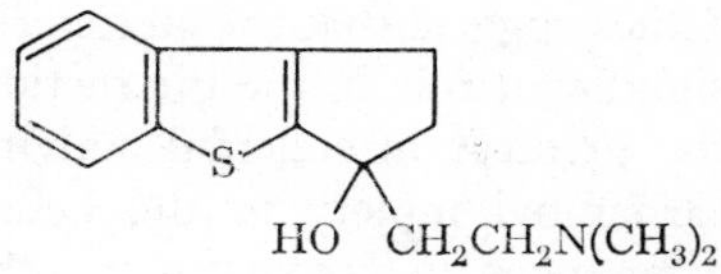 (96)

5.6 PESTICIDAL AGENTS

The presence of pesticidal activity among benzo[b]thiophene derivatives has been well documented, particularly for Mobam®, 4-benzo[b]thienyl-methylcarbamate (16). Numerous reports have appeared, attesting to the insecticidal properties of 16 towards a variety of pests. Table 15 summarizes these reports.

TABLE 15

Studies of the insecticidal properties of Mobam® (16)

Insect(s)	Reference
Gypsy moth larvae (*Porthetria dispar*)	Tomlin and Forgash (1972)
Body lice (*Anoplura: Pediculidae*)	Steinberg and Whitlaw (1969)
	Steinberg *et al.* (1972)
Mosquitos (*Anopheles stephensi* and *Aedes oegypti*)	Hadaway *et al.* (1970)
Mosquitos (*Anopheles, Aedes, Culex*)	Taylor and Schoof (1971)
Mosquitos (*Anopheles gambiae, A. funestus, Culex pipiens fatigans*)	Hudson (1971)
Grasshopper (*Acrididae*)	McEwen *et al.* (1972)
Stable flies (*Stomoxys calcitrans*)	Campbell and Hermanussen (1971)
Spruce gall aphid (*Adelges abictis*)	Cameron *et al.* (1973)

The anticholinesterase and insecticidal properties of the 3-,5-,6- and 7-isomers of 16 in the housefly (*Musca domestica*) have been studied (Kilsheimer *et al.*, 1969; Mahfouz *et al.*, 1969). They found the I_{50} values for the cholinesterase enzyme to be: 16=7-isomer, 3×10^{-8} M; 3-isomer, 1×10^{-7} M; 6-isomer, 4×10^{-7} M; and 5-isomer, 9×10^{-7} M. These

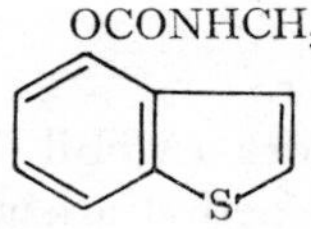

OCONHCH$_3$

(16)

values suggest that the steric orientation of the benzo[b]thienyl ring plays a significant role in the interaction with the enzyme. They also showed that the greatest insecticidal activity was associated with attachment of the carbamoyl moiety to the benzene portion of the heterocycle and that differences in activity may reflect differing rates of detoxification (ring hydroxylation) by mixed-function oxidases (Mahfouz *et al.*, 1969).

Several new benzo[b]thiophene-containing pesticides have also appeared in the literature. Gough (1969) has claimed that 4-benzo[b]thienyl ethyl 2,2-dichlorovinyl phosphate (97) possesses pesticidal activity, and Bock-stahler (1970) has similarly claimed broad pesticidal activity for a series of

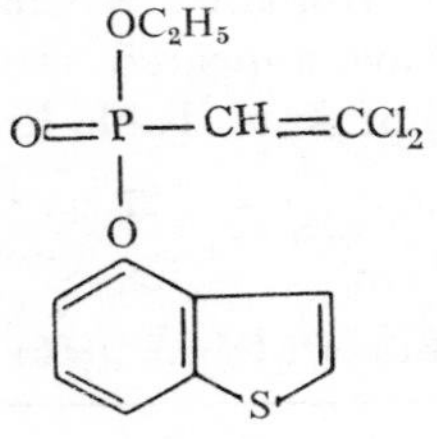

(97)

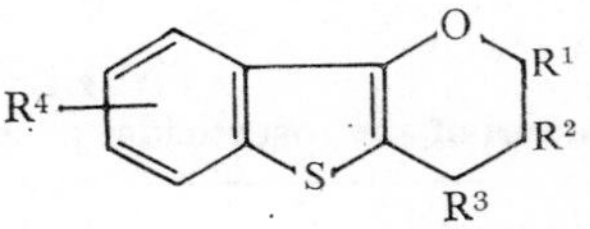

(98) R^1=piperidino, morpholino
       R^2=CH_3; C_2H_5
       R^3=C_2H_5; n-C_3H_7
       R^4=H; 7-Cl

substituted 2-amino-3,4-dihydro-2*H*-(1)benzothieno[3,2-*b*]pyrans (98). Derivatives of 2-hydroxybenzo[b]thiophene have been reported to exhibit pesticidal activities (Maravetz, 1974). For example, Compound 99 at 2 lb per acre was 100 per cent effective against pre-emergent crabgrass. A series of substituted benzo[b]thiophenes related to Mobam® (16) have been found

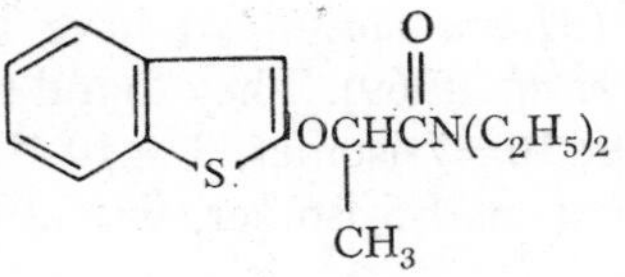

(99) 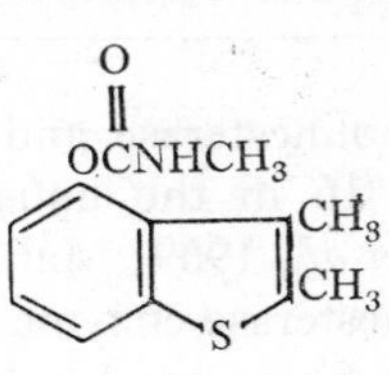   (100)

to be general action insecticides (Mobil Oil Corporation, 1974). 2,3-Dimethyl-4-benzo[b]thienyl *N*-methylcarbamate (100) was found to completely control *Aphis fabae* and *Epilachia verivestis* on beans at a concentration of 50 ppm.

5.7 OTHER ACTIVITIES

It is known that some of the more potent radioprotective substances are found among indole derivatives, i.e., 5-hydroxytryptamine (11) and 5-methoxytryptamine (101). Deanovic *et al.* (1970, 1971) evaluated the radioprotective activities present in the corresponding benzo[*b*]thiophene derivatives of 11 and 101, 13 and 102, respectively. The compounds were administered ip to mice 10–15 minutes prior to whole body irradiation

(11) X=NH; Z=OH
(13) X=S; Z=OH
(101) X=NH; Z=OCH$_3$
(102) X=S; Z=OCH$_3$

(103)

with a lethal dose, 950R (LD$_{100}$/30 days), or a supralethal dose, 1250–1400 R. The results of these studies appear in Table 16 and reveal 13 to be as active as 11 in lethally irradiated mice and 50 per cent as active at supralethal irradiation levels. Compound 102, in contrast to 101, exhibited no radioprotective activity.

The synthesis and pharmacological evaluation of a benzo[*b*]thiophene derivative, 4-oxo-4*H*-[1]benzothieno[3,2-*b*]pyran-2-carboxylic acid (103), possessing significant antiasthma activity has been reported (Wright and Johnson, 1973). In rats, comparison of 108 to disodium cromoglycate for the ability to inhibit the passive cutaneous anaphylaxis produced I$_{50}$ values of 5·0 mg kg^{-1} and 2·5 mg kg^{-1}, respectively. In the Rhesus monkey (*Macaca mulatta*), 103 was found to be 3·2 times as active as disodium cromoglycate in its ability to inhibit the Prausnitz–Kustner reaction. In the same species 103 was shown to be 18 times as active as disodium cromoglycate in inhibiting the active cutaneous anaphylaxis reaction resulting from intradermal administration of extracts of hog *Ascaris suum*.

Attention has also been focused on the hypochlolesterolemic properties of select benzo[*b*]thiophene compounds. Crenshaw *et al.* (1971) found that serum cholesterol levels were reduced in rats treated 4–30 days with 6 - methoxy - 3{*p* - [2 - (*N* - pyrrolidyl)ethoxy]phenyl} - 2 - phenylbenzo[*b*]thiophene (47). Rats dosed at 2·5 mg kg^{-1} for 4 days exhibited a 46 per cent decrease in serum cholesterol levels with no weight changes of testes or accessory sexual organs. In a 30-day study, no significant effect was observed even at doses of 5 mg kg^{-1}. Hypocholesterolemic activity has also

TABLE 16

Radioprotective effectiveness of some indole and benzo[b]thiophene derivatives

Compound Name	Number	Number of animals	Dose mM kg⁻¹	Radiation dose (R)	Number of survivors after 30 days (%)	Mean survival time (±S.E.M.) days
5-Hydroxytryptamine	**11**	120	0·28	950	120 (100%)	30·0
		40	0·28	1250	38 (95%)	28·9 ± 0·7
3-(2-Aminoethyl)-5-hydroxybenzo[b]-thiophene	**13**	20	0·28	950	20 (100%)	30·0
		20	0·28	1250	8 (40%)	18·8 ± 2·2
		20	0·56	1250	15 (75%)	24·4 ± 0·6
5-Methoxytryptamine	**101**	20	0·28	1400	15 (75%)	23·9 ± 2·0
3-(2-Aminoethyl)-5-Methoxybenzo[b]-thiophene	**102**	20	0·28	1400	0	5·3 ± 0·6

From Deanovic et al (1970, 1971).

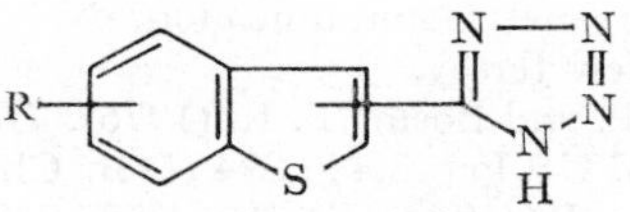

(104)   R=H; 5-Cl

been found for some 5-tetrazolyl-2- and -3-benzo[b]thiophenes **(104)** (Buchanan and Partyka, 1969).

Campaigne (1976) had a series of benzo[b]thiophene analogs **(107–110)** related to ellipticine **(105)** and olivacine **(106)** screened for their anti-tumor activity. When screened against L1210 lymphoid leukemia tumors in mice, compounds **107–110** were found to possess very weak antitumor activity (Wood, 1967, 1976).

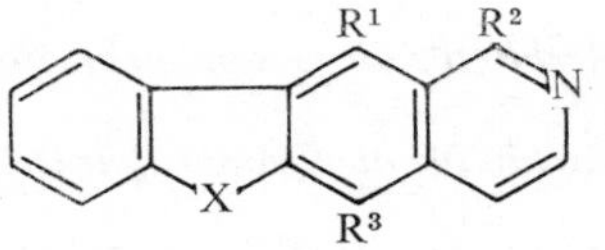

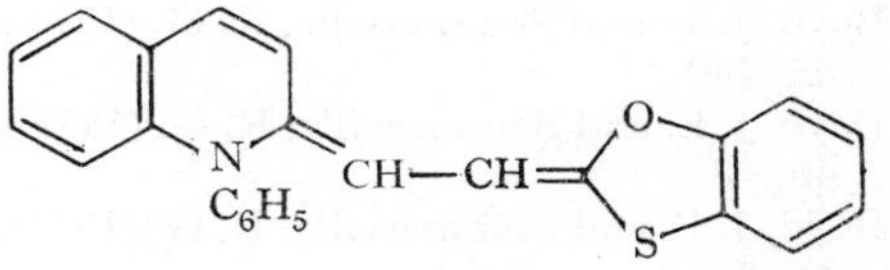

(105)   X=NH; R^1=CH$_3$; R^2=H; R^3=CH$_3$ (111)
(106)   X=NH; R^1=H; R^2=R^3=CH$_3$
(107)   X=S, R^1=CH$_3$; R^2=H; R^3=CH$_3$
(108)   X=S; R^1=H; R^2=R^3=CH$_3$
(109)   X=S; R^1=R^2=H; R^3=CH$_3$
(110)   X=S; R^1=R^2=R^3=H

Finally, the merocyanine dye, 2-(1-phenyl-1,2-dihydroquinolylidene)-3-oxo-2,3-dihydrobenzo[b]thiophene **(111)** has been claimed to be useful as a growth stimulant for spring barley (Pilyugin *et al.*, 1972).

References

Areschka, A., Mahaux, J.-M., Verbruggen, F., Houben, C., Descamps, M., Werbenec, J.-P., Broll, M., Simiand, J. and Eymard, P. (1975). *European Journal of Medicinal Chemistry*, **10**, 463.

Axelrod, J. (1962). *Journal of Biological Chemistry*, **237**, 1657.

Axelrod, J. (1971). *Science*, **173**, 598

Barrass, B. C., Coult, D. B., Pinder, R. M. and Skeels, M. (1973). *Biochemical Pharmacology*, **22**, 2891.

Baumgarten, H. G., Everts, K. D., Holman, R. B., Iversen, L. L., Vogt, M. and Wilson. G. (1972). *Journal of Neurochemistry*, **19**, 1587.

Beck, R. A. (1973). Personal Communication. New Jersey Neuro-psychiatric Institute, Princeton, New Jersey.

Bickers, R., Maickel, R. P. and Bosin, T. R. (1976). *The Pharmacologist*. In press.

Bockstahler, E. R. (1970). US Pat. 3,499,894 (Dow Chemical Co.).

Boissier, J. R. and Ratouis, R. (1970). Fr. Pat. 1,585,930 (Société Industrielle pour la Fabrication des Antibiotiques).

Bosin, T. R., Maickel, R. P., Dinner, A., Snell, A. and Campaigne, E. (1972a). *Journal of Heterocyclic Chemistry*, **9**, 1265.

Bosin, T. R., Campaigne, E. and Maickel, R. P. (1972b). *Life Sciences*, **11**, 685.

Bosin, T. R., Buckpitt, A. R. and Maickel, R. P. (1974a). *Life Sciences*, **14**, 899.

Bosin, T. R., Hathaway, D. R. and Maickel, R. P. (1974b). *Archives Internationales de Pharmacodynamie et de Thérapie*, **212**, 32.

Bosin, T. R., Hathaway, D. R. and Maickel, R. P. (1975). *American Journal of Physiology*, **228**, 496.

Bosin, T. R., Campaigne, E., Dinner, A., Rogers, R. B. and Maickel, R. P. (1976a). *Journal of Toxicology and Environmental Health*, **1**, 515.

Bosin, T. R., Hixson, E. J. and Maickel, R. P. (1976b). *British Journal of Pharmacology*, **56**, 25

Boyd, J. E. and Sommerville, R. G. (1974a). *Archiv für die Gesamte Virusforschung*, **45**, 249.

Boyd, J. E. and Sommerville, R. G. (1974b). *Archiv für die Gesamte Virusforschung*, **46**, 78.

Boyd, J. E. and Sommerville, R. G. (1974c). *Archiv für die Gesamte Virusforschung*, **46**, 86.

Buchanan, R. D. and Partyka, R. A. (1969). US Pat. 3,452,049 (Bristol-Meyers Co.).

Buckpitt, A. R., Bosin, T. R., Morris, J. B. and Maickel, R. P. (1976). *Federation Proceedings*, **35**, 803.

Burkard, W. R. and Kettler, R. (1975). Personal Communication, F. Hoffman-LaRoche and Co., Basel, Switzerland.

Cameron, E. A., Campbell, R. L. and Adams, L. E. (1973). *Journal of Economic Entomology*, **66**, 811.

Campaigne, E. (1976). Personal Communication, Indiana University, Bloomington, Indiana.

Campaigne, E., Neiss, E. S. and Bosin, T. (1969). *Quarterly Reports of Sulfur Chemistry*, **4**, 229.

Campaigne, E. and Dinner, A. (1970). *Journal of Medicinal Chemistry*, **13**, 1205.

Campaigne, E., Knapp, D. R., Neiss, E. S. and Bosin, T. R. (1970). *In* "Advances in Drug Research" (Ed. A. B. Simmonds), vol. 5, pp. 1–54. Academic Press, London and New York.

Campaigne, E. and Rogers, R. B. (1973a). *Journal of Heterocyclic Chemistry*, **10**, 297.

Campaigne, E. and Rogers, R. B. (1973b). *Journal of Heterocyclic Chemistry*, **10**, 963.

Campaigne, E., Maickel, R. P. and Bosin, T. R. (1973a). *In* "Proceedings of the Third International Symposium on Medicinal Chemistry" (Ed. P. Pratesi), pp. 65–81. Butterworth, London.

Campaigne, E., Rogers, R. B., Donelson, A. C. and Bosin, T. R. (1973b). *Journal of Heterocyclic Chemistry*, **10**, 979.

Campbell, J. B. and Hermanussen, J. F. (1971). *Journal of Economic Entomology*, **64**, 1188.

Centre d'Etudes pour l'Industrie Pharmaceutique (1971). Fr. Demande Pat. 2,035,768 (Centre d'Etudes pour l'Industrie Pharmaceutique).

Chandler, A. D., Jr. and Florestano, H. J. (1971a). US Pat. 3,592,907 (Dow Chemical Co.).

Chandler, A. D., Jr. and Florestano, H. J. (1971b). Ger. Pat. 1,926,522 (Dow Chemical Co.).

Chandler, A. D., Jr. and Florestano, H. J. (1971c). Gr. Demande Pat. 2,043,479 (Dow Chemical Co.).

Chapman, N. B., Scrowston, R. M. and Sutton, T. M. (1972). *Journal of the Chemical Society*. Perkin I, 3011.

Chapman, N. B., Clarke, K. and James, J. W. (1974). US Pat. 3,855,242 (Aspro-Nicholas Ltd).

Charlier, R., Delanois, G. and Bauthier, J. (1973). *Archives Internationales de Pharmacodynamie et de Thérapie*, **201**, 234.

Charlier, R., Bauthier, J. and Richard, J. (1975). *Arzneimittel-Forschung*. **25**, 46.

Chiu, P., Harrison, S. D., Jr., Maickel, R. P. and Bosin, T. R. (1973). *The Pharmacologist*, **15**, 184.

Chodnekar, M. S., Crowther, A. F., Hepworth, W., Howe, R., McLoughlin, B. J., Mitchell, A., Rao, B. S., Slatcher, R. P., Smith, L. H. and Stevens, M. A. (1972). *Journal of Medicinal Chemistry*, **15**, 49–57.

Claeys, N., Goldenberg, R., Wandestrick, R., Deray, E., Descamps, M., Delaunois, G., Bauthier, J. and Charlier, R. (1972). *Chimica Therapeutica*, **7**, 377.

Clements, A. N. (1975). Personal Communication, Sittingbourne Research Centre, Sittingbourne, Kent, England.

Colot, M., Van Damme, M., Dirks, M., Beersaerts, J. and Charlier, R. (1974) *Archives Internationales de Pharmacodynamie et de Thérapie*, **208**, 328.

Costa, J. L., Kirk, K. L. and Murphy, D. L. (1976). Personal Communication, National Institutes of Health, Bethesda, MD.

Crenshaw, R. R. and Luke, G. M. (1969). *Tetrahedron Letters*, 4495.

Crenshaw, R. R., Jeffries, A. T., Luke, G. M., Cheney, L. C. and Bialy, G. (1971). *Journal of Medicinal Chemistry*, **14**, 1185.

Crenshaw, R. R., Luke, G. M., Jenks, T. A., Bialy, G. and Bierwagen, M. E. (1972). *Journal of Medicinal Chemistry*, **15**, 1162.

Crenshaw, R. R., Luke, G. M., Jenks, T. A., Partyka, R. A., Bialy, G. and Bierwagen, M. E. (1973). *Journal of Medicinal Chemistry*, **16**, 813.

Crenshaw, R. R., Luke, G. M., Jenks, T. A. and Bialy, G. (1974). *Journal of Medicinal Chemistry*, **17**, 1262.

Crenshaw, R. R. (1976). Personal Communication, Bristol-Meyers Co., Syracuse, NY.

Crowther, A. F., Howe, R., McLoughlin, B. J., Mallion, K. B., Rao, B. S., Smith, L. H. and Turner, R. W. (1972). *Journal of Medicinal Chemistry*, **15**, 260.

De Angelis, G. G. and Hess, H. J. E. (1972). US Pat. 3,706,747 (Pfizer Inc.).

Deanovic, Z., Pericic, D. and Supek, Z. (1970). *Strahelenterapie*, **140**, 749.

Deanovic, Z., Pericic, D. and Supek, Z. (1971). *Experientia*, **27**, 1448.

Descamps, M., Van Durme, E., Colot, M. and Charlier, T. (1973). *Chimica Therapeutica*, **8**, 536.

Dickinson, R. P., Iddon, B. and Sommerville, R. G. (1973). *International Journal of Sulfur Chemistry*, **8**, 233.

Dobson, T. A., Humber, L. G. and Charest, M. P. (1975). Personal Communication, Ayerst Research Laboratories, Montreal, Canada.

Donelson, A. C. (1975). PhD Thesis, Indiana University, Bloomington, Indiana.
Eberspacher, F., Uesseler, H. and Lingens, F. (1970). *Hoppe-Seyler's Zeitschrift für Physiologische Chemie*, **351**, 1465.
Elslager, E. F., Haley, N. F., McLean, J. R., Potoczak, D., Velosa, H. and Wheelock, R. H. (1972). *Journal of Medicinal Chemistry*, **15**, 61.
Freter, K., Weissbach, H., Redfield, B. G., Udenfriend, S. and Witkop, B. (1958). *Journal of the American Chemical Society*, **80**, 983.
Gaind, B. and Mathur, V. S. (1971). *Journal of Reproduction and Fertility*, **27**, 459.
Goldenberg, C., Wandestrick, R., Van Meerbuck, C., Descamps, M., Bauthier, J. and Charlier, R. (1974). *European Journal of Medicinal Chemistry*, **9**, 123.
Gough, S. T. D. (1969). US Pat. 3,468,909 (Mobil Oil Corporation).
Gubin, J., Claeys, N., Deray, E., Descamps, M., Bauthier, J., Richard, J. and Charlier, R. (1975). *European Journal of Medicinal Chemistry*, **10**, 418.
Hadaway, A. B., Barlow, F., Grose, J. E. H., Turner, C. R. and Flowers, L. S. (1970). *Bulletin of the World Health Organization*, **42**, 369.
Hall, L. E., Hegeman, G. D. and Bosin, T. R. (1974). *Research Communications in Chemical Pathology and Pharmacology*, **9**, 145.
Harrison, S. D., Jr., Bosin, T. R. and Maickel, R. P. (1974). *Drug Metabolism and Disposition*, **2**, 228.
Heikkila, R. E. and Cohen, G. (1974). *Research Communications in Chemical Pathology and Pharmacology*, **7**, 539.
Hess, H. J. E. and Nelson, R. P. (1971). Ger. Pat. 2,106,038 (Pfizer Inc.).
Holmberg, C. G. and Laurell, C.-B. (1948). *Acta Chemica Scandinavica*, **2**, 450.
Hudson, J. E. (1971). *Bulletin of Entomology Research*, **61**, 267.
Humber, L. G., Demerson, C. A., Asselin, A. A., Charest, M.-P. and Pelz, K. (1975). *European Journal of Medicinal Chemistry*, **10**, 215.
Kaltenbronn, J. S. (1970). Ger. Offen. Pat. 1,941,543 (Parke, Davis and Co.).
Kaltenbronn, J. C. (1971a). US Pat. 3,558,655.
Kaltenbronn, J. S. (1971b). US Pat. 3,598,839 (Parke, Davis and Co.).
Kaltenbronn, J. C. (1972). US Pat. 3,706,767 (Parke, Davis and Co.).
Kiechle, F. L. (1974). PhD Thesis, Indiana University, Bloomington, Indiana.
Hadaway, A. B., Barlow, F., Grose, J. E. H., Turner, C. R. and Flowers, L. S. (1970). *Bulletin of the World Health Organization*, **42**, 369.
Hall, L. E., Hegeman, G. D. and Bosin, T. R. (1974). *Research Communications in Chemical Pathology and Pharmacology*, **9**, 145.
Harrison, S. D., Jr., Bosin, T. R. and Maickel, R. P. (1974). *Drug Metabolism and Disposition*, **2**, 228.
Heikkila, R. E. and Cohen, G. (1974). *Research Communications in Chemical Pathology and Pharmacology*, **7**, 539.
Hess, H. J. E. and Nelson, R. P. (1971). Ger. Pat. 2,106,038 (Pfizer Inc.).
Holmberg, C. G. and Laurell, C.-B. (1948). *Acta Chemica Scandinavica*, **2**, 450.
Hudson, J. E. (1971). *Bulletin of Entomology Research*, **61**, 267.
Humber, L. G., Demerson, C. A., Asselin, A. A., Charest, M.-P. and Pelz, K. (1975). *European Journal of Medicinal Chemistry*, **10**, 215.
Kilsheimer, J. R., Kaufman, H. A., Foster, H. M., Driscoll, P. R., Glick, L. A., and Napier, R. P. (1969). *Journal of Agricultural and Food Chemistry*, **17**, 91.
Kikugawa, K. and Ichino, M. (1973). *Chemical Pharmaceutical Bulletin*, **21**, 1151.
Krupinski, V. M., Robbers, J. E. and Floss, H. G. (1976). *Journal of Bacteriology*, **125**, 158.

Kyburz, E. (1974). Personal Communication, Hoffman-LaRoche and Co., Basel, Switzerland.

Lagno, Z. Y. and Sviridor, S. M. (1972). *Khim. Seraorg. Soedin. Soderzh. Neftyakh Nefteprod.* **9**, 580.

Lerner, A. B., Case, J. D. and Heinzelman, P. V. (1959). *Journal of the American Chemical Society*, **81**, 6084.

Lombardino, J. G. and Wiseman, E. H. (1970). *Journal of Medicinal Chemistry*, **13**, 206.

Lwoff, A., Sy, M., Maillet, M., Pages, J. and David, P. (1970a). Ger. Offen. Pat. 2,020,230 (Agence Nationale de Valorisation de la Recherche and Institut National de la Recherche Agronomique).

Lwoff, A., Sy, M., Maillet, M., Pages, J. and David, P. (1970b). Ger. Offen. Pat. 2,023,551 (Agence Nationale de Valorisation de la Recherche and Institute National de la Recherche Agronomique).

Mahfouz, A. M. M., Metcalf, R. L. and Fukuto, T. R. (1969). *Journal of Agriculture and Food Chemistry*, **17**, 917.

Maickel, R. P., Bosin, T. R., Harrison, S. D., Jr. and Riddle, M. A. (1974). *Life Sciences*, **14**, 1735.

Maickel, R. P., Baldwin, J. R., Campaigne, E. and Bosin, T. R. (1975). *Federation Proceedings*, **34**, 293.

Manhas, M. S., Sharma, S. D. and Amin, S. G. (1972). *Journal of Medicinal Chemistry*, **15**, 106.

Maravetz, L. L. (1974). US Pat. 3,836,542 (Mobil Oil Corporation).

McEwen, L. C., Knittle, C. E. and Raymond, M. L. (1972). *Journal of Range Management*, **25**, 188.

Miller, F. P., Garski, G. and Gauger, D. (1971). *The Pharmacologist*, **13**, 207.

Mobil Oil Corporation (1974). Fr. Demande Pat. 2,203,590 (Mobil Oil Corporation).

Neidlein, R. and Gehringer, C. (1974). *Archiv der Pharmazie*, **307**, 232.

Pendleton, R. G., Kaiser, C., Gessner, G., Finlay, E. and Green, H. (1974). *The Journal of Pharmacology and Experimental Therapeutics*, **190**, 551.

Pilyugin, G. T., Verteletskaya, N. I., Perepecko, N. P. and Lepikhova, S. V. (1972). USSR Pat. 361,780 (Chernovtsky State University).

Pinder, R. M., Green, D. M. and Thompson, P. B. J. (1971). *Journal of Medicinal Chemistry*, **14**, 626.

Ramsden, E. N. (1970). *Biochemical Journal*, **120**, 12P.

Reed, B. L. (1968). *Life Sciences*, **7**, 961.

Reed, B. L. (1974). Personal Communication. Victoria College of Pharmacy, Brisbane, Australia.

Robbins, J. D., Bakke, J. E. and Feil, V. J. (1969). *Journal of Agriculture and Food Chemistry*, **17**, 236.

Robbins, J. D., Bakke, J. E. and Feil, V. J. (1970). *Journal of Agriculture and Food Chemistry*, **18**, 130.

Saraf, S. D. (1971). *Pakistan Journal*, **14**, 341.

Shaskan, E. G. and Snyder, S. H. (1970). *Journal of Pharmacology and Experimental Therapeutics*, **178**, 404.

Shetty, R. V. (1969). Personal Communication, Pharmaceutical Division of Pennwalt Corporation, Rochester, New York.

Sproessler, B. and Lingens, F. (1970). *Hoppe-Seyler's Zeitschrift für Physiologische Chemie*, **351**, 967.

Steinberg, M. and Whitlaw, J. T. Jr. (1969). US Clearinghouse Federal Science and Technology Information, No. 859440.

Steinberg, M., Cole, M. M., Miller, T. A. and Godke, R. A. (1972). *Journal of Medical Entomology*, **9**, 73.

Suh, J. T. (1970a). US Pat. 3,494,528 (Colgate-Palmolive Co.).

Suh, J. T. (1970b). US Pat. 3,492,294 (Colgate-Palmolive Co.).

Suh, J. T. (1972). US Pat. 3,663,702 (Colgate-Palmolive Co.).

Taylor, R. T. and Schoof, H. F. (1971). *Journal of Economic Entomology*, **64**, 1173.

Tomlin, A. D. and Forgash, A. J. *Journal of Economic Entomology*, **65**, 953.

Tucker, R. K. and Hargele, M. A. (1971). *Toxicology and Applied Pharmacology*, 57.

Vaughan Williams, E. M. and Polster, P. (1974). *European Journal of Pharmacology*, **25**, 241.

Von Schmeling, B., Davis, R. A. and Relyea, D. I. (1970). Ger. Pat. 2,002,801. (Uniroyal, Inc.).

Webber, J. A., Huffman, G. W., Koehler, R. E., Murphy, C. F., Ryan, C. W., Van Heyningen, E. M. and Vasileff, R. T. (1971). *Journal of Medicinal Chemistry*, **14**, 113.

Williams, P. P. and Stolzenberg, R. L. (1972). *Applied Microbiology*, **23**, 745.

Wood, H. B. (1967, 1976). Personal Communication, National Cancer Institute, Bethesda, MD.

Wright, W. B. and Brabander, H. J. (1970). Ger. Pat. 1,936,721 (American Cyanamid Co.).

Wright, W. B., Jr. and Brabander, H. J. (1972). US Pat. 3,646,047 (American Cyanamid Co.).

Wright, J. B. and Johnson, H. G. (1973). *Journal of Medicinal Chemistry*, **16**, 861.

Wright, W. B., Jr. and Brabander, H. J. (1973). US Pat. 3,734,915 (American Cyanamid Co.).

Subject Index

233

Cumulative Index of Authors

Cumulative Index of Titles

239

DATE DUE